Experts Catastrophe

Chronic fatigue, tiredness, autism, anxiety,
depression, sleep and memory problems,
indecision, phobias, bipolar, schizophrenia,
fibromyalgia, MS, ME, CFS....

Robin P Clarke

Best Books Press

~

Note: This book was written
before the "Covid" crisis.

First published 2020 by BestBooks Press
11923 NE Sumner St, STE 745011, Portland, Oregon 97220, USA
www.bestbookspress.com

Note: This book was written
before the "Covid" crisis.

ISBN: 978-0-9995780-0-1 paperback
ISBN: 978-0-9995780-1-8 kindle
ISBN: 978-0-9995780-2-5 hardback

Disclaimer notice 1: We are not aware of any definitive proof that
any of the experts specifically identified in this book have been
actually lying in the sense of trying to deceive others.
(But credibility certainly gets strained to within a hair's-breadth of
breaking at various points.)

Disclaimer notice 2: Nothing in this book should be construed as
expert health or medical advice. For medical advice you are advised
to consult a properly competent professional expert. The author and
publisher disclaim all liability for any liability, loss, or risk, of any
nature, that might result from use or application of any contents of
the book.

~

www.pseudoexpertise.com

www.robinpclarke.com

With this book I attempt to follow in some footsteps of......

Hal Huggins D.D.S., 1937-2014,
de-licenced for telling the truth

and

Jeff Bradstreet M.D., 1954-2015,
assassinated for asking the right questions

and

Hans Eysenck 1916-1997 and Bernard Rimland 1928-2006,
who laid many of the foundations on which this book rests

and

Adelle Davis, 1904-1974,
the 'quack' without whom none of this would have been possible.

Contents

1. The strange facts they aren't telling you about expertise   1

2. Experts evidencelessly parrotting about a "disorder"   47

3. A suppressed report of millions of (non-autistic) victims   78

4. Expert excuses from "Neurotoxicology" journal   115

5. Expert excuses from other "scientific" journals   135

6. Nonsense and yet more nonsense about vaccines   166

7. The peer-reviewed publication of a still-unfaulted theory   200

8. Years and years of careerlessness caused by official expertise   240

9. The NHS complaints-denial system and the PHSO   262

10. The hideously ugly *un*-truth about bloodletting and leeches   266

11. "Did the UK Committee on Toxicity lie to the government about vitamin B6?" (co-authored with Bernard Rimland)   273

12. Is Cambridge's Simon Baron-Cohen a charlatan too?   288

13. Robert Whitaker's "Anatomy of an Epidemic"   306

14. A "pause" for reflection, as in Schumann's Carnaval   308

15. What can be done about the failed institutional systems?   313

16. Update review of the published theory (with some surprises!)   324

Afterword for concerned environmental experts   344

Afterword for the cleverest IQ experts   346

After-Afterword for our most expert leading intellectuals   349

Acknowledgments   354

References (sources cited except in Appendix of Chapter 3)   355

Index   372

~~~~~~~

1

The strange facts they aren't telling you about expertise

The information in this book is likely to make a majorly positive difference to your life and the lives of your friends and family. But it's like taking the red pill in the famous Matrix movie – once you have entered in here you can never go back to your previous ignorance. So beware!

This is not yet another book for people who just want to be told what "facts" to believe, by some "properly-qualified" "authority" person blankly asserting, in effect, "Believe me, I'm the expert".

Instead, this book is designed to *demonstrate to you* what is the genuine expertise and what is not. And to *empower you* to develop enhanced competence of your own for discerning what is true expertise rather than false.

It is mainly about health/medical expertise, but also has much relevance to many other areas (though not all equally).

In our current information age there are many "doctors" and "professors" asserted to be medical experts, but their expertise can't *all* be well-founded, because they disagree hugely on so many of the most important questions. And then there are some yet more important questions that aren't allowed to be asked anyway. This book reaches the parts that no other information source does.

In these pages you will learn that there is a huge extent of false expertise, causing devastation of the lives of millions of disinformed victims – quite possibly including yourself or your friends. And the false expertise is not so much from "quacks" but rather from some of the supposedly most "authoritative" "experts" dead or alive.

The greater part of this information is not available from anyone else, for reasons that will become obvious in later pages.

Most of the millions of cases with which this book is concerned are conditions other than autism, but that a- word gets much mention herein because the research about it opens a surprising door to also understanding what is causing various other conditions.

I have made some seriously bold assertions in the opening paragraphs here. But you don't have to blindly trust me about them, because this book will show you the proof – starting here with some words of what others have been saying.

Please consider first this quotation from Armstrong & Green (2017), which testifies that something rather weird is going on:

"Incentives for scientists should encourage the discovery of useful findings. However, [....] the incentive structure present at universities and journals is detrimental to the scientific value of research. [Thus we found that] to improve their chances of getting their papers published, researchers should *avoid* examining important problems, *avoid* challenging existing beliefs, *avoid* obtaining surprising findings, *avoid* using simple methods, *avoid* providing full disclosure, and *avoid* writing clearly."

.....and *ALL* of those "sins" will be committed in this evil book!

And I should meanwhile point out that I am not alone in having changed my mind about various things:

"Like most people, and almost all doctors, I just believed what the 'experts' said. I have long since learned my lesson."
      – Malcolm Kendrick M.D. in *Doctoring Data*

"It wasn't until I retired and began reading in more depth that I realised just how 'brainwashed' many doctors are"
      – Paul Travis M.D.

"If this is the expert why can't he answer my questions?"
      – Suzanne Humphries M.D., author of *Dissolving Illusions*

"Among all our contemporary experts, physicians are those trained to the highest level of specialised incompetence for this urgently needed pursuit."
      – Ivan Illich in *Medical Nemesis* (1975)

And the following further quotations will be useful here to advance your understanding of some key facts about expertise. ("Peer review" is the system by which science bureaucrats decide which scientific discoveries are allowed to be published in "scientific" journals.)

"There are many problems with the peer review system. Perhaps the most significant is that the truly imaginative are not being judged by their peers. They *have* none! .... what has been demonstrated by this study is .... reviewer and editorial incompetence. .... In my Nobel lecture, I published the initial letter of rejection by the *Journal of Clinical Investigation* of

work that was to prove to be of fundamental importance to the development of radioimmunoassay."
– R.S. Yalow, Nobel Laureate in Physiology/Medicine

"The concept of peer review is based on two myths..... [of which the second is] that in those rare instances in which someone who is exceptional does appear, the ordinary scientist always instantly recognises genius and smooths its path. No one who knows anything at all about the history of science can believe for one second in either myth....."
"Peer review is an open invitation to the crooked...."
– David F. Horrobin, Editor, Medical Hypotheses

"....a gravely pathological situation, calling for further serious inquiry and radical remedy."
– John Ziman, H. H. Wills Physics Laboratory, Bristol

Those quotations are from Harnad, ed., (1982), as detailed in the reference list at the end of this book.

Note that in the preceding sentence I have included a reference to a source ("Harnad, ed., (1982)"). If you are to make good progress in learning to unpick the true expertise from the sham, then you will need to learn to pay attention to such references, also called citations. I'll say more about this further on. Meanwhile here's two more quotes you might usefully ponder (Smith, 2014; Horton, 2000):

"Things are badly wrong with journals and the research they publish." "The problem doesn't arise from amateurs dabbling in research but rather from career researchers."
– Richard Smith, editor of the British Medical Journal

"We know that the system of peer review is biased, unjust, unaccountable, incomplete, easily fixed, often insulting, usually ignorant, occasionally foolish, and frequently wrong."
– Richard Horton, editor of the Lancet

In later chapters I will show actual detailed examples of things which in this first chapter I only suggest or assert as being true.

I should also mention here that in my experience most people, even the highly-qualified, are too much prone to categorise both things and people into false simplistic categories of "good" or "bad". For instance, some people declare as their expert knowledge that "mercury is a *toxin*", categorically *bad* for health, and that the only acceptable level of mercury is zero. And yet the real zero here is the amount of evidence they cite in support of that notion – a notion of which I will show the theoretical and evidential precariousness further on.

No less unsoundly, the persons and institutions involved in some matters covered in this book tend to get categorised as either evil deceivers whose claims are consistently lies or else wonderful saintly heroes whose information is consistently truthful. Depending on which side we are hearing from in this warfare of words, either the official authorities are evil and the dissidents are heroes, or else it is those quack dissidents who are evil and the vilified official experts are heroes for actually working hard to help reduce illness. Again, I consider the reality to be altogether more complicated and that there is truth and falsehood and honesty and treachery to be found in all quarters to some extent. This is not a book of "our side" versus "theirs".

With these preliminary comments out of the way, I will now move on to the main content here.

~~~~~~~

Information relating to many aspects of health and illness is available from many books, websites, and other sources. But there is radical disagreement on many important points.

So wise persons will necessarily find themselves asking the question of how they should decide between these conflicting assertions.

Some will think I am posing a rather stupid question here. It is obvious, they will reason, that the views of a person with a relevant doctorate or professorship must outweigh the views of a person with only meagre qualifications or none. And that a peer-reviewed report in a prestigious scientific journal must outweigh the assertions of a group of ordinary people who consider themselves victims of some sort of medically-caused harm. The hierarchy of such expertise is well-known, with professor ranking above PhD doctorate ranking above graduate ranking above non-graduate and suchlike.

Do you see how that makes sense? Well, if you do, then you might wish to consider the facts of Lysenkoism in Stalin's Russia.

Trofim Lysenko is now universally understood to have been a charlatan, a purveyor of pseudo-science rather than of genuine biology and agricultural science. And yet for three decades he and his acolytes prevailed unchallenged in all the universities and institutes of the great USSR, honoured as the most distinguished professors and so on. So it must have been they that were surely the experts, just as for instance Professor Simon Baron-Cohen must be the real autism expert today as he is the head of the Autism Research Centre at Cambridge University. Meanwhile, the genuinely outstanding geneticists, agronomists and other biologists were either executed or sent to slave-camps in the bone-chilling wastelands of Siberia. Or perhaps they surely weren't the experts, rather the charlatans. You aren't going to find the true, most out-standingly distinguished scientific experts recognised only as status-less barely-surviving salt-miners, are you? And yet the great biologist Vavilov, who created the first ever seed bank, starved to death in prison. This corruption of science did not end until years after the death of Stalin, by which time the false science of Lysenko had caused immense damage to Soviet agriculture.

But could it be that Lysenkoism was just something that happened in a peculiar far-off country 70 years ago, under a total-itarian regime in the grip of a false ideology – whereas of course now we have the modern uncorrupted world in which everything has been sorted into its proper place? Well, I invite you to consider some further historical facts which I have excerpted from the book *Genius* by the late Prof. Hans J. Eysenck, the most-cited-ever scientist (back then at least). The excerpts are in the frame below.

Planck's experience with other leading physicists was no different. ... "I found no interest, let alone approval, even among the very physicists who were clearly connected with the topic. Kirchoff expressly disapproved. I did not succeed in reaching Clausius. He did not answer my letters, and I did not find him at home when I tried to see him in person in Bonn. I carried on a correspondence with Carl Neumann, of Leipzig, but it remained totally fruitless" (Planck, 1949, p.18). ".... A new scientific truth does not triumph by convincing its opponents and making them see the light, but rather because its opponents eventually die, and a new generation grows up that is familiar with it."

.... even after the publication of *De Revolutionibus* most astronomers retained their belief in the central position of the Earth; even Brahe (Thoren, 1990) whose observations were accurate enough to enable Kepler (Caspar, 1959) to determine that the Mars orbit around the sun was elliptical, not circular, could not bring himself to accept the heliocentric view. Thomas Young proposed a wave theory of light on the basis of good experimental evidence, but because of the prestige of Newton, who of course favoured a corpuscular view, no-one accepted Young's theory (Gillespie, 1960). ....

Similarly, William Harvey's theory of the circulation of the blood was poorly received, in spite of his prestigious position as the King's physician, and harmed his career (Keele, 1965). Pasteur too was hounded because his discovery of the biological character of the fermentation process was found unacceptable. Liebig and many others defended the chemical theory of these processes long after the evidence in favour of Pasteur was conclusive (Dubois, 1950). Equally his micro-organism theory of disease caused endless strife and criticism. Lister's theory of antisepsis (Fisher, 1977) was also long argued over, and considered absurd; so were .... . [ ]   Priestley (Gibbs, 1977) retained his views of phlogiston as the active principle in burning, and together with many others opposed the modern theories of Lavoisier, with considerable violence. Alexander Maconochie's very successful elaboration and application of what would now be called 'Skinnerian principle' to the reclamation of convicted criminals in Australia, led to his dismissal (Barry, 1958).

Another good example is Wegener's continental drift theory, which was given short shrift when he first announced it (Wegener, 1915), but which is now universally accepted. .... most geologists rejected it out of hand. Many of them refused to take it seriously and simply ignored it.....

Here I will rather cite in a more detailed manner a particularly interesting case, that of Ignaz Philipp Semmelweis (Slaughter, 1950). .... An almost ten-fold reduction in mortality might have been expected to provoke praise, interest and imitation. Nothing of the kind. .... Professor Klein, his boss, driven by jealousy, ignorance and vanity, put all sorts of obstacles in Semmelweis's way, underhandedly prevented his promotion, and finally drove him from Vienna.

Another victim of mindless medical orthodoxy was the great Andreas Vesalius, who pioneered modern anatomy 450 years ago. .... Embittered by the harsh condemnation of his work, Vesalius gave up scientific work, burnt his notes, ... Vesalius was made to undertake a pilgrimage to Jerusalem .... he was shipwrecked and perished.

.... it would be quite wrong to imagine that this is the sort of thing that happened in ancient, far-off days, and that nowadays scientists behave in a different manner. .... It is odd that books on genius seldom if ever mention this terrible battle that originality so often has when confronting orthodoxy.

[Excerpted from pp 148-152 of Eysenck (1995).]

(One of the numerous cases which Eysenck did not mention here was that of Ludwig Boltzmann, whose discovery of statistical thermodynamics – fundamental to most modern technology – was ridiculed by professors for ten years till he took his own life.)

It should be apparent from these facts that a similar situation to Lysenkoism, in which the foremost experts were likewise side-lined and oppressed into obscurity by second-rate "distinguished experts", has prevailed in many times and places throughout history. And should we be so confident that our here-and-now scientific communities are somehow different? In this book I will present evidence and reasons to the contrary.

For that purpose let us first step back to the important basics of how our world, of us and knowledge and other people, works. About the first thing we learn as a child is the immensely important fact that some people are more knowledgable (expert) than others, and that the way to get on in life is to learn from those more know-ledgable people. We learn this on our first day at school, but we learn it before then from our parents, and indeed, arguably we have already been programmed to assume it by our genes.

And thus we start our climb up the Ladder of Knowledge. The child learns from the teacher. The teacher learns from the college lecturer. The college lecturer learns from the university teaching professor. The teaching professor learns from the research professors. But at this point, the sequence breaks. From whom do the research professors learn? Do they receive Tablets of Truth handed down from God?

Well of course the research professors learn directly from the reality don't they? The history researchers learn from direct studying of dusty ancient archives and muddy archeological excavations, and likewise the medical researchers learn from direct studying of the reality of healthy and unhealthy people and the molecular processes involved. Or is it really so simple?

One reason it might not be so simple could be that the researchers are not well-engineered truth-discovering robot devices, but instead human beings with dodgy psychologies sometimes deflected from the truth by personal motivations and quirks and societal incentives or pressures. In connection with those distorting factors, it could be useful to consider how persons come to become research professors (e.g. "Principal Investigators") in the first place, or how they get selected. So let us examine a further notional ladder up from childhood, this time the ladder of developing expertise, or at least the ladder of growing authorisation.

The way it works in the UK is similar in essence to most other modern countries. A child progresses through school up to age 16 to take GCSE exams, and only after success in those exams can they move on to take A-levels, and only after success in those further exams can they enter a university to take first year exams, and only after success in those first-year exams can they take second-year exams, and only after success in those second-year exams can they take their finals exams to get a first degree, and only after success in the first degree exams can they then progress to a masters degree, and only after success in the masters exams can they enter to study for their doctoral "thesis", and only after success in their doctoral thesis (which is the obligatory minimum qualification to be a researcher) can they progress to a postdoc position, and only after that can they hope to become a lecturer or thereafter a professor.

Many people talk about the "top universities" and the "best graduates", as if this system is self-evidently a well-founded means for selecting the best minds for the job. But is it? Where is the criterion of validity of "best"? In reality, there is reason to believe that something has gone very wrong here. And yet this system of "meritocracy" is rarely if ever subjected to any coherent criticism or even questioning. And that could be because it is in the nature of the resulting society that those in a position to be heard and to be influential are those who have themselves found success in that "meritocratic" selection process, and consequently are strongly inclined to admire it. The awarding of a degree can be seen as a biasing bribe, incentivising its recipient to believe that it is some sort of valid indicator of their hard-earned intellectual superiority over others less deserving.

The exams system does indeed at first appear to make sense. It is rather obvious to any child that their parents and teachers do indeed have more knowledge and understanding than themselves, and are not teaching them a load of rubbish. And it is rather obvious to the child that those exams do indeed give fair indications of those who have "worked harder" and or learned more or less of what they are being taught, or have become more or less skilled in solving mathematical problems, playing musical instruments and so on. I recall my own pride / smugness about my own easy excellence in grammar school exams, and my notion that anyone who didn't have a maths A-level must be somehow mentally handicapped. I'm glad that gas heating fitters are required to score 100% in their exams. The system of exams clearly works in many ways as an essential component of seemingly every advanced civilisation in memory.

And yet.

Scientific research is very different from maintenance of gas heaters. Ideally the gas fitter will confine their creativity to dealing with the customer, and will do the actual technical work with resolutely uncreative rule-following avoidance of interesting experimentation in your home. By contrast, competent research requires extreme creativity, at every turn thinking up the questions that no-one has ever asked before, and questioning every sacred assumption they have dutifully learnt. Myself being a person to whom scientific research was as inevitable a "career choice" as composing must have been to a Beethoven or Bach, I recall only too well the BPS advice booklet saying that research posts would require the "highest intellectual standing". And yet it made no attempt to unpick that psychological atom into its sub-component electrons or protons.

In all manner of respects, our modern societies have far advanced from one or two thousand years ago. And yet the fundamental social mechanism of selection by exams is virtually unchanged over those millennia, except in that writing and box-ticking now predominates over face-to-face viva-voce interrogation and defence.

What talents do exams measure? Arguably they almost entire-ly measure the ability to learn the facts and notions and standard skills being taught. They reflect the ability to read, remember, recall, and rewrite, with sufficient speed and facility between 9am and 1pm on one particular hot summer day not of one's choosing. But you don't have to take my word for it, because here it is "from the horse's mouth":

"As a Cambridge medical graduate it always saddened me to see so many able-minded people struggle through our medical course. The sheer volume of information we were expected to memorise was mind-boggling." (Gundroo, 2014)

"The medical curriculum is so overloaded with information that you just have to learn what you hear, as you hear it." (Humphries & Bystrianyk, 2013)

"I was good at exams, and so I bloody well should have been. The system was set up for people like me – thorough, plodding, uncreative, capable of taking in great mounds of received wisdom and regurgitating them, undigested, unquestioned, unprocessed in three-hour bursts of neat handwriting." (Mangan, 2014)

"The school system is now finely focussed only on exam success and the exam game has very very little to do with success in real life. In business and other parts of the real world the skills that get you on in chosen area are ones such as:
- admitting you don't know something and going out to find it out;
- finding someone who knows more than you and working with them to create something bigger and better;
- going out on a limb, flying a few kites, taking a bit more time over the really difficult issues.

In an exam situation this is either called cheating or will ensure you fail. Life is very very rarely like an exam situation – it is surprisingly a lot more like the coursework that is being consigned by Gove and his fellow conservatives to the scrap-heap." (Edwards, 2014)

((Some readers are claiming that the information quoted above is out of date, so I'll add yet more here. Firstly some words from the brand-new book *"So You Got into Medical School... Now What?"* (Paull, 2015): *"....the sheer amount of information....";* *"A popular analogy likens the medical student's efforts to absorb all the information presented in class to trying to drink from a fire hose."* *"Every medical student feels the strain of information overload. So what to do with the colossal amount of information being forced upon you daily?".* And finally some latest words from a 16-year-old (Vogt-Vincent, 2015): *"Suddenly, the creativity I'd brought to all my school projects wasn't accepted anymore. Instead I had to memorise facts and statistics." "One bad result makes you a failure. Success is measured by how well you remember".*))

And now, what talents are demonstrated by a person obtaining a doctoral PhD qualification? Generally the candidate has to be able and willing to stick for several years to a particular project or at least field of research, and at the end of it produce a sufficiently long sequence of words to impress the existing experts, while not contradicting any established beliefs too uncomfortably.

And meanwhile what talents are required for excelling in genuinely scientific research and discovery? Or at least functioning as a competent researcher? Arguably the ability to question one's prior learning and assumptions, to creatively think of new questions and possibilities, and to make reasonable judgements of what is more likely to be truer or more credible or effective.

And arguably the best researcher is one who is constantly open to the possibility that the line of research they are following may not be the best, and so they should dump it and move to something better. And they should learn to present their work in not too many words. Because whereas the PhD thesis will fail if it isn't more or less book-length, in contrast the journals demand that their papers be kept below a rather tight length. For instance as the geniuses at the Lancet state, "If you can't express your idea [and by implication a useful amount of evidence and explanation] in less than 1500 words it probably isn't a *Hypothesis* [and so we will bin it]". (And note that you have just now read the 4055th word in this book, and Chapter 2 is approx 12,600 words, and Chapter 7 is approx 18,000 words.)

In my experience, the predominant intellectual shortcoming of the human race is not deficient ability to *learn*, but instead is deficient ability to *unlearn* that which has already been learnt in error. Once your brain has got a faulty notion etched into its neurons, it can be much harder for that faulty notion to be removed and a corrected notion to be substituted in its place. And the education and selection systems of exams strongly favour uncritical learning unencumbered by too much inefficiency-creating doubt giving capability for unlearning.

There probably hasn't been any research on the question, but it seems rather self-evident anyway that a disposition towards questioning and doubting of information would tend to interfere with the headlong rush of hyperactive memorising which has evidently become a prime preoccupation of those in the business of supposedly nurturing the world's greatest intellectual excellence. It's a bit like a cycle race going up a mountain pass, in which having no brakes on your bike would give you a faster time up the hill. And yet in a real world which includes the corresponding downhills your bike without brakes would soon result in your death rather than any time records.

Thus the extreme relentless selection of supposed excellence falsely defined in terms of hyperactive learning would also be extremely selective *against* any talent for *unlearning*.

And it is arguably that *unlearning* ability which is the path to wisdom and to competence as a great researcher and discoverer, and hence a great true expert. I see so many persons of high intelligence who have taken one or more intellectual wrong turnings early on and consequently ended up far from the truth they thought they were heading towards. Their "super-bike" without brakes left the road to reality on one of those downhill bends.

One of the most important wrong turnings appears to be that "fact" which we learn first and most persistently. That is that the experts, namely the more "qualified" more senior people, know best and that any less-qualified inferiors who challenge them can be dismissed as wrong. All through childhood and formal education we get reinforced in that notion. And those of us who are awarded degrees and the like are all the more strongly reinforced (effectively bribed) into this cultist belief. All this time we lack a proper appreciation of the flaws in the Ladder of Knowledge pointed out in the preceding paragraphs here. The thing is that some of what we learnt from our teachers may have been wrong, because the researchers or discoverers it came from were wrong in the first place.

In conclusion then, there is reason to believe that our academic selection procedures, far from selecting the most suitable intellects for research careers, ironically instead block at every turn those most talented to be researchers and discoverers. Producing even a great discovery does not in the slightest require being able to read at the highest speed, learn "facts" at highest speed, recall at high speed, wake up and attend a course or exam before 10 am yesterday, or stick at completing a rubbishy boring thesis with sufficient tenacity.

The greatest genuine creative geniuses would be particularly unlikely to be found getting firsts in such centres of hyperactive parrotting excellence as Oxford and Cambridge medical schools.

To the extent that any competent researchers still manage to emerge through the multi-hooped talent-excluding system described above, they still then face the social context of the research career.

I see a certain personal irony in my writing those words. Measuring the carbon content of steel samples has been an important function in hi-tech societies, and my father W. E. Clarke F.R.I.C. invented a means of doing it without need for an oxygen supply, in respect of which some people in India wrote in appreciation. At other times I had heard him express regret that much of his work at the cast iron research association had been under commercial confidentiality.

At age 16-17 we grammar-school pupils had to choose what degree subjects we would apply to universities to study, and discuss it with the headmaster. I was superbly talented in maths and physics and so the headmaster was very concerned at my wish to not study science of the maths/physics/chemistry sort. My reluctance was based on a vague notion as a very naïve youth that a career as a scientist entailed being a cog in the wheels of machinery controlled by others for not necessarily the purposes one would choose oneself. And not so many decades after the Hiroshima atomic bombing it seemed to me that the main problems were in social rather than physical sciences. Meanwhile of course many thousands of my contemporaries did just carry on getting further entangled in those social mechanisms and ultimately becoming visible as "distinguished" cogs therein.

I don't believe that many people go into medical research with an intention of becoming charlatans. But, like my abovementioned contemporaries, they probably don't really understand what they are getting into. This is especially the case in respect of medical schools. Getting into med school is thought of as the highest achievement of a school-leaving university applicant. Just about any normal 17-year-old would assume that med school is where you learn the truth, and most useful truth, about health and illness. They are rarely told the crucial fact that med schools long ago became the pawns of the hugely-profitable big pharma industry. Rather than institutions of education, they should properly be recognised as institutions of propaganda brainwashing for corporatised medicine (that is patented drugs and expensive surgical technologies). (I won't give any sources in proof of these points here because if you don't want to believe them they have anyway been well-explored by others elsewhere such as Healy (2012) and Gøtzsche (2013) and my main concern in this book is to show my own new contributions to knowledge rather than encyclopedise the work already done by others. But note the Cambridge medical graduate's comment above here for a very large hint that the students may not be operating in higher scepticism mode during their "higher education".)

It does appear that a lot of what students learn in medical schools is true, but I've also seen a remarkable amount of deathly claptrap emerging therefrom, and I would hesitate to make a judgement of which is the greater in volume or impact.

I am told that the corruption of medical students already begins in their first days, with freebies and inducements of various sorts being handed to them by corporate interests. No less importantly, how best to succeed at med school? To conveniently agree with most of what your professors tell you, or instead to challenge them as mistaken? And how did they get to be professors anyway? (see above and below).

I've never been enrolled in a medical school course, but someone who has, and indeed graduated therefrom, is Dr Malcolm Kendrick. And on page 194 of his excellent book *Doctoring Data* (Kendrick, 2014) he makes it clear that the students are very emphatically taught that they must never question the existing "knowledge", or else their career will come to a bad end. (And this sort of thing doesn't end on graduation. David Healy, author of *Pharmageddon*, was dismissed from a professorship due to telling people of the evidence that antidepressants were causing suicides; they have also caused America's epidemic of "gun" massacres and probably the suicide airliner crash in France.)

Having successfully completed the 20-year high-jumping marathon of exams and got your PhD doctorate at last, you still have no chance of being recognised as a *leading expert* until you have first developed a sufficiently extensive and impressive *publication record*. And the published items have to be not self-published but instead accepted by "leading" "prestigious" "peer-reviewed" journals or else they don't count at all in the authoritarian bureaucracy-loving pecking-order competition that is institution-alised academia.

Building up your publication record usually requires some succeeding in the "peer preview" system of assessing research grant applications, and invariably requires sufficient succeeding in getting your publications accepted into journals through the "peer-review" system of volunteers the journals operate. And it helps if your publications don't later get "retracted" – retrospectively asserted to be unfit for publication.

There is so much wrong in this context, so much fallacy, that it is difficult to know where to start on demuddling it.

The mythology is that genuine science is that which comes from universities and is published in peer-reviewed journals, while anything else is merely unproven rubbish from a nobody. The universities were all personally founded by God/Allah for the accurate enlightenment of His subjects, and peer-review involves sending verification emails up from the universities to Heaven and back.

In reality, human beings tend to gather into convenient ideological lobbying groups (universities and their departments) and devise systems for efficient back-stabbing of rivals and for mutual back-scratching of collaborators ("peer-review" and "peer-preview").

Not the least of the myths about "peer review" is that scientific publication has just about always used it. In reality "peer review" did not exist until recent decades, with the rise of the mass-production professionalised publish-or-perish career "publication record" corporatised science that now dominates every field. Einstein's ultra-famous non-professional publications were not subject to "peer review" (so we'd better dump them in the trash for a start). Indeed when one of his later papers was sent to a reviewer Einstein objected and got another journal to publish it instead (without "peer review").

"Peer review" and "peer preview" have a number of severe faults in common. But basically, if you have made a great discovery, you can only get it meaningfully published (or get a research grant to progress it) if your anonymous deadly enemy rivals first give their anonymous endorsement of it being worth the bother. Consider the following scenarios which are *precisely* analogous to how the so-called "peer-review" system works in scientific publishing.

The Uruguay football team are selecting their players for the 2014 World Cup, and they obtain an anonymous peer-review from Wayne Rooney who anonymously says that Suarez is really lacking in any ball-kicking skill and not talented enough to play in a national team. (Oh, but it was from an expert unpaid peer volunteer!) So Suarez receives a letter telling him he's not hot enough to participate in international football.

The Democrats party are selecting their presidential candidate and obtain an anonymous peer-review from Hillary Clinton which anonymously tells them that Barack Obama is far too foolish and incompetent to ever function as a US president. (Oh, but it was from an expert unpaid peer volunteer!) So Obama receives a letter telling him he hasn't qualified for the presidential contest.

Wimbledon are sorting out who should play the 2014 games

and they seek an anonymous peer-review from Venus Williams who anonymously says that Maria Sharapova is really past it and not remotely competent to play tennis any more. (Oh, but it was from an expert unpaid peer volunteer!) So Sharapova gets a letter saying that she isn't good enough at tennis and won't be allowed to play there.

A record label seeks an anonymous peer review from Mick Jagger which anonymously informs them that Paul McCartney really has no talent for music such as is worth making recordings of. (Oh, but it was from an expert unpaid peer volunteer!) So McCartney gets a letter telling him his music isn't good enough for recording.

A classical music recording company seeks an anonymous peer review from Karajan who anonymously says that his contemporary Sir Georg Solti is vastly overrated and his conducting is worse than an average drunk. (Oh, but it was from an expert unpaid peer volunteer!)

The international chess federation are sorting out the upcoming championships and obtain an anonymous peer-review from Bobby Fischer who anonymously informs them that Kasparov is too thick to play chess even with babies. (Oh, but it was from an expert unpaid peer volunteer!)

And the means by which the genuinely most excellent science gets published (or more likely is *prevented from* getting published) (in any meaningful form) is exactly like those examples above.

You may of course think that those examples are bonkers. But yes, indeed the "peer review" system is an absolutely stark raving bonkers way for supposedly selecting the best discoveries in science for publishing.

Consider it from another angle. You may have heard of the Olympic Games, in which the world's top sportspeople compete. Anyone who attends or watches the Olympics can see for themselves who runs the fastest, jumps the highest, and so on. They can see for themselves what the scores are and who is actually the world's greatest. Meanwhile there could be what we might call the "Science Olympic Games". To be a champion in the Science Olympics is a much more important achievement than all those sports golds and silvers put together. A great scientist's work is creative and valuable whereas no-one really needs high jumpers and fast runners (who can't even do that after about age 30 anyway). And yet, the way the "science olympics" (aka "peer review") works is rather peculiar. That's because – we are required to believe – the only persons capable of "seeing the score" and discerning who is the champion are the deadly rivals of that potential champion. So it's exactly like as if Wiggins could only win the 2012 cycling gold medal if Cavendish testified that Wiggins had indeed been faster than himself. And what any "non-qualified" person claimed about who cycled fastest was of no consequence.

Now let's have a guess as to why the great scientific geniuses of the past ceased to keep emerging at exactly the same time as corporatised "peer-reviewed" science developed.

Peer reviews are not 100% bad. I have been invited to do six myself and in the process seen the reviews from six others, and also seen numerous reviews of my own papers including of course the ones which got them accepted. Often the unpaid volunteer peer reviewers do contribute to improving published papers and weeding out defective ones. But that positive is utterly outweighed by the vast negative that my examples above here should make clear. The most important thing in science publishing is that the most groundbreaking discoveries should not be completely suppressed from entering the scientific discourse and public record. And yet that outrageous outcome is what the so-called peer review system is perfectly set up to achieve. It is completely unaccountable and wide open to abuse and that abuse very regularly happens as I will show you in detail further on. And I remind you of the five quotations at the start of this chapter.

Not only is there that problem of corrupt hostile rivals suppressing great discoveries, but also there is the problem of even well-meaning "peer" colleagues being unable to make the mental adjustments to appreciate great new "paradigm shifts" replacing flawed conventional wisdoms with radically improved ways of seeing the same things. And there are also bad commercial reasons for disfavouring inconvenient discoveries.

Another fault of the peer review system is in the opposite direction, giving favourable treatment to outright rubbish. I myself was requested to peer-review a paper about the "Fractional Autism Triad Hypothesis". I recognised this (non-)concept as the complete and utter dis-logicality it was and explained this in detail in my review (Clarke, 2012). But strangely the other two reviewers went on about how "important" and "valuable" the paper was and that it should therefore be published. (The editor decided to refuse the paper despite those two favourable reviews, presumably because of my own outrightly terminal critique.) The problem is that the "expert" specialists on the "Fractional Autism Triad Hypothesis" would be those working as specialists on that same particular pseudic theme and therefore inclining to say(/?pretend?) what "important" "valuable" research it was. I think the editor was canny enough to see that my own, "non-fractional", viewpoint about autism would mean I could give an alternative (if not entirely disinterested) view of the matter. So you can see that not only can the peer review system hideously block the most important discoveries, but it meanwhile can allow through the most timewasting of rubbish unchallenged if there is a professional community of publish-perish "specialists" to support it.

My comments above about peer review don't come out of a vacuum. Numerous *published* authors have complained about the absurdity of the system. (I'm also such a published author myself I should make clear.) Numerous articles have been published discussing the same, such as for instance Eysenck & Eysenck (1992) and Horrobin (1990). Others have commented how Einstein would have had no chance of getting his famous works published nowadays. And here are the words of Dr. Marcia Angell, the editor of the New England Journal of Medicine for 20 years:

"It is simply no longer possible to believe much of the clinical research that is published, or to rely on the judgment of trusted physicians or authoritative medical guidelines. I take no pleasure in this conclusion, which I reached slowly and reluctantly over my two decades as an editor of The New England Journal of Medicine." (NY Review of Books, January 15, 2009)

A further severe problem in medical research is a huge hostility to new ideas. There has accumulated an enormous amount of data (e.g. 98,000 studies of glutathione alone) and yet a great paucity of presentation of ideas to tie it together into meaningfulness. And yet the vast majority of putatively "scientific" journals in the medical sphere still will not even consider publishing anything theoretical or even marginally theoretical. For instance I noticed that some studies of distance from highways were suggesting that traffic pollution was causal of autism, and so I sent to Simon Baron-Cohen's journal a "Brief Report" of data showing that the increase of autism was rather obviously unrelated to the increase of vehicle miles travelled, rendering that theory highly improbable. It made sense for me to briefly mention in that report my proposed explanation in terms of indoor mercury vapour from parents' amalgams. And yet Dr Baron-Cohen would only publish it if that were cut out and the readers left in the dark as to what the explanation could be.

This theory-hostile perversion of science was complained about more than fifty years ago by the great medical discoverer Emmanuel Revici (1961)(who lived to be 101 by the way):

".... the relationship between theory and experimentation has been progressively distorted. An unrestrained exaggeration of the role of the experiment, the erroneous view that pure facts represent the aim of research, has led to an entirely unbalanced approach"; "data alone do not generate ideas"; "science cannot progress without theory".

A symptom of this anti-theory perversion is that many academics routinely abuse the word *"hypotheses"* to refer to what are in reality *theories*. I shall elaborate about this in a later chapter.

Anyway, let's imagine that at last you have got your PhD and wish to apply for a research grant. A problem is that the money comes from a big grant-making institution which in turn gets its money from the most profit-making medical industries of patented drugs and surgery and high-tech in general. Not the least of those huge profit-making lobbies is dental amalgam (50% neurotoxic mercury), which is inserted in millions of teeth every year partly because the use of other materials requires much more skill and patience of the dentists (so they can't earn as much). And an equally huge profit-making industry is psychiatric drugs (such as antidepressants, antipsychotics, and sedatives), the increasing use of which might just possibly have a huge amount to do with the health consequences of those same profitable amalgams, as you may see in a later section here.

If you seek to study a question which is inconvenient or embarrassing for the funding sources, or study it in an inconvenient way, you are liable to get your funding refused or terminated. Just one example of many of this corruption in the US government's NIH has been detailed by Cathy DeSoto (2014).

You might think that medical research charities would help by funding research that is not attractive to commercial or professional objectives. To some extent that may happen, and yet by the time a charity gets big enough to make a significant impact it easily becomes prey to entryism and the forces of the vast wealth of the medical corporations and professional unions, for whom a million dollars is peanuts. And just imagine the huge extent you could influence things with even just one such "peanut". Another part of the problem with the charities is that even if they are controlled by well-meaning non-research people, those non-professionals then just naively assume that they should look for guidance exclusively from the professional "proper experts" anyway – so they end up as just more of the same anyway. Gøtzsche (2013) has some further discussion of the corruption of medical research charities, not least the telling observation that they frequently campaign stridently for the government to find the money for an expensive new drug but never campaign for the manufacturers to reduce the price (duh?!).

And if you try to get journals to publish such inconvenient research, you will find the editors of the journals refusing to accept it. (Further on I will show you some of the cheap rubbish that issues from those journals in that connection.)

And even if they do accept it, the authors (and editors) are liable thereafter to be bullied into "retracting" it – of which I'll show you more further on here.

A further testament to the abysmalness of the "peer review" / "publication record" system for discerning the "leading experts" is the case of Peter Higgs, the 2013 Physics Nobel Laureate. He is widely thought of as being the greatest living physicist, having forty years ago predicted the "Higgs boson", only recently confirmed. And yet he and others have commented that if he had come a generation or more later, he would have had no career at all, because he did not have a sufficiently high output of publications to remain qualified for a research post.

The last few pages here have been less than entirely positive about the peer review system. As a matter of fairness I should perhaps point out that my unflattering evaluation is not universally shared. Some prominent organisations such as the Royal Society say of peer review only how valuable and important it is to the advancement of science. Well, they would do, because they are the organisations of the corporatised hierarchised science establishment, and the peer review system does a "great" job of favouring their "correct" "sensible science" establishment views and rejecting everything else, so their enthusiasm is to be expected? So far in this book I have quoted six people including a Nobel prizewinner and the editors of the three most prestigious journals (Lancet, BMJ, and NEJM) all speaking very condemnatorily about peer review. The institutional establishment's only response to these highly-qualified critics is to ignore their comments and pretend they don't exist. This is typical "cherry-picking" behaviour, of which I will say more further on here.

Anyway let's suppose that at last you have got some publications of outstanding discoveries accepted in peer reviewed journals. Surely you are *now* qualified as a *leading expert* at last!? But no, because you still don't have a *citation record*. Such a citation is when researcher B's paper cites (i.e. mentions) researcher C's paper as being relevant to their own. Effectively researcher B thereby gives a career "point" to researcher C (even if actually they are citing them as being flawed rubbish – yes please don't blame me for this crackpot system). Published papers have typically 30 to 200 such citations (references) listed at the end.

This citation ranking system is basically as bonkers as the peer review system. It's like waiting for Venus Williams to give Sharapova a point, for Rooney to give Suarez a point, for Bobby Fischer to give Kasparov a point, and so on. But why the hell would a hostile rival want to bother to give you *any* points? Especially if you have made a massive discovery but are a "nobody" in the field. Or even more if you are a "nobody" who has somehow managed to publish something embarrassing or inconvenient to others in that line of business. You have to bear in mind that modern health research is extremely competitive, with many times more "postdocs" constantly coming up than there are jobs for them to get.

And there is *a very special sort of citation* which has a vital importance here. Under the lunatic publish-or-perish system, there are so many papers getting published that researchers do not have time to ponder even all those papers which have been peer-reviewed and PubMed indexed even in or relevant to their own specific field such as autism or bipolar. So they often have to rely on "review articles" to provide an overview of a particular question, or at least provide them with a decent reading list – and especially when they are newly entering the field. Those review articles cite (or at least are *supposed to cite* and *assumed to cite*) all the relevant previous papers and books on that subject, for instance on ....

.............."theories of autism".

In a later chapter here is reprinted a theory of autism which was published in a peer-reviewed journal some years ago. You can see that it is a substantial document. The editor HJ Eysenck, the most-cited-ever scientist (back then at least) wrote that it was *"well-worth publishing"*, and Bernard Rimland, the founder of Autism Research Institute and Autism Society of America and demolisher of the Bettleheim "refrigerator mothers" theory and pioneer of the modern bio-genetic concept of autism, wrote of it as *"excellent"*, *"fine work"* and *"Robin P Clarke is one of those rare souls with the ability to assimilate and synthesise large amounts of information and generate new and interesting ideas"*. It is the only autism theory to actually explain *why* autism exists, and to explain the presence of such strange features as the handflapping and unusual facial symmetry and spinning without dizziness, and to do that in terms of well-established biological concepts. And it was back then the only paper to indicate the relevance of gene-expression, whereas now just about everyone recognises that gene-expression is absolutely central to the causation of autism. It already recognised that many genes and environmental factors contributed to the causation. And much more. And not a single fault of reasoning or evidence has been raised in the two decades since - which is very exceptional for any psychiatric theory (as they just about always have something clearly wrong with them). The point is that this theory was not and is not just some speculative lightweight drivel to be rightly ignored without even a mention.

Review papers (reviewing for instance the existing autism theories) are usually authored only by the topmost "leading experts" in a field, effectively as guidance or teaching documents for other upcoming researchers. And this comes in the context of the comment of the physicist Planck in 1949 that:

" .... *a new scientific truth does not triumph by convincing its opponents and making them see the light, but rather because its opponents eventually die, and a new generation grows up that is familiar with it.*"

(a notion since confirmed by Azoulay et al. (2015).)

And of course that new generation will only become "familiar with it" if the older generation of "leading experts" bother to let them know it exists anyway.

Lorna Wing [1928-2014] has been widely considered a hero of autism research, and supreme leading expert. She kindly wrote to me a letter in which she stated: *"As a social psychiatrist I do not have the expertise to comment on your* [supposedly] *genetic theory of autism."*

It is in that context that she nevertheless found herself somehow able to have the expertise to write and publish the key overview reviews of theories of autism causation. In her reviews she did not even mention the existence of that published paper. And that can hardly be because it was just any old rubbish that could rightly be dismissed with a wave.

Perhaps the preceding paragraph is giving an impression of bad faith by Dr Wing. Which might not be justified. The thing is as I said earlier that people are very poor at un-learning their previous faulty learning. And Dr Wing's overview reviews adopted a standard form of neatly sorting the autism theories into "genetic theories", "environmental theories", and "psychological theories" – which was all very well until a certain Clarke came along and proposed to upset this tidy arrangement with a theory which was genetic *and* environmental *and* psychological *and* also molecular *and* evolutionary *and* at the level of actual weird symptoms. Any decent theory does need to address all of these. But it did not fit in with Dr Wing's pre-existing conceptual scheme, and to make matters worse had at its centre an entirely novel concept of "general suppression of gene-expression" (antiinnatia), which is not always a wise thing to do. Basically being too far ahead of one's time may be worse than being behind it. And if a person can't understand something they are liable to assume the error lies in that which they don't understand and consequently assume it can be ignored as rubbish anyway. Especially if they are already being worshipped as the leading expert. Such is the repeated history of science as indicated in those excerpts from Eysenck's book. I recall Rimland's words over the phone that "You should be celebrating that your work is being ignored". Which would be fine if I was a computer rather than a would-be member of society with a don't-bother-marrying-after-date attached.

Subsequent to the honourable non-mentions by Dr Wing and others, I have encountered various people reasoning along the lines of "Baah baah, no-one else is trotting over to your corner of the field so I don't see any reason why I should either, baah!". This does of course indicate independent-minded thinking on their part.

If I were to present you with a new painting, or new music video, or new style of coat, you would not respond by saying "But I'm not an expert on coats (or music or art) - what do the experts think?" And yet that is exactly how "non-experts" invariably respond to the presentation of a great new scientific discovery: "What do the experts think?". But then why would any "distinguished expert" have any motivation to admit that he had been out-"experted" by some nobody other person's work? So what should you seriously expect by way of answer to "What do the experts think?"? In the face of such a comprehensive "Catch-22" situation, where neither "experts" nor "non-experts" are willing to grant any recognition, hence logically no-one is, it is not really surprising that so many great scientific discoveries have had such a struggle to gain any recognition. Or that creativity research professor Dean K Simonton (1989) wrote:

"what I worry about most is whether all the commotion of big science obscures the voices of a few homeless people who are today's versions of the great geniuses of old."

I will have more to say about these stone-age selection systems in the later chapter about what changes could be made.

And so the Ghost of Lysenko lives on

Again I think we should be wary of embracing false absolutist stereotypes. Not everything the medical establishment says is untrue, and not everything it advocates is harmful. My own experience is that there are some professors who do indeed talk much sense and probably are the genuine leading experts in their fields, even in aspects of health science. But there are also too many of whom the reverse is the case. In the preceding pages here I have described the abysmal systems of selection and suppression which make that just about inevitable. The processes are very much still in place which enable control by a medical establishment of charlatans and suppression of any dissidence from certain established dogmas. This situation has been extensively written about by for instance Henry Bauer in his book "Dogmatism in Science and Medicine" (Bauer, 2012), and numerous earlier books cited therein.

A recent article by Aseem Malhotra (2014) indicates that medics are far from uniformly mindless dogma-following parrots. But on the other hand, at least in respect of certain important but "taboo" questions there appears to be near-absence of dissidence from the official quackery. Telling the truth gets you persecuted.

And I will show you in later sections the detailed workings of the powerful system which completely prevents any successful challenge to the false expertise, no matter how utterly absurd its defences may be and no matter how gigantically scandalous its misconduct may be.

Finally here I recommend an informative article by a professor of medicine which you can find on the web titled "Academia Suppresses Creativity" (Southwick, 2012).

Finding your way through the minefield of "expertise"

In this section I am going to have to disagree with just about everyone on one thing or another. Not a great route to increased popularity! On the internet there are some very valuable websites such as (most prominently) *Mercola.com* and *NaturalNews.com,* and also the website of the UK-published magazine *What Doctors Don't Tell You.* I consider that these (and some similar) sources contain much very valuable information which is often insufficiently highlighted by the more prominent mainstream media. But there are also major respects in which I disagree with them all. I could at this point resort to declaring that they are all fools and they could in turn use such words about myself. But instead I shall just say that I think they have been mistaken for the reasons I will explain further on. They may or may not agree with me, but I still respect their honourable intentions and conscientious work and hopefully they will be persuaded by my arguments or alternatively we can at least agree to disagree. I suspect it is myself who is more correct, but so what?! The bottom line as I see it is the following. If you were to slavishly follow the entire advice of any of those three sources I've stated above here, you would certainly find yourself in vastly better health than if you followed the deadly ruinous claptrap issuing from the medical schools of the "leading" "universities" and from the official "expert" "authorities" of the various controlling regimes in all or most of the corporatised-capitalismocracies.

I also need to preface here with some comments about terminology. Roughly-speaking, there are some people who tell you mostly the truth, and some who tell you major untruths. Some of the latter tell you outrageously nasty absurd untruths while with gross hypocrisy asserting that it is the (truth-telling) others who are really the liars. And elaborate tricks are set up to aid in the process of misleading you. I could show you an impressive collection if I have space in this book. And you can discern the major commercial and selfish motives behind those untruths and tricks. It is tempting to conclude that *all* these people should rightly be called liars or criminals (though some certainly should as you will see further on). However, I remind you of the human deficiencies stated a few pages back. And of the systems whereby incompetents get promoted to positions of high authority.

Some people have a great capacity for believing utter rubbish and for becoming blind to contrary information – "confirmation bias" in action. A great example of this is the 9-11 "truth" movement. There are (or were) many websites trying to tell us that the World Trade Center towers were felled deliberately by insider conspirators using pre-installed explosives to cause controlled demolitions (and all that stuff about planes crashing into them was just a smoke-screening sideshow). The "truthers" tell us that (a) WTC1, 2 and 7 all "fell into their own footprints", (b) "at freefall speed", and (c) WTC7 was virtually undamaged before it also suddenly fell down for no reason in one piece, and that we can see and hear the explosions and so on in various videos. In reality there are plenty of video recordings showing that the towers buckled at the level of the fires and then pancaked downwards under the tremendous weight of the upper floors. And far from falling into their own footprints, large parts crashed onto surrounding buildings causing extensive damage to those other ones. And huge damage had been caused to WTC7 such that it was not at all surprising that it also collapsed - but not before its penthouse fell in first. And yet if you show this evidence to the "truthers" it just goes in one eye and out the other. And that can't be because they are earning any great amount for promulgating their ideas, or because they feel in any prospect of winning physics Nobel prizes for them. They can't seriously be considered liars or crooked deceivers, even though they talk such obvious utter rubbish.

So people sometimes talk utter rubbish. They turn blind eyes to blaringly obvious facts. They say one thing while doing exactly the opposite. They tend to do these things in a context of serving their own self-interest. But we often have no way of knowing whether they are deliberately lying to us. They may be "in denial".

Those who have been the greatest suckers for the education system as outlined in earlier pages here may especially be so convinced of the sacred infallibility of all those tokens of "properly authorised" expertise that they feel it their sacred duty to say absolutely any conceivable nonsense in defence of their delusions of what they see as the truth. All the more so as all those powerful wealthy institutions are telling them they are right. So I am not here intending to say whom I consider is a nasty liar or a vile crook. I will try to just state the facts from which you may or may not wish to draw your own conclusions.

One of the most laughable of myths is the notion that suppression of inconvenient information only happens in "bad" countries such as – I am told – North Korea, Russia, and China. But even more laughable is the comment that the problem with the internet is that "anyone could put anything there". Sure, exactly! Yes, anyone can, in contrast to the other media where only those with huge finances and connections can get access for their "authoritative" profitmaking propaganda. And unlike the managed media, the internet (outside of corporate-controlled sites) is a 24/7 global argument-board in which untruth constantly faces exposure as what it is. My own life for one was transformed by the crucial information I got from the internet. It's just a shame I had to survive through so many years of "authoritative" criminal disinformation before it was developed.

I do not see any 100% guaranteed easy principle by which to distinguish genuine expertise from dangerous charlatanism. It helps if you can study all the details of information for yourself and thereby become your own expert yourself. But of course there are only so many hours in your day, and there are a great many studies of x or y health question you would need to read and understand.

Anyway, firstly, perhaps you could take note of the ancient wisdom of Matthew 7:15: *"Beware of false prophets, who come to you in sheep's clothing, but who inwardly are ravenous wolves."* Truth-tellers rarely present themselves as deceivers, but deceivers habitually present themselves as truth-tellers, and present the truth-tellers as deceivers themselves. You need to see through these pretences. You need to seek out alternative points of view and alternative sources of information, and then consider them together. And bear in mind that there can be more than two possible positions on a question. For instance in autism, the question "did vaccines cause an autism increase?" can be answered either with "the increase was caused by vaccines" (Age of Autism people), or with "autism hasn't increased anyway" (NHS etc). But there is also the answer I myself favour which is that the increase has been caused by a certain something else.

A favourite trick of deceivers is to make out that it is the truth-tellers who are the charlatans. They will point out supposed faults in the positions of the truth-tellers. You will see examples of such pseudo-faults in later chapters here. You have to use your wits to tease out whether the criticisms are sound or bogus. You can't properly just assume that because a particular position has been subjected to a barrage of criticisms that therefore that position must be faulty. But on the other hand, just because advocates of position B present a faulty criticism of position E, it doesn't follow that position B is indeed wrong or position E is right. Everyone has the potential for making mistakes in their rationales even if their conclusions may be correct. But when a party presents a whole load of false criticisms as some supposed proof of their proudly-proclaimed superiority then you should hear a bell ringing out that "this is probably a charlatan here".

But then again, there is a propaganda trick I have seen deployed which we might call the "deliberate own goal". I noticed that a UK national newspaper had a pro-car article by the head of the AA, falsely claiming that UK motorists pay the full social cost of their motoring (when in reality they gigantically underpay for the enormous costs of injury and death and inconvenience and environmental damage). Then the next week it had an "anti-car" article by some guy going on about how wonderfully practical he personally found his life without a car. So that must be balance there – one pro-car and one anti-car? On the surface the "deliberate own goal" article appears to be advocating position G, but it does so with carefully-judged rather stupid arguments. You are thereby tricked to "see through" that stupidity and therefrom then conclude — as they wanted you to — that position G is actually a load of rubbish. The article meanwhile carefully omits to mention the sound reasons and facts that actually do justify position G.

One important basis for distinguishing false from true is the scientific (and common-sense) plausibility, though this can require some education and judgement. For instance no amount of clinical evidence would ever persuade me that there is any validity in homeopathy, acupuncture, applied kinesiology, "energy fields", or some other such systems. As far as I can determine, no one has ever been able to find any actual evidence of the alleged meridians which are supposed to mediate acupuncture treatments. And no plausible mechanism by which the needles would help has been shown. But there are intelligent others who see acupuncture as having a rational evidence-base and you will have to judge for yourself which view is the sounder. As for homeopathy, the whole concept appears to have been discovered, or perhaps more accurately, invented, by Hahnemann out or thin air and with no relation to any other aspect of the huge scientific canon before or since. And indeed it stands in bizarre defiance of all common sense and canonical scientific notions of causality. So it looks to me and other "hard nosed" scientists that homeopathy is just a make-believe or hoax invented by Hahnemann for his convenient purposes. I think another thing that should arouse suspicion about homeopathy and acupuncture and similar alleged systems is that we are expected to believe they only have beneficial effects and never have any harmful effects.

To my mind, many standard pharmaceutical drugs have barely any more credibility than homeopathic preparations. The basic paradigm of pharmaceuticals tends to involve first identifying some substances that could be profitable (due mainly to novelty and practicalness of production) and then throwing millions of dollars into a determined attempt at "proving" them able to suppress one or other symptom (or pseudo-symptom such as cholesterol) while having scant regard to their effect on the patient as a whole. Others (such as Healy, 2012, Gøtzsche, 2013) have written about the extreme lengths of falsehood to which pharmaceutical advocates have sometimes gone in their quest to persuade that the benefits out-weigh the harms. I for one have no regret about the choice I made at age 15 – after one final aspirin – never to take any pharma drug again (and I discreetly binned some previous pharma-tech at age 10). I consider most to be third-rate junk medicine. At least homeopathics don't poison you.

(You may wonder how even the most brilliant of ten-year-olds could have any competence to reject drugs as the pseudoscience they often are. My answer is that it's rather obvious that humans can have difficulty making machines work correctly even when humans have designed them themselves and consequently understand the princ-iples of their functioning. And yet the human mind and body are vastly more complicated and mysterious than anything designed by people. So if anyone was claiming some decades ago to know that this modern liquid or pill will be the proper cure of this or that disorder, the odds would be almost certain that they would be merely pretending rather than in reality having that competence. And generally it is best not to mess with something if you don't really understand what you are doing. And no education or qualifications are needed for recognising and understanding this.)

Mike Adams of NaturalNews sums up the pharma paradigm as follows: "See how this works? Big Pharma invents a drug that causes cancer, then hires a bunch of fraudulent P.R. firm scientists to slap together a series of fictional 'science' papers, then the FDA approves the drug and doctors start pushing it. The drug companies bribe the doctors with free vacations to Hawaii, then prescriptions skyrocket, earning billions for the pharma giants. As the cancer rates start to skyrocket, the cancer industry cashes in on all the cancer surgery, radiation and chemo-therapy profits."

Meanwhile, some people will tell you that while some drugs do more harm than good, there are nevertheless some that are useful or even valuable. And I'm not in a position to say I have studied all these drugs and found them all useless. But what I can say is that there has been so much proof of dishonesty in drugs research and the portrayal of its conclusions, that a wise person views the entirety of it with deep suspicion. Why search for food in a smelly rubbish tip when you can buy it in a shop instead? Sure, perhaps relatively reasonable would be for instance a drug for Rett syndrome seeking to replace the missing MeCP2, but the odds of finding a useful such agent look to me far lower than the odds of someone overhyping the evidence in support of a harmful one. Perhaps some well-justified uses of drugs are for extreme pain, or last resort in life-threatening or otherwise intractable conditions, or for calming some psychotic persons who would otherwise harm themselves or others.

Compared to pharmaceuticals, nutrition by contrast has a far more sound scientific rationale, in its paradigm of first identifying substances likely to properly belong in your body and benefit your health as a whole, and then working out how to supply them in optimum doses.

You need to bear in mind that for at least five decades there has been very heavy propaganda designed to discredit nutritional therapies, because they provide solutions which are much cheaper and effective than profitably-patented pharmaceuticals and the like. For instance drug treatments for epilepsy, anxiety, insomnia, and deadly heart attacks are big business, and yet the prevention (often but not always) by correcting the magnesium deficiency with a bit of epsom salts every day costs hardly a penny so salespeople have more financial incentive to deride it rather than promote it. (I myself have taken epsom salts several times a day without fail since age 24; and one soon learns how not to "overdose".) The anti-nutrition propaganda operations have included studies deliberately mal-designed to give misleading results suggesting that nutritional therapies are either ineffective or harmful or both. One example of the level of tricks used was the book "Let's Stay Healthy", published after the death of Adelle Davis and pretended to be her last book, but which in reality contained advice almost the exact opposite of what her genuine books had done. My chapter here about vitamin B6 shows another <u>example of the deceitful tricks deployed</u> against nutrition. When you see a purported health guru being critical of nutritional therapies it should immediately ring alarm bells about the competence of their advice.

But there is an additional complication to expert views about nutrition. This is exemplified by, among others, the book "Deadly Medicines and Organised Crime" by Peter Gøtzsche (2013). The one and only point where that book gets mistaken is in its opening paragraphs about the supposed worthlessness of nutritional supplements. And yet the author of that book has considerable expertise combined with extreme criticalness towards medical orthodoxy. Many doctors such as Gøtzsche will resolutely assure you that nutritional supplements are a waste of money and that "you can get all the nutrients you need from food". But I don't think they are lying there. What they don't understand is the following.

Medically-qualified people are highly unrepresentative of the population in general. To get qualified as a medic you have to score very highly in one mega-parrotting exam after another, and you can only do that if you have very high capacity for memorising of mounds of information. As quoted earlier in this chapter: *"The sheer volume of information we were expected to memorise was mind-boggling."* And you can only excel in that if you are very healthy and not particularly stressed-out by anything (and certainly not mercury-poisoned). Such an unstressed person can indeed succeed very well with minimal nutrition for years. Eventually after some decades the lack of nutritional optimisation is liable to impact in rather predictable ways (e.g. creaky joints, need for specs, circulation getting dodgy), but by then it can be falsely attributed to some proper timing of natural ageing processes with no thought that nutrition could have made any difference. The medics and their medic colleagues all infer from their own experience of getting on fine without those supplements. But they err in presuming that that can be correctly assumed to also apply in respect of people who have suffered significant stresses or who have some different genetic makeup. Stressful conditions such as adverse life events and toxic exposures can cause illnesses which are very much dependent on whether the victim has access to optimised nutrition obtainable only from supplements.

The medics then make a further error in their perception of the literature. They see that the evidence for drugs is biased in favour of exaggerated usefulness and understated harm. It doesn't occur to them that the propaganda biases tend to be exactly the opposite way round in respect of nutrients. The studies are largely funded by big organisations which wish to belittle the value of nutrients rather than hype them. So for instance they use too little vitamin C, or use an unnatural form of vitamin D, or they fail to have regard to the fact that nutrients do not work like drugs, in glorious isolation, but instead as a coordinated orchestra to build health. For instance, vitamin D needs to be balanced with vitamins E and A, and zinc needs to be in suitable ratio to calcium and copper. No amount of vitamin C can substitute for immune weakness caused by deficiency of zinc or copper, or vice versa.

Meanwhile there ia a seemingly endless stream of prominently-published anti-nutritional propaganda articles such as: *"The truth about 'miracle foods' – from chia seeds to coconut oil"* (Mohammadi, 2015). From which I quote: "If you see a claim on a blog, and if it's persuasive and looks good, ask yourself why has the company not used it in their marketing? If the product really did prevent cancer or heart disease, do you not think it'd be plastered all over the packaging?". To which I reply to the evidently genius Nottingham University Professor Duane Mellor behind that pearl of quasi-wisdom: Those companies haven't used it in their marketing because freedom of speech is so, so, supremely important in the free world, and so it has been made a criminal offence to tell people what life-saving benefits your product has, unless you have first managed to find the millions of dollars to get your health claims approved by the health fascist nannying system. Was that complex enough for you to understand, Professor? Because it is necessary that big organisations constantly bully small organisations into silence, because the big organisations (not least Nottingham University) are notoriously honest whereas the small ones are mostly crooks.

Another gem from that same article: "Coconut oil is predominantly a medium-chain triglyceride which, proponents state, might carry benefits for weight loss, but this claim has not been shown in human studies." But more to the point is that farmers long ago gave up trying to fatten their animals with a harmless food which sadly only makes them thinner instead, and no company has any incentive to risk $millions on re-proving the point in humans. (And the writer usefully prefaced there with the so-so- practically useful point about being a "medium-chain triglyceride" so as to ensure we would be aware that this was a proper scientific expert educating us about it.) (And you will see the same *"Look how much cleverer we are than you!"* trick being used against vitamin B6 in Chapter 11.)

Another trick I should mention relates to the declaration you will find on some sun-creams that they are "PABA-free". Thank sod, I hear the purchaser thinking, I wouldn't want to get any of that nasty Para-Amino-Benzoic Acid on my face! The great thing about the words "PABA-free" is that they aren't actually a lie, but they can nevertheless do exactly the same job as a lie. PABA is a natural vitamin, which was recognised decades ago as useful in topical application as a natural way to prevent sunburn and skin cancer. But some people would of course prefer to sell you something more profitable (and with any luck causing more profitable skin and other problems further down the line). Meanwhile progress must take place in the capitalist world, with outmoded "truthful" science replaced by more modern profitable science. The fact that the greatest free capitalism nation in history now has some of the worst health stats on the planet may have some connection to that.

Another vitally important nutrient which has become the subject of major disinformation is iodine (Abraham, 2005). Basically any natural substance which genuinely helps to cure or prevent cancer gets subjected to such disinformation (another example being cannabis) so as not to undermine the huge profits of the chemo'therapy' scam industry.

There nowadays also exists something of an intermediate between pharma and nutrition, in terms of what are called nutriceuticals, such as compounds related to but not identical to specific actual nutrients. This is also a sensible scientific paradigm and I guess may be one of the most powerful of ways forward.

Herbal remedies I would place on a continuum between nutrition and pharma. This ranges from the superlatively enhancing (curcumin, ginseng) to the sometimes valuable but sometimes harmful in incompetent hands (gingko, liquorice root, coriander, chlorella). I myself was unable to take even a quarter of a tiny gingko tablet without getting inflamed gums (but then I did also have half a ton of mercury stored right there too). And chlorella can cause ruinously injurious (and even fatal) iron overload.

Vaccines appear to fit into the same third-rate paradigm as other issuings from the pharma trade. As with other drugs, first an exclusive patented profitable product is identified and then money is invested in persuading everyone that it is crucially important. I think you should consider a recent book titled "Dissolving Illusions: Disease, Vaccines, and The Forgotten History" (Humphries & Bystrianyk, 2013). And a more recent one by Tetyana Obukhanych, who got a PhD in immunology then on reflection decided her education had been very defective anyway. On the internet you can see some of the fanatical personal attacks such non-conforming authors get subjected to by corporate-aligned people.

You could also consider these comments from a study recently published in a top peer-reviewed journal (Wang et al., 2014).

"*The reported coverage of the measles–rubella (MR) or measles–mumps–rubella (MMR) vaccine is greater than 99% in Zhejiang province. However, the incidence of measles, mumps, and rubella remains high. .... measles, mumps, and rubella remain common diseases throughout Zhejiang province. .... Therefore, the elimination of measles and control of mumps and rubella are urgent public health priorities in local regions.*"

Note that this report is telling us that not just one but all three famous infections (measles, mumps and rubella) have not been effectively countered even by 99% double-coverage of those vaccinations in a population of 50 million. This huge study alone suffices to cast large doubts on the vaccine industry's scientific credibility.

But maybe you are thinking that that Wang report is just a one-off anomaly, like the famous anecdotal report of men landing on the moon. Well, here are three more I have learned of from Tetyana Obukhanych:

Nkowane et al 1987 Measles outbreak in a vaccinated school population: epidemiology, chains of transmission, and the role of vaccine failures. Am J Public Health.

Boullane et al 1991 Major measles epidemic in the region of Quebec despite a 99% vaccine coverage. Canadian J Public Health.

Sutcliffe et al 1996 Outbreak of measles in a highly vaccinated secondary school population. Canadian Med Assocn.

The evidence highlighted by Dr Obukhanych and others shows that measles vaccines do indeed generate some sort of immunity, but that it usually lasts only a few months or years, in contrast to the lifelong immunity created by having a relatively trivial natural measles infection in childhood. And this has two adverse consequences. Firstly it increases the risk of measles in older people, for whom it can be more harmful. And secondly it prevents mothers passing on their immunity to their babies, with the result that those infants lack that natural protection and are thus at risk of an infection which can be deadly at that unnatural age.

Four further things reflect this dubiousness of vaccine science. Firstly that their manufacturers have been granted some peculiar exemption from the normal legal liability for harm caused. Secondly that they are not required to prove actual effectiveness, but merely that they generate some antibodies, even though there is a lot more to the immune system than those antibodies which clearly don't have effects equivalent to those of the infections themselves. Thirdly that people are often bullied into enforced acceptance of them. Fourthly that those who refuse are not challenged with any scientific arguments but instead are vilified as supposedly evil criminals putting others at risk. So I find vaccines to be at best very dubious. I speak as someone who hasn't had an infection ("common" cold etc.) for about 20 years, because there are less dubious alternatives based on building natural immune functioning.

Note that I haven't mentioned autism anywhere here. I'll come to that in a later chapter.

I am aware that I will have alienated almost all the varieties of healthcare people with the views I have stated in various paragraphs above here. The corporate illness industry will condemn me for challenging vaccines, but also most of the anti-corporate health people will condemn me for dismissing some "alternative" medicines such as homeopathy and acupuncture. Well, ...

At this point I should remind you of the point I made in the opening pages, that I do not see a neat contrast between one side which tells all the truth and the other side which tells all the nonsense. But it is my experience that other people do tend to reckon in such terms. Even some very competent health gurus tend to over-react when they discover that official "experts" have been talking rubbish about matters x, y, or z, and covering up major sound science such as the value of vitamins and suppressed cures for cancer. They then over-react by going to the opposite extreme. They mis-reason to a false inference that in that case the establishment "experts" must be also be lying to them about all the other derided ideas such as homeopathy, acupuncture, "energy medicine", applied kinesiology, and so on, and they thereby come to a false conclusion that those alternative approaches are valid and that criticisms of them are just more unsound corporate propaganda.

Sadly, I find that in consequence the health expertise world is largely divided into two camps neither of which are quite correct. The alternative gurus rightly challenge the official pseudoscience, and champion sound science such as nutrition and exercise, but then spoil it by also endorsing all the unsound "alternative" therapies. Meanwhile, the corporate establishment people rightly decry those alternatives, but then err themselves in defending the harmful drugs and surgery approaches. Well, at least thousands of people aren't being killed or poisoned by homeopathy or acupuncture.

Part of the problem here is that the alternative thinkers tend to forget to apply scientific criticalness to their unconventional ideas (not that the conventionals do any better).

For instance some people are claiming that the Fukushima earthquake was deliberately caused by radio waves from the HAARP transmitter in Maryland US, by its beaming at the ionosphere over the earthquake epicentre and also sending out low frequency waves of 2.5 Hz (approximating to earthquake resonances). The evidence they present is at first glance impressive.

But it rather clearly does not stand up to examination by the numerically-literate, as follows. Firstly, a ground-based transmitter cannot send even a moderately focussed beam (in a straightish line) to the ionosphere more than about 30 degrees away around the Earth, but Japan is more than 90 degrees around from Maryland. Secondly, a radiowave of 2.5 Hz frequency has a wavelength of about 300 million kilometers, and consequently it would be impossible to focus it on a single entire planet let alone on a single continent. It would be just as likely to trigger the long-expected California earthquake as one somewhere else.

For this sort of reason I strongly recommend that you put some time and effort into studying maths, physics, chemistry, and biology preferably up to GCE A-level level (i.e. students at 18 years old), even though going on to study a medical degree is a serious waste of time unless you really do want a career as a corporate pawn spouting FDA/MHRA/GMC-approved claptrap all day long.

But you also need to learn the separate ability to ask whether an idea might be simply daft. Some people who ought to know better tell you that there is a conspiracy to poison whole populations in the USA by spraying chemicals from aircraft, in so-called "chemtrails" which you can see in the sky as allegedly being different from the normal contrails. I dismiss that theory on the simple basis that even if someone did want to poison millions of people, a huge secret system of chemtrails would be a stupendously inefficient and indiscriminate way to do so. It would be a lot neater and easier to put some poisonous industrial waste in the public water supply, such as sodium hexafluoride (as is indeed done under pretence of benefitting health). Or sell poisonous junk in food stores (as is indeed done everywhere). The "chemtrails" can be easily understood to be just contrails which behave differently due to changes in aviation or the modern atmosphere. No more clinching evidence has ever emerged.

Anyway, back to the principles of discerning the genuine from the false. You need to look out for "cherry-picking" of evidence, people telling you only the evidence or reasoning that supports one position, while omitting to mention other important information that doesn't fit in (though in the process they also make out an impression that they are *not* failing to mention anything important).

For instance in my peer-review-published autism theory paper herewith, you can see that I cited and provided easy explanations for a number of seriously "weird" facts about autism (not present in all cases but certainly in some, hence their getting into the list of Wing (1976)). Spinning without dizziness. Bursts of alternating hand-flapping and posturing. Reversals of "I"/"me" with "you". Low seating of ears, wide spacing of eyes, and webbing of toes. "A springy tip-toe walk without appropriate swinging of the arms." "An odd posture when standing, with head bowed, arms flexed at the elbow and hands drooping at the wrist." "Unusual symmetry of face." "Attractive appearance, intelligent appearance". Peculiar associations with high IQ and high SES (social class). "An unusual form of memory: ability to store items for prolonged periods in the exact form they were first experienced".

While all these "weird" facts about autism fitted easily and perfectly into the theory presented in my own paper, they continued to present an inconveniently baffling mystery to autism researchers holding onto other lines of belief. So they just conveniently ignored them all, failed to ever mention them, and instead concentrated on imagining that the defining symptomology of autism equals solely the Holy Triad of Impairments handed down by the Prophet Wing to which no more needs be added. And notably none of these autism "experts" (other than Rimland) have ever mentioned (cited) that that peer-reviewed PsycInfo-indexed paper even exists, despite its being fundamentally relevant to many of the papers they themselves publish. A wise competent truth-seeking reader keeps an eye out for those things which are "weird" (anomalous), even though sometimes of course they can be just wrong observations anyway.

Other gross examples of cherry-picking have been the various official reports asserting there is "no evidence" that dental amalgam causes any harm (other than minor local allergy). They just ignore the many reports of people having "miraculous" recoveries from their long-term disabilities after removal of amalgams, some of which featured in the various studies reviewed in Hanson (2004). And you can also see in my later chapter about vitamin B6 how the "experts" failed to mention the counter-evidence of safety and usefulness.

A complication to discerning the cherry-picking principle is that some studies are not very competent so should indeed be left unpicked, or at least explicitly rejected. Again, you need to use judgment and knowledge and wits to discern whether the studies are genuinely useless or you are just being fooled into thinking so. For instance some defenders of amalgam assert that the many reports and studies of recoveries after amalgam removal are merely "anecdotal" and or "placebo effects". They conveniently fail to mention (let alone discuss) any actual details about these recoveries. I invite you to decide for yourself whether one can validly just laugh off as merely anecdotal or merely placebo thousands of such observations as 40 years of unretractable depression "miraculously" ended within days of amalgam removal, or cancerous tumours on the cheek clearing away after amalgam removal, many other recoveries documented on the youtube channel of the London dentist Hesham el-Essawy, and so on.

You will also see in Chapter 4 how Reviewer #1 seeks to discredit the study by Holmes et al, and how I proceed to demolish that discrediting in turn. And you can see how Reviewer #3 cites studies by Bellinger, DeRouen, and Maserejian as supposedly proving that amalgams cause no harm, and my rebuttals there again.

Another major trick of deceivers (or mere muddle-makers) is to misrepresent a study or position, by means of a "straw man argument", attacking a position that is not being proposed anyway. You can see an example in how that same anonymous Reviewer #1 makes a false assertion about the Bradstreet study, starting with his/her misleading words "The fact that....".   (Dr Bradstreet has since been assassinated by the Pharma pseuds.)

Another characteristic of pseudo-experts is that on the one hand they tend to be extremely critical and dismissive of studies which go against their position, and yet on the other hand wonderfully positive about those trashy studies which just happen to support what they are saying. You can again see some of this in the vitamin B6 and the amalgam discussions. The rubbish rolled out to supposedly justify criminalising British people from buying harmless life-saving vitamins would be particularly laughable were it not also so criminal. Worse, in the exact same year that the "distinguished" volunteers of the "independent" Committee on Toxicity were declaring that the British should not be allowed to buy "dangerous" vitamin B6, they were also declaring that there was no evidence at all that storing big lumps of dental amalgam mercury in your mouth might be harmful or that anyone should be given any suggestion it might be.

Another hint of whether or not information is honestly competent is the extent to which it reflects what I could call "the gradient of knowledge". Propaganda will tend to tell you that we "know" xyz to be "true" and we "know" xwv to be "untrue". But an important part of being a competent scientist, and even more a competent science writer, is to recognise that claims do not simply dichotomise into "true" and "untrue". Competent presentation of information reflects an infinite gradation of "trueness" versus "untrueness", such as "conceivably", "quite possibly", "it has been suggested that", "the results seem to imply", "some researchers think", "it can't be ruled out that", "almost certainly", and so on. If you find instead the "true"/"untrue" sort of thinking then you may be better advised to not waste your time further with that particular source.

There are some books by other authors which contain much detailed guidance on the ways in which scientific studies and reports can be greatly flawed, e.g. Kendrick (2014) and Goldacre (2012). You may find it useful to study these books if you are not already familiar with this sort of thing.

The teasing out of whether you are reading truth or falsehood can be a rather time-consuming and tedious task even once you have picked up some background knowledge. Some people will decide they are just too busy, and in that case they are effectively gambling on their luck as to whether their chosen options are life-saving or life-ruining. I'd like to think that a wise person would learn the basics of biology and chemistry and physics and maths at least to the level that teenagers do at school. And learn some of the basic terminology of health, such as proteins, enzymes, neurons, gene-expression, controlled study, significance level. Without such knowledge you are effectively a health-illiterate, as childishly dependent as someone who can't read or write or do sums. There is now a wonderful resource in the internet in that you can just type in a word and immediately find free lectures and guides as to what all these words mean. I've learned a lot that way myself. The internet is very useful also in that if some expert tells you that a new study in the Lancet shows that statin drugs instantly double your IQ, you can search out the authors and title of that study and then obtain it for yourself (often for free) and see for yourself how strong the case is, and also check what others are saying about it, and even ask questions of other internet users or even the authors themselves.

One thing you need to be wary of is that the internet is being abused by corporate propagandists. This is especially the case with Wikipedia, of which the health pages have been specially targetted by Pharma shills in order to block editing by those who challenge the official pseudoscience. See these links: www.naturalnews.com/053869_science_skeptics_Wikipedia_guerrill a_propaganda.html   *and*   http://bolenreport.com/mike-adams-natural-news-attacks-skeptics-center-point/

Also a particularly famous search engine ("G..."?) have a project underway to "improve" their health-related search results. So you may be best advised to beware of their results rankings, and or use other search engines such as goodgopher.

A bit of a shortcut can be obtained by getting a general impression of the credibility and any biases of a particular writer or source. The Age of Autism website is highly unlikely to publish an argument that vaccines never cause any autism. And the LBRB blog or Pediatrics journal or the NHS are equally unlikely to publish anything suggesting that they ever *could* cause autism. Likewise certain individuals can be seen to be riding on certain hobbyhorses. Rightly or wrongly. If you see that they regularly deploy unsound arguments for the positions they purport to be experts in, then you can reckon them to have low credibility in anything else they say in that direction of the debate. But if they ever say anything in the other direction, going against their own established position, then all the more reason to consider that they may for once be making a valid point.

You will observe that there is much material being published which seeks to undermine the credibility of particular individuals. For instance the attacks against Andrew Wakefield, whom I consider to be a basically honest and conscientious person whose expertise in gastroenterology has sadly not been matched by any expertise in epidemiology or due cynicism about the decency of official authorities. My experience is that such *ad hominem* attacks are almost always deployed by those who do not have the actual scientific facts on their side and so seek to distract from that with the personal attacks instead. However, those who are thus attacked commonly find it necessary to attack back at those who attack them. So it again gets complicated. And some foolish people can complicate the picture by going in for ad hominem even when they are supporting a valid position.

Another indication of the soundness of a source is the nature of the documentation proof they provide. Simple "information" leaflets in a clinic may just state things as if they are self-evident truths, such as "Statins will always make your nose adjust to the correct length eventually". These are written for an audience of people who just believe what the authorities tell them. Their claims aren't necessarily untrue, but neither would I assume anything they say is remotely true either (in rather obvious consequence of the information documented in later chapters).

The situation is rather different in respect of those books and other publications which are purporting to be addressed to a critical, discerning, audience. In such media, it is not normal just to assert things and expect them to be found credible. Instead such important contentions as "Statins *will* adjust your nose to its correct length" are expected to be backed up with citation of some evidential basis. In the "primary literature", that is papers published in "scientific journals", the norm is that every statement of much importance has to be supported by one or more citations indicated in the text, which link to a list of all the cited documents included at the end.

Two citation systems are commonly used in health-related writing: the name-date system, e.g. Clarke (2015) or (Clarke, 2015);

and the Vancouver system which would just have a number such as [23] or in superscript as [23], with that reference no. 23 in the list then being Clarke's 2015 paper or whatever. Either of these are reasonable and have their advantages and disadvantages. You can see from them if the author has failed to provide any supporting documentation or what it is if they have provided it. But even then you can't safely assume that the citations do actually justify the conclusion being asserted. If the assertion in question is crucial and in doubt, then you might want to critically read any cited source documents for yourself.

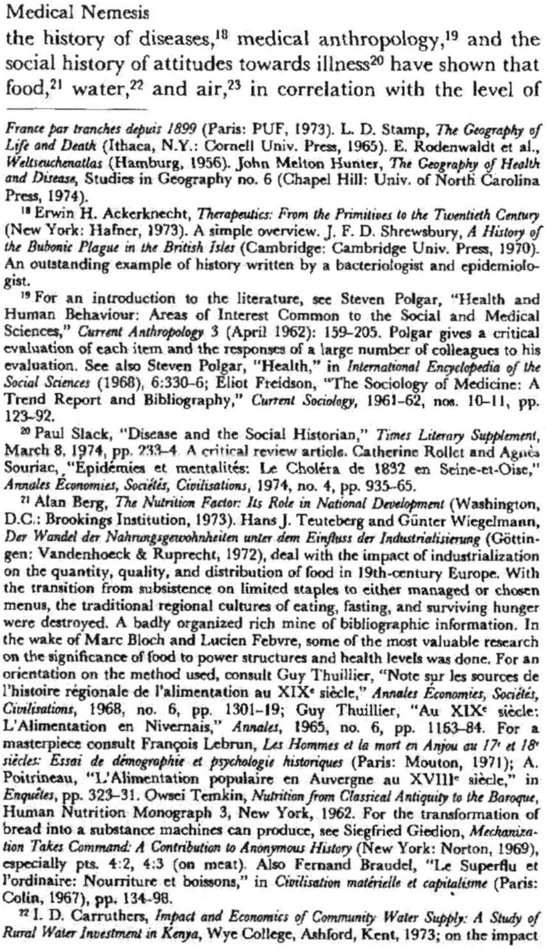

Medical Nemesis

the history of diseases,[18] medical anthropology,[19] and the social history of attitudes towards illness[20] have shown that food,[21] water,[22] and air,[23] in correlation with the level of

France par tranches depuis 1899 (Paris: PUF, 1973). L. D. Stamp, *The Geography of Life and Death* (Ithaca, N.Y.: Cornell Univ. Press, 1965). E. Rodenwaldt et al., *Weltseuchenatlas* (Hamburg, 1956). John Melton Hunter, *The Geography of Health and Disease*, Studies in Geography no. 6 (Chapel Hill: Univ. of North Carolina Press, 1974).

[18] Erwin H. Ackerknecht, *Therapeutics: From the Primitives to the Twentieth Century* (New York: Hafner, 1973). A simple overview. J. F. D. Shrewsbury, *A History of the Bubonic Plague in the British Isles* (Cambridge: Cambridge Univ. Press, 1970). An outstanding example of history written by a bacteriologist and epidemiologist.

[19] For an introduction to the literature, see Steven Polgar, "Health and Human Behaviour: Areas of Interest Common to the Social and Medical Sciences," *Current Anthropology* 3 (April 1962): 159–205. Polgar gives a critical evaluation of each item and the responses of a large number of colleagues to his evaluation. See also Steven Polgar, "Health," in *International Encyclopedia of the Social Sciences* (1968), 6:330–6; Eliot Freidson, "The Sociology of Medicine: A Trend Report and Bibliography," *Current Sociology*, 1961–62, nos. 10–11, pp. 123–92.

[20] Paul Slack, "Disease and the Social Historian," *Times Literary Supplement*, March 8, 1974, pp. 233–4. A critical review article. Catherine Rollet and Agnès Souriac, "Epidémies et mentalités: Le Choléra de 1832 en Seine-et-Oise," *Annales Économies, Sociétés, Civilisations*, 1974, no. 4, pp. 935–65.

[21] Alan Berg, *The Nutrition Factor: Its Role in National Development* (Washington, D.C.: Brookings Institution, 1973). Hans J. Teuteberg and Günter Wiegelmann, *Der Wandel der Nahrungsgewohnheiten unter dem Einfluss der Industrialisierung* (Göttingen: Vandenhoeck & Ruprecht, 1972), deal with the impact of industrialization on the quantity, quality, and distribution of food in 19th-century Europe. With the transition from subsistence on limited staples to either managed or chosen menus, the traditional regional cultures of eating, fasting, and surviving hunger were destroyed. A badly organized rich mine of bibliographic information. In the wake of Marc Bloch and Lucien Febvre, some of the most valuable research on the significance of food to power structures and health levels was done. For an orientation on the method used, consult Guy Thuillier, "Note sur les sources de l'histoire régionale de l'alimentation au XIXᵉ siècle," *Annales Économies, Sociétés, Civilisations*, 1968, no. 6, pp. 1301–19; Guy Thuillier, "Au XIXᵉ siècle: L'Alimentation en Nivernais," *Annales*, 1965, no. 6, pp. 1163–84. For a masterpiece consult François Lebrun, *Les Hommes et la mort en Anjou au 17ᵉ et 18ᵉ siècles: Essai de démographie et psychologie historiques* (Paris: Mouton, 1971); A. Poitrineau, "L'Alimentation populaire en Auvergne au XVIIIᵉ siècle," in *Enquêtes*, pp. 323–31. Owsei Temkin, *Nutrition from Classical Antiquity to the Baroque*, Human Nutrition Monograph 3, New York, 1962. For the transformation of bread into a substance machines can produce, see Siegfried Giedion, *Mechanization Takes Command: A Contribution to Anonymous History* (New York: Norton, 1969), especially pts. 4:2, 4:3 (on meat). Also Fernand Braudel, "Le Superflu et l'ordinaire: Nourriture et boissons," in *Civilisation matérielle et capitalisme* (Paris: Colin, 1967), pp. 134–98.

[22] I. D. Carruthers, *Impact and Economics of Community Water Supply: A Study of Rural Water Investment in Kenya*, Wye College, Ashford, Kent, 1973; on the impact

Figure 1.1. A page from Ivan Illich's *Medical Nemesis*.

An even better, particularly transparent, method of showing citations was exemplified in Ivan Illich's book *Medical Nemesis* back in 1975, in which he put the citations right there as footnotes on the text pages. Many of the pages of Illich's book have more such sourcing footnotes than text, as illustrated by the sample page here. (Footnotes were normal practice until recent decades.)

But there is another method of citation which has started happening in some health-related books as society becomes increasingly superficialised and lazy and corrupted. This "shy" method of citation puts nothing in the text pages themselves and relies on the reader constantly checking the reference list at the back, where the cited sources are listed in terms of which page of the text they are not being mentioned on. So in the course of just reading the text you have no idea which assertions are based on some source and which of the assertions are merely blank assertions with no supporting basis. This is of course an excellent arrangement if you wish (deliberately or unconsciously) to deceive your readers into assuming that some of the rubbish you are writing is true when it isn't.

A particularly notable book making some remarkable use of this system of shy citations is "Autism's False Prophets" written by the millionaire vaccine-patentee Paul Offit, and which I consider to be a leading contender for the most evil book published in the last 70 years. (And I say that even though I agree with some of it.) I will have more to say about that book in the chapter about vaccines, where you can see some illustrations of its pages using the shy citations system.

Perhaps you could compare Offit's shy citation systems with Illich's out-front footnoting approach and then work out for yourself whether intellectual standards have risen or fallen in the 40 years since Illich's condemnation of the medical authoritocracy.

Another very important hint for distinguishing truth from falsehood is as follows. Truth does not need criminalisation or persecution of opposing or doubting views to defend itself. Only organisational propaganda lies do. Likewise if someone starts angrily threatening and shouting at you or expressing moralising contempt for your supposed evilness when you raise a thought, then you should ask yourself what was the evidence that had earlier persuaded that angry person who claims to resolutely know so much better than you. After all, they appear to think that being threatened or shouted at and accused of being a vile person will be sufficient evidence for yourself to be persuaded to believe those "facts", so it is difficult to avoid the conclusion that that is all that their own "knowledge" was actually founded on too. "Oh but there's tons of evidence as everyone knows." "And in that case could you perhaps tell me just one bit you found persuasive?" "!!![Angry threat to xyz-iate you if you don't stop civilly requesting some actual evidence.]".

Another trick is as follows. The authors start off by telling you a lot of true things. You become impressed by their competence and honesty. And then, once you have thus been induced into a state of uncritically trusting that author, only then they introduce their whopping big lie. I'll leave you to guess the titles of some books which might use that trick. (Am I using it here?)

Finally, I shall now tell you about what is probably the most powerful propaganda technique of all. It could be called the "unmentioned pseudo-obvious". A simple example of this is something you will often encounter in the media, in which the ruling people in countries x, y, and z are routinely referred to as "regimes", whereas the ruling people in countries a, b, and c are routinely referred to as "governments". And meanwhile those media never address the question of what evidential justification there could be for that difference of terminology.

A more developed example is a radio program just today about the difficulty of obtaining some cancer drugs. It goes on for 45 minutes about all the difficulties of some drugs only working for situation x or y, the NICE committee being very stingey with their funding decisions, and so on. It's all very impressively critical and logical and by goes-without-saying implication soundly evidence-based. Listening to it you would easily assume that it is accurately presenting a proper sound scientific discipline. It impresses you by carefully-managed mentioning of some of the methodological points I've made above here. And yet it makes not the slightest mention of any of the damning facts pointed out in the books by Gøtzsche, Healy, Goldacre, Davis, Kendrick and many others. Nor does it even begin to address what evidence there is that any of these drugs are at all good for anyone. The deceiving surface of criticalness is carefully designed to avoid penetrating to the real problems which show the entire drugs industry "science" to be utter baloney unworthy of any characterisation as science.

Anyway a good rule of thumb is that if media are going on about something being good, then it is probably very bad, and if they are going on about it being bad, then it is probably vitally health-enhancing, and worth looking into further.

And key questions you should always ask about any document are: (1) What actual evidence is raised? (2) How sound and decisive is it? and (3) what evidence has been misrepresented or omitted from mention?

In conclusion then, there are no hard-and-fast easy rules by which you can consistently discern truth from falsehood in purported information about health, but the more you can work at applying these principles and studying and thinking for yourself, the less you are depending your life and welfare on big gambles on Expert Dr X or Institute Y being truthful or otherwise in what they tell you. I for one consider it well worth putting some time and effort into making my life and health less of a lottery.

You may be wondering whether some preceding pages here could justify rejection of seeming expert consensus thinking in respect of other fields of science, for instance climate change. Not necessarily. I will say more about that in an afterword.

Other books about false and genuine medical expertise

Numerous others have written books about the major corruptions of medical expertise and the products and procedures which are doing more harm than good. It would be easy to assume that they are all or mostly just repeating the same content, at least in factual terms if not style. But in reality, such is the extent of the defectiveness of the medical authoritocracy that numerous books have been written about it with relatively little overlap. Such books vary in their soundness, but some recent ones which could usefully supplement this one would include *Doctoring Data* (2014) by Malcolm Kendrick, *Deadly Medicines and Organised Crime* (2013) by Peter Gøtzsche, *Dissolving Illusions* (Humphries & Bystrianyk, 2014) and *Bad Pharma* (2012) by Ben Goldacre. Others more specific to psychiatry would include *Pharmageddon* (2012) by David Healy and *Cracked* (2013) by James Davies. However, I myself have since childhood considered pharma drugs to be a load of pseudic rubbish anyway, so none of those books has had much practical relevance to my own healthcare. Instead of reading those books just read my lips when I say "Medical drugs are poisonous pseudo-scientific c....p".

Of more practical value would be various books about nutrition, including the books by Adelle Davis which are decades outdated now but still mostly very informative, with the exception of "Let's Stay Healthy" which was falsely attributed as her "last book" in yet another of the pharma-lobby's propaganda tricks. Unfortunately there are also plenty of misconceived books laying in wait to confuse you or at least waste your time, including *The China Study* and *The End of Illness*. I also consider Robert Whitaker's *Anatomy of an Epidemic* to be at least mistaken about the cause of that epidemic, as I explain in later chapters here.

Continuing from here

I should here first reiterate a point I made on the first page – that this is not primarily a book about autism. It just so happens that the information about autism opens the door to understanding a much larger catastrophe involving entirely non-autistic problems. Most of the victims of the false expertise are non-autistic (and <u>I am not autistic either</u>). Anyway.....

Before starting on this book I had written three main scientific papers about autism (and some lesser ones). In the chapters that follow I will include two and a bit of those papers. In order of the original writing, the first was "A theory of general impairment of gene-expression manifesting as autism", which you can now read in Chapter 7 here. Please note that this was written years ago for a very different audience and I would present it somewhat differently nowadays. Not least I would change the title to "A theory of *evolution-biased suppression.....*" because the "impairment" word gives a false impression that autism (all autism, and autism *per se*) entails that "something has gone wrong", which has now become the most malign of myths about autism. And that "general" word confuses too.

At the time of publishing that theory, autism was little-known and the nature of its causation a rather marginal "academic" question. No one was talking back then about autism being some puzzling mystery or considering *What causes autism?* to be any sort of important let alone urgent question. But in years that followed, autism became the focus of many media headlines, with the questions of what was causing autism and an alleged increase thereof becoming the centre of one of the most prominent and heated scientific controversies in recent history (and ongoing).

Then later I became aware of three crucial facts about dental amalgams – the "silver" metal fillings mainly used in back teeth. Firstly that amalgams emit neurotoxic mercury vapor. Secondly that mercury randomly binds to DNA and dose-dependently reduces gene-expression – a fact which "rang a bell" very loudly given that I had said in the theory paper that things randomly binding to DNA and thereby reducing gene-expression would thereby cause autism. And thirdly that in the 1970s there had been a change to a new sort of amalgams, which emit far more mercury vapour (and which would thus be a potential cause of the autism increase). A website by Ulf Bengtsson titled "The instability of amalgams" was particularly helpful in respect of this matter. And I had also in the meantime noticed a number of reports of peculiar findings which confirmed predictions of the published theory paper.

This new information inspired me to investigate the possibility that the change of dental amalgam had been the (or a) cause of the autism increase. This looked very likely, so I started work on researching an update review of the autism theory paper, which eventually became titled "The causes of autism: a theory confirmed by four predictions; why dental amalgams caused the autism increase; and why mercury pollution caused the Flynn effect IQ increase". But I had hardly started work on writing that update review when a horrendous harassment operation was launched against me, the house where I had established my home being overrun by unregulated violent lifestyle-alcoholic lifestyle-criminals as detailed at my website www.2020housing.co.uk. Nevertheless, in between episodes of having bricks thrown through my windows and so-on I eventually managed to sort-of-complete the update review and send it out to some relevant readers a year later, and thereafter send to some journals. After two years of coping with the criminals, I was suddenly evicted into homelessness on entirely false grounds by the more than thirty cheap (not even clever) lies these sentences temporarily redacted these sentences temporarily redacted these sentences temporarily redacted these sentences temporarily redacted these sentences temporarily redacted these sentences temporarily redacted these sentences temporarily redacted.

Anyway, somewhat belatedly the city council eventually designated me as officially homeless, thereby getting me to the front of their waiting list of 20,000 others; and after some further years of semi-chaos (and continuing untreated mercury poisoning and NHS lies) I eventually managed to get started on the update review again. My attempts at getting it published were met with the same sort of rubbish rationales as had prevented my theory paper from being published for some years previously. Then, three years later, I discovered evidence that exactly concurrently with the autism increase there had also been a fourfold increase of non-autistic adult disabilities of the sort that dental mercury would cause. Note that while the autism increase has not been a minor occurrence, it is very much over-shadowed in numbers by this other increase of adult non-autistic disabilities which the data suggests to be about four million victims in the UK alone (and with new victims being disinformed and clinically assaulted every day).

Two years later, still finding my update review being blocked from publication with cheap excuses, I began to wonder whether part of the problem might be the word "theory", which seems to arouse a knee-jerk bigotry from science academics, along the lines of not asking "in what ways could this be correct?", but instead "in what ways can we fob this off as yet another load of rubbish?"

Indeed the majority of "scientific" medical journals won't even consider theory papers for publication, or at best only under the stupid conditions of "If you can't express your idea in less than 1500 words it probably isn't a *Hypothesis*" – "hypothesis" being the standard word to cheaply belittle a theory via a misleading contemptuous pejorative. Your idea (even if it is a great revolutionary breakthrough logically argued and documented with *14,000* words of evidence) is only a "hypothesis", pah-hah-hah! (Of which more in the next chapter.)

So I guessed there might be more hope of getting a paper published if it was more oriented to presenting the *facts* of the two increases, while keeping the theory aspect in the background. So I re-worked parts of the update review into a new paper, titled "Autism, adult disability, and 'workshy': Major epidemics being caused by non-gamma-2 dental amalgams". And I sent it to a journal. Now, two years later, it has been sent to at least 17 putatively appropriate journals. In some following chapters you can judge for yourself the merits or otherwise of the reasons these journals gave for refusing to publish this information I sent them. Those chapters show you the insides of the supposedly wonderful so-called peer-review system in operation, something which non-authors usually never get to see. The two-legged entities discharging this filth assumed their words were never going to be published for reading by the public. I'll just state the facts and leave to you to decide for yourself how colourful any adjectives ought to be. But bear in mind that these faceless nameless entities were not there merely writing anonymous yet public critiques of published evidence, but were rather writing their non-public "reasons" why that evidence should not even be allowed into the public scientific record (for you or the victims to learn about) anyway. And evidence about a crime against millions of victims at that. And with that crime still devastating newly-deceived victims right now. So much for the "open dialogue" of science which you will hear various people enthusing about in high places.

In the preceding paragraphs I have indicated the chronological order in which I wrote those papers. But it might be more useful or desirable for you to read them in a different order. The later papers cite and build on the initial paper. But not so extensively as to be impossible to make progress on independently. If you are not already familiar with the realities of autism, or are under a delusion that you *do* have that familiarity due to having learnt the rubbish being taught by others, then the original theory paper would give you a useful introduction to the nature of the autistic syndrome. But on the other hand that first paper is somewhat harder going because it presents radical unfamiliar ideas and combines them into one great whole. By contrast the "epidemics" paper is more a presentation of facts, with a sparser amount of ideas being needed to join them together into a conclusion. There's also the consideration that the epidemics paper purports to show the discovery of the greatest catastrophe in the history of medicine, whereas the theory paper merely answers the boring question of "why is autism". On the other hand, from a history-of-science perspective, the latter is the purportedly great historical paradigm shift of understanding whereas the epidemics paper is merely a current affairs frontpage headline or two.

So there is no clearly correct order in which you should read those chapters. Anyway I am here presenting these papers more or less exactly as published or sent to journals. Though I may add some intro or commentary to make them more public-friendly.

Much of the material of the update review was incorporated into the epidemics report (and then further updated or improved). So to avoid duplication I will in Chapter 16 include just some parts of the update review which have not found their way into the epidemics report (/review).

The epidemics review in Chapter 3 presents this catastrophe in mostly impersonal, population-scale, abstract, theoretical terms. Chapters 8 and 9 give an alternative perspective on exactly the same phenomenon, in terms of one individual's experience of encountering the relevant charlatanism which naturally pretends to be competent and honest expertise. Those chapters also similarly relate rather obviously with the analysis in this first chapter about the processes whereby genuine expertise more often that not does not become duly recognised as such.

Meanwhile the Chapter 2 which follows on from here presents some further useful preliminaries prior to those Chapters 3 to 7 which I have been explaining about above here. So Chapter 2 is the next thing you should read following from here anyway.

P.S. to Chapter 1:

Many (perhaps most) researchers and other experts are hard-working honest people woefully overworked, underpaid, and under-appreciated. As is very extensively explained in the excellent https://www.quora.com/What-glamorized-career-path-is-actually-a-complete-nightmare/answer/Huyen-Nguyen-111 But that does not change the importance of the unflattering facts which are documented in this first chapter and the ones which follow it.

~~~~~~~

2

Experts evidencelessly parrotting about a "disorder"

[[Afterthought to this chapter: Some readers may feel that my talking of "experts parrotting" is cheeky language symptomatic of too much conceit and too little respect. And indeed, who am I to speak thus? I too read things and then repeat them to others. Nevertheless, I suggest that the majority of research professionals are still somewhat rightly criticised here, as they often treat their own parrotting much more seriously than they ought to. There's a difference between merely saying "researchers have found that xyz" and insisting that that xyz is an established fact which doubters only doubt because they are stupid or ignorant non-professionals.]]

~~~~~~~

"New scientific ideas never spring from a communal body, however organized, but rather from the head of an individually inspired researcher who struggles with his problems in solitary thought." — Max Planck

In a previous chapter I have explained how research professionals are highly selected and trained to become very skilled at mindlessly parrotting the received pseudo-wisdoms without the inefficiency of stopping to think whether they might actually be a load of rubbish anyway. The results of these defective social arrangements are all too substantial in the outputs of almost all the professional researchers in the autism causation field (even though many have with some ingenuity and honesty discovered many things despite the handicaps of their defective educations).

Competent science is absolutely dependent on competent, careful use of language. Terminology must not be used in ways which presumptively imply that there is greater knowledge than is in honest reality actually known. And while it would be generally preferable for the language used to be pleasant and positive, it most certainly should not be euphemistically clouding over some realities or other, nor underhandedly steering the reader to one or other hoped-for interpretations of the facts.

The matters to be explained in this chapter are not some mere trivialities of "mere semantics" or personal taste preference of labelling. Rather the terminology used by these autism experts indicates that they have not even grasped the basic essence of what autism "is", but have instead encased their thinking in a fallacious misunderstanding. There is little prospect of ever understanding the causation of autism if you haven't even reached the most basic starting point of understanding what sort of thing autism *is* anyway. And autism is hard enough for the public to understand without experts talking rubbish language to complicate the matter even more.

Words mean different things to different people, and vitally fundamental proper meanings tend to get overlaid by more simplistic ones as the intellectual decadence of academia continues. This muddling has been happening to the vitally useful word that is "syndrome" but I shall continue here anyway.

The word *syndrome* derives from the classical Greek σύνδρομον, meaning "concurrence". A syndrome is a descriptive-observational sort of thing – the observation that certain symptoms or features or characteristics tend to be associated together. One might thus talk of the "biggic syndrome", of greater tallness, longer arms and legs, larger hands, larger feet, larger chest, larger head, and so on. That "biggic syndrome" does not exclude the fact that some people have large heads but average feet, and so on, but such persons would be recognised as being relatively atypical, only marginally biggic, rather than typical or central examples of "biggism".

Within health science, various syndromes have been recognised. For instance, carpal tunnel syndrome tends to involve numbness, tingling, or burning sensations in the thumb and fingers and loss of grip strength. Such a syndrome does not necessarily correspond to a single causality. But meanwhile a number of syndromes have indeed been identified as caused by particular genetic abnormalities, such as Down syndrome, Turner syndrome, and Williams syndrome. In those cases the syndrome word is used in the usage manner of modern genetics to indicate that specific causality.

Note that a syndrome (in its traditional descriptive meaning) is a statistical characteristic of a population rather than something which a particular individual can "have". By contrast, a person may indeed have the abnormality of a genetic syndrome (in the word's modern genetics meaning), for instance may have the relevant deletion from chromosome 7 and consequently be properly said to *have* Williams syndrome. Or they may have an extra chromosome

21 and consequently be properly said to *have* Down syndrome. But note that in respect of autism there is not any such genetic or molecular characteristic which autistic individuals *"have"*.

Which brings us to an even more problematic word, namely "diagnosis". In respect of the autistic syndrome this word causes much more confusion than enlightenment. In just about all other fields of medicine a diagnosis means the identification or at least inference of *the cause* (or at least some aspect thereof). For instance you don't diagnose that "you have a headache" but rather you diagnose that that headache is caused by a blow to the head, or nervous tension, B-vitamin deficiency, or whatever. The diagnosis thus goes beyond mere observation to a deeper understanding, hopefully not too inaccurate. The diagnosis word could also be properly applied in respect of Down syndrome, because the causation by trisomy 21 can be established.

Unfortunately it has become customary to use the exact same word – "diagnosis" – with an entirely different meaning in psychiatry. Psychiatry is notorious for its controversial syndromes, such as schizophrenia, bipolar, depression, and of course the autistic syndrome (and or "Asperger syndrome" of which more further on). From my own studying I am satisfied that all the main syndromes are more-or-less valid observations of real-world phenomena. And in that respect I am very much a non-heretic here, unlike a significant number who insist that those labels correspond only to social constructs. But the notion that individuals can be "diagnosed" as "having" these conditions I find to be nonsense. The diagnosis word thereby insinuates what is not true. Such psychiatric "diagnoses" do not identify any originating cause or even any aspect of causality. All they do is sort the individual's behavior into one or other of the syndrome clusters. They are purely descriptive and unenlightening of anything deeper. The statement that "your child has been diagnosed as autistic" really means little more than that "your child behaves the non-standard way he does, and some other children also behave somewhat similarly". It doesn't mean they've seen some worms crawling around in his brain, some gene has "mutated", or necessarily anything more. (It probably would indicate that the child would better benefit from certain specialised educational provisions, but you would almost certainly have concluded that already anyway regardless of the "diagnosis".)

And this brings us to the most seriously unhelpful misuse of language about autism, namely the constant parrotting that "autism is a disorder", which some people supposedly "on the spectrum" supposedly "have" or are "with".

Just about every proudly PubMed-indexed paper about autism starts off with the required declaration of faith that autism is a "disorder" or even a "severe disorder", which certain persons "have" or are "with".   No evidence is ever cited for this supposed fact. Which doesn't surprise myself as there isn't any such evidence but instead considerable evidence pointing in the alternative direction of autism very definitely *not* being a "disorder", as I will now start to explain.

Autism can be disabling and can be distressing. But so can an IQ of 100 by comparison with a more useful IQ of 130. It doesn't follow that the 100 IQ must be a disorder or disease or pathology or caused by something "gone wrong" in the brain.

Autism can be *caused by* a disorder such as viral infection, or may sometimes be *associated with* disorder, but it doesn't follow therefrom that the autism *itself* is a disorder *per se*.

I inquired on this point of one of the autism researchers who has contributed the most to our knowledge of the brain atypicalities associated with autism, namely Prof Manuel Casanova. He's not been particularly fanatical about the "disorder" concept himself, but anyway he suggested in response various observations such as:

> *"When neurons do not migrate from the periventricular germinal zone they form nodular heterotopias. These are unorganized islands of neurons present under the ependyma of the ventricles."*

But even if that were established as being a manifestation of disorder, it would still not follow that that abnormality was itself the autism, or that autism itself is a disorder per se. All that the various researchers have shown is that autism can *involve* or be *caused by* disorder.   (I should emphasise that I don't think Dr Casanova has been personally responsible for originating or promoting this "disorder" language.)

Two clarifications on the above. Firstly, many people have been interested in finding whether there was something different about the brain of Albert Einstein. And yet if they did find such a difference they would not then conclude that it showed Einstein had a brain "disorder". The brains of Obama and Trump are almost certainly visibly different from one another, but it doesn't follow that one or other of them must have a "disorder". Secondly, all humans have a shrunken, non-functional appendix. But it doesn't follow that they can be properly described as having "shrunken appendix disorder". And the gaps between our fingers are created by death of the cells between those fingers. These sorts of "gone wrong" facts in no way evidence let alone prove that a "disorder" or even maladaption is involved.

I am not here making an impossible demand for evidence. If all autistics were shown to have some clearly pathological biological marker in common, such as high levels of a toxin, a specific gross genetic abnormality, a part of the brain rendered dysfunctional by a circulatory stoppage, or whatever, then the standard declarations that "autism is a disorder" would be justified. But even after 70 years of autism research no such marker has been identified, and that is why the "diagnosis" still consists merely of looking at the person's behavioral features and expressing an opinion about them.

And I here confidently declare that no such marker will ever be found anyway, because all the evidence tells me that autism is not a disorder anyway. Rather it is merely, or more accurately, it IS an important part of the non-pathological variability of being human (or alive more generally). Indeed I will go further and explain why autism can never be defined solely in terms of the brain, or even the body, but only in relation to the environment outside of the person or other organism. I emphasise this: autism is not a characteristic of the brain or of the body, but only of the organism (person or animal) *in relationship to a specific environment.*

I'll first just point out some facts that don't sit comfortably with the notion of autism being a disorder *(per se).*

Some of these facts were already pointed out years ago in my theory paper (Chapter 7 here), even though at that time I did not have any thoughts of this "disorder" dogma which only got canonised into Holy Writ later on. I quote (in which *SES* means Socio-Economic Status, and *bimodal* means like a graph with two peaks on the same curve.):

> "The only epidemiological survey of the IQ of parents (Lotter, 1967) found substantially above-average scores on the Mill Hill Vocabulary Scale ($p < 0.005$) and the Standard Progressive Matrices ($\chi2(2, N = 15) = 98.7, p < 10^{-20}$). The other studies of parental IQ have given similar, though less marked results (Cantwell, Baker, & Rutter, 1978). Members of Mensa (IQ > 148) have been found to have three to six times the normal frequency of autistic siblings and children (Sofaer & Emery, 1981). though the significance of this is somewhat limited by the small number of cases. Because there is a substantial correlation between IQ and SES, and because this theory proposes similar bimodal distributions for both, these findings must be set in the context of the preceding discussion of evidence concerning SES."

And that evidence concerning SES involved substantial and highly significant associations of autism with high SES including peculiar bimodal distributions (i.e. double-peaked graphs), none of which can be merely dismissed in terms of sampling (reporting) bias. (Fuller details are in Chapter 7.) The lower-SES peak of the bimodal graphs can be understood as being caused by pre-natal or peri-natal adversities suffered by lower class mothers (and the next chapter here will be discussing a "health" technology which is very much forced on the lower classes to this day).

Those associations with high IQ and high SES are perfectly in line with the central concept of the antiinnatia theory of autism (Chapter 7). Namely that antiinnatia factors in the normal range of intensity cause high IQ (and tend to raise SES) and are exactly the same factors which cause autism in a higher range of intensity. Certain other observations which further support that concept were also cited in the published theory paper, such as:

"Immaturity of general appearance and unusual symmetry of face. (Attractive appearance, and intelligent appearance....")

(this in the context that as predicted by the antiinnatia theory, facial symmetry has since been found to be correlated with high IQ, as referenced in Chapter 16.).

And:

"Skills that do not involve language, including music, arithmetic, dismantling and assembling mechanical or electrical objects, fitting together jigsaw or constructional toys. (Some very retarded can read words out loud.)"

And a study of 137 parents of autistic children found that 28% believed their children met the criteria for a savant skill, defined as a skill or power "at a level that would be unusual even for 'normal' people" (Howlin et al., 2009).

And:

"An unusual form of memory: the ability to store items for prolonged periods in the exact form they were first experienced."

Meanwhile some professors such as Temple Grandin have been "diagnosed" as or otherwise considered to be autistic. And there have frequently been suggestions that creative geniuses have some elements of autism. Indeed the antiinnatia theory was from its very start a theory of IQ, genius, and autism, with all being caused by one or other level of antiinnatia factors.

And add to this the finding of autistics being more rational than non-autistics (Allman et al., 2005; DeMartino et al., 2008).

Plus the findings that in the first two years they have larger brains and more neuron connections in those brains. (Their brain growth later slows down but that would be expected to happen in consequence of the grimly unstimulating but stressful lives the more severe children tend to experience.)

Plus the fact that many autistics strongly object to being described as having a "disorder" or even "having" or being "with" anything for that matter. Instead they are proud to be what they are, namely autistic, and thereby as they see it often superior to what they see as the inferior normals.   Regarding which maybe this would be a good place to tell you about my discovery of Neurotypicalism Spectrum Disorder ("neurotypical" being a word invented by autistics to refer to "normal" people). I quote from my account on the 2009 Awares autism online conference:

> "Neurotypicality is a disorder with desperately tragic symptoms, some of which are indicated below.
>
> Many neurotypicals, especially male ones, spend endless hours obsessed in intense fascination at people they will <u>never meet or even communicate with</u> kicking leather spheres around an area of grass for hours at a time.
>
> Meanwhile the female neurotypicals spend endless hours in intense fascination reading about people who <u>don't even exist,</u> or avidly watching tv series about such non-existent people. Another neurotypical symptom is a great preoccupation with which group, "class", movement, etc, which they or others supposedly belong to. Some even become obsessed with the obsessions of others about which groups etc the others are obsessed about...."

And note that the autism pride (neurodiversity) movement is a peculiar anomaly.   There's never been any "psychosis pride", "neurosis pride", "depression pride", "attention deficit pride", etc.

And here is another quotation about the autism "disorder", this time from a newsletter email I got from Karen Simmons of AutismToday.com on 30th Aug 2014:

> "In fact, I thought Jonathan was extraordinarily bright since he began reading at the age of 2 1/2, when he read the word "recycle" off of a truck. At 3, he would memorize songs like it was nothing too. One song in particular included all the letters of the alphabet."

And recent-ish research has found superior pitch discrimination hearing (Bonnel, Mottron, et al., 2003; O'Riordan & Passetti, 2006; Heaton et al., 2008). And superior touch sensitivity (Blakemore, Sarfait, et al., 2006). And greater ability to detect odours (Ashwin, Chapman, et al., 2014). There have also been reports of greatly enhanced visual acuity though there are contrary views as to whether they have been well-founded or not.

Meanwhile, autistics have also been found to be far cleverer than they seemed (which goes strangely harmoniously with that theory I published years ago claiming that autism was caused by exactly the same factors as high IQ, and involving exceptionally low levels of "IQ impairers"....). The Raven's Progressive Matrices (RPM) is considered the ultimate measure of the most essential, general aspect of intellectual ability involved in problem-solving and other processing tasks. Hayashi et al. (2008) found that Asperger autistics had RPM scores higher than controls, leading them to suggest "that individuals with Asperger's disorder have higher fluid reasoning ability than normal individuals, highlighting superior fluid intelligence." And various other studies have reached similar conclusions (Dawson, Soulieres, et al., 2007; Soulieres et al., 2011) and that autistics solve the RPM items much faster, and also had 31% faster performance on "inspection time" tasks compared to controls matched on the WISC IQ test (Barbeau et al., 2013). The studies I have cited here are web-accessible and will point you to others which find more or less the same. And notably the Dawson, Mottron, Soulieres, et al. team share my own rejection of the "disorder" terminology along with the hypocritical "persons with autism" nonsense, as does Jim Sinclair (1999).

And now putting all those preceding facts together, namely special skills, abnormally accurate memory, better-looking, more symmetrical, more rational, less emotionaically jerkic, larger brains with more connections, superior hearing, touch, and smell, high fundamental intelligence, faster brain speed, no pathological criterion found after 70 years of research, association with higher IQ and higher SES, and being something which many of the "victims" consider themselves proud to _be_ (rather than be "with" or "having" or "on") anyway.... on what basis can this be ASSUMED to be obviously a "disorder" such as to justify just about every "scientific" paper ever listed in PubMed beginning with that evidence-free recitation that "Autism is a disorder........." ? ("Well we all got our PhDs at Harvard so it must be true....")("Baah!")

In a later chapter here you can read the only theory of autism (and IQ and genius) which actually successfully grapples with all the key facts and questions. And it has no need to resort to any far-fetched presumption that autism is a disorder, indeed rather its neglect for so many years could raise a question of whether *Academism* Spectrum Disorder is very much more the real disorder.

By way of moving on to what I suggest to be a more competent understanding of the matter, here's another quote from my first published paper:

"the existence of a continuum ranging from severe autism through the much milder and more common Asperger's syndrome (Gillberg & Gillberg, 1989; Frith, 1991) to normality."

Re which please consider the dimension of personality from extraversion to introversion, specifically in people who are a bit inclined also to above-average neuroticism. An extremely extravert person would tend to be "pathologically" impulsive and consequently doing stupid things such as reckless criminal offences or dangerous acts. And an extremely introverted person would tend to be "pathologically" shy and averse to commonplace noise and excitement. Both these extreme persons have serious problems but they are in no way due to a "disorder" they "have". They just are as they are, by reason of natural variation (due to genes and or environment or something in the water).

Likewise some people have lower IQs than others. Yet there is no level of IQ which can be said with scientific justification to be a boundary between "having" or not "having" of "low IQ disorder" ("mental retardation" or whatever the latest squirm-word is nowadays). Rather if we look at progressively lower levels of antiinnatia factors the brain becomes progressively slower and more error-prone, hence the lower IQ, as explained in Chapter 7. And conversely, with progressively higher levels of antiinnatia factors, the brain first becomes progressively faster and error-free, and then other things start happening which give us firstly a narrow window of creative genius-potential merging into marginal autism (including "Aspergers"), and then onwards to severe autism and ultimately non-viability manifesting as stillbirth.

In the first chapter here I explained how just about all academics have a severe unlearning disability, and consequently many of them are going to be unable to unlearn their parrotting of the "disorder" word and the faulty notions underlying it. They will soothe their cognitive dissonance by claiming that the conception I have outlined above is wrong in some way or other.

One of the points they will raise to rationalise away their denial of their inability to unlearn will relate to yet another problematic terminology commonly used about autism, namely *"de novo mutation"*.

You probably already know that a mutation is a change in an organism's DNA sequence of genes. If you don't already know about this it would be best if you study about it via a biology textbook or encyclopedia or equivalent online information before continuing here.

A *de novo mutation* is a mutation which is not present in either parent, hence has arisen "de novo", that is newly, in the individual in question. Actually in this case the terminology is not being incorrectly used. What is incorrect is what is being implied about and inferred from those de novo mutations.

Certain sectors of autism research have as their greatest preoccupation the finding out of "what has gone wrong" to cause the "disorder" which is autism/ASD/ Aspergers. From the perspective of a career-cautious researcher, it makes a lot of sense to try to blame a gene or a virus for "what has gone wrong", because genes and viruses cannot get angry at you for blaming them and cannot start legal action for libel compensation. By contrast if you blame some product put in peoples' mouths, then the makers and marketers of that product might indeed get angry at you and start legal action and other bother against you. So there's a very important principle in medical research that it's far better if you can blame a gene or virus.

Indeed it gets much better. If you can blame one or more genes, not only can those genes not sue you but you can then patent everything about them and the tests to detect them and ways to change them and patented drugs to block them, and thereby make a recurring income-stream fortune of trillions of dollars. Not to mention all the research jobs created in the process.

In respect of autism, there has for many years been evidence that a virus such as rubella can increase the risk of becoming autistic. But only in a minority of cases. So for the researchers it's very important that we go on to find those evil (but highly profitable) genes which are hoped to be behind "what's gone wrong" (even though in reality nothing has "gone wrong" in the autistic brain anyway).

In my published theory paper I indicated my conclusion that most or much autism before that time (before the increase) had been mainly due to genes, and that a great many different genes would be involved. *And* that they would be exactly the same genes which cause raised IQ and raised SES and in some rare circumstances also cause creative genius. I'll now suggest there was much wisdom in the comment many years later from Simon Baron-Cohen that seeking to abort autistics could be greatly misconceived on account of it also tending to eliminate rare valuable talents from our populations.

But meanwhile most research money has been staked on finding the evil genes causing this "disorder". A few years back, a huge study was published in *Nature*, the most prestigious of all journals. The list of authors alone filled several pages. And yet the genes and genetic anomalies they (reckoned to have) found could only account for a very small minority of autism cases.

An important part of the evidence which researchers assume to be supporting their "bad genes" theory of autism relates to ages of parents. It has been found that older mothers and older fathers tend to have a higher probability of autistic children. But curiously the studies in question give notably differing results in different countries (Sandin et al., 2015), which should hint to us that there may be something partly or entirely cultural going on rather than entirely or partly genetic. (A very competent review of the evidence is given by Zhou (2015), who with much understatement concludes: "All this suggests that social factors may be more at play in these figures than it simply being a question of paternal or maternal age.")

But why let an inconvenient fact get in the way of a convenient one? The convenient fact in question is that the number of de novo mutations increases with age of the father. Which seems certainly true. But it does not follow that those de novo mutations are mainly causing or a main cause of autism, and even less that they represent a bad thing happening to the genes anyway.

Cutting-edge science is difficult to get perfect and it makes fools of even the cleverest of other people from time to time. There is a well-known concept of evolution by natural selection as follows. There is first the accidental generation of random changes in the DNA, that is random de novo mutations, and then the resulting slightly-changed organisms are subjected to the filtering effect of natural selection such that those with disadvantageous mutations get rarer or even eliminated.

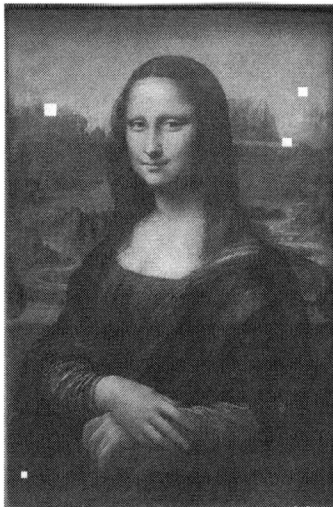

The Mona Lisa after modification
by a few "de novo mutations"?

It would be useful to think here of a famous painting such as Leonardo's Mona Lisa portrait. The mutation process could be thought of as analogous to a blind child randomly dabbing a paintbrush at that painting. The point is that the Mona Lisa painting has been the result of much patient work and developed skill, and so just about any random change to it would be a deterioration rather than an improvement. Likewise randomly loosening or tightening bolts on a car engine would be much more likely to make it less functional than more functional. And the standard (assumed by most scientists) reasoning about mutations proceeds likewise reasonably to the conclusion that mutations will almost always be deleterious (bad) rather than advantageous (good), considering that our existing genomes are the result of millions of years of constant natural selection towards "perfection". The familiar talk of radiation tending to cause harmful mutations is seen in this same light of mutations being bad.

But..... (with sincerest apologies to those Cambridge medical graduates) But...., well, to explain this I will use another of my analogies. This involves two elderly Bechstein pianos of my acquaintance, the one made in 1890 and the other in 1893. Various springs, strings, and weakly brass bridgepins died many years ago and have had to be carefully replaced. But their soundboards live on, sounding extremely much like high-quality new ones would.

And yet piano soundboards are noted for often degrading over the years (even some from S...you-know-who). The sound can be dependent on some very precarious engineering, where a difference of less than a millimetre can make the difference between excellent and abysmal. Anyone who's played around many pianos knows that even new ones can have poor tone, and that many have turned into key-controlled drum-kits or worse a long time before they reach 80 years old let alone more. Yet these two pianos have certainly not had a cocooned pampered life, but on the contrary been grievously abused by previous ungrateful owners.

The secret of these pianos as I see it is that by 1890/1893 Carl Bechstein had been progressively refining his design (the cheapo Model 5 upright in this instance) through 40 years and through the experience of many thousands of instruments produced, and as a result he had "evolved" a production formula which was robust and would still sound good even with the occasional random change of something or other.

And the relevance of this analogy about those pianos is that the DNA's production formula of the human body has likewise been refined by evolution, but not merely over 40 years and 30,000 serial numbers, but for vastly longer and more. And it is to be expected that the human body would, like those pianos, have evolved to be something that is robust and not easily defuncted by just a bit of change. I'll now go into this in more detail.

The first thing is that genes are not all equal units. Some genes have vitally important effects such as relating to sickle-cell anemia. Many other genes appear to have much more marginal importance or even none at all. It follows that mutations cannot be all equally important either.

The second thing is that not all changes of genes are equally likely to occur.

And a third, key, thing is that by reason of the stabilising refinement (in humans as in Bechstein's pianos), the genome *itself* will have evolved, such that easy but bad changes are few and far between, whereas easy but non-deleterious changes are very common.

And a fourth, even more key thing is that there is no such thing as the ideal "perfect" person with "perfect" genome. As I explained back in the published theory paper if more than a handful had bothered to read it, there are reasons why genetic diversity (and hence genetic change, hence those nasty *de novo mutations*) can be actually *advantageous*.

Here another illustration may be useful, this time an actuality rather than mere analogy. Anyone with experience of Olympics-level fly-swatting will be well aware that flies do not all behave the same. Some keep crawling around on the window-pane, others jiggle around a bit then have a rest below on a book instead, and so on in various variations. Clothes moths have even more diverse personalities despite their flour-grain-sized brains. Without such unpredictable behavior the flies and any other such species or group would quickly get eliminated by predators or other enemies who could easily anticipate what they were going to do next. There is also advantage in not having all individuals competing to fill exactly the same niche (locationally, occupationally, or food preference etc.).

So evolution can be expected to actually *favour* some appropriate de novo mutations, especially in respect of behaviour, and the notion that they are most likely to be deleterious (under normal conditions such as without intense radiation) is unsound.

This positive importance of genetic change is reflected in the work of Nobel laureate Werner Arber (2014), who refers to "natural strategies of genetic variation", and "a multitude of specific molecular mechanisms to contribute to the overall spontaneous genetic variation.", and "reports on cross-species gene transfer, as well as recent DNA sequence comparisons, speak clearly in favor of a general validity of the relevant natural laws of genetic variation for all living organisms."

Some further elaboration about this corrected understanding of genetics and mutation is provided in an appendix to this chapter.

~~~~~~~~~~~~~~~~~~~~~~~~~~~~~~~~~~

(You may at this point wish to turn to that appendix to this chapter, pages 70-77, then return back here thereafter.)

~~~~~~~~~~~~~~~~~~~~~~~~~~~~~~~~~~

The appendix shows that the latest research confirms that my understanding is correct, and that the outdated but still-predominant would-be wisdom is mistaken.

Thus the evil genes autism theory is unsoundly founded on a false assumption of how mutations fit into the processes of evolution.

I indicated above that one should expect the main reasons for the associations with parental age to be cultural rather than genetic. But let's first take a silly idea to its logical conclusion. The idea swimming around is that older parenthood causes inferior offspring and so parents should be encouraged to have their children earlier. There's a slight problem with this advice, because the age association with autism and with those de novo mutations goes near-linearly right back to age 15 or earlier. So on this logic we should be advising 15 year-old boys and girls to have families straight away before legal adulthood so as to avoid those supposedly horrible autistics being born. Meanwhile in the real world.....

In the real world I explained many years ago that autism is associated with higher IQ, higher SES, more beautiful faces, and higher biological superiority generally, because the antiinnatia genes tend to produce all of those. Oh.... and "immaturity of general appearance" (Wing, 1976, cited in my theory paper). The average 45-year-old man in many countries is an ageing slob who (a) is no longer attractive to youngish women, (b) probably has enough on his hands already children-wise (in terms of energy and money earning means), (c) is probably not physically up to any more fatherhood anyway, or at least not much bothered, and (d) quite likely dead and buried already anyway. Meanwhile the high-SES (and "immature-looking") 45-year-old is just getting into his stride as a self-made zillionaire, or semi-celebrity, or starting a second family after a first has flown. Thus the reason why the older father has more autistic children is not because his genes are inferior but precisely because his genes are (biologically) *superior*. And likewise the under-privileged teenage schoolkidparents family have fewer autistics precisely because they have less of the antiinnatia genes for biological superiority. By the way, I haven't said anything about moral/ethical/cultural superiority here. I am merely referring to biological propensities to successfully continue the lineage to grandchildren and onwards.

For those whose brains did not stretch sufficiently to take on board the previous paragraph, I shall add here that I have just now entirely by chance encountered an article about Jeffrey Skoll, a 47-year old billionaire, who says *"I don't have kids yet, but when I do, there's only so much I think they should have. They can make their path their own."* (Grant, 2012).

And here's another. Al Pacino, described as "one of the greatest actors in all of film history". His three children were born when he was 49 and 61 years old. "The joy of work is what keeps me going."

And "Millionaire nightclub owner Peter Stringfellow is to become a father again at the age of 72."

And add these too: Frank Skinner (55), Gordon Brown (55), Sir Paul McCartney (61), Rod Stewart (66), Clint Eastwood (66). And Rupert Murdoch having two children in his seventies.

Reality dawned yet?

And so by marrying that cute guy in the same student year as yourself you may minimise the risk of your children turning out to be geniuses or superstars, or even just really nice guys and gals.

In summary about this supposed "disorder", there is no evidence that autism is a disorder, there is huge obvious evidence that it is not, and the only theory that actually accounts coherently for the syndrome explicitly endorses the concept of autism as being just a part of the normal variation of human (and non-human) life.

Interestingly Simon Baron-Cohen shares my disinclination towards the disorder word, preferring to refer to Autism Spectrum Condition, ASC. This probably reflects that he like myself has come to autism from studying psychology rather than psychiatry. The psychiatrists have trained at med schools so they see every difference as a disease to be treated, whereas the psychologists see it as part of the multi-dimensionality of human diversity to be treasured and wondered at.

Not everything the autism researchers do is wrong. The latest edition of the Diagnostic and Statistical Manual (DSM-V) has made some progress, eliminating Asperger syndrome and adding five or so levels of severity to the "diagnosis" of autism. This is properly justified because there is no scientific basis for a distinction between autism and Asperger's. It was merely a historical accident that Kanner and Asperger made simultaneous rediscoveries of approximately the syndrome described by JL Down in 1887. But the DSM-V is still light-years off course in still containing the pseudo-scientific notion of "Autism Spectrum Disorder" aka "ASD".

Here's two last paragraphs about the "disorder" word, namely of why such inexcusable baseless false language is being used.

Parents who have autistic children are in many cases very upset about them (and very tired by the extra demands involved). They hoped their children would grow up to be clever and social and get on in life but instead they find them problematic in various ways. They think that their child ought to have been "normal" and that something has "gone wrong" such that they "have" this something "wrong" with them which is not what they should have been. We have to sympathise with the parents using this language but it is simply not factually correct. And so it must be rejected, even though the situation is not entirely that simple as I will now explain.

I will present in a later chapter the evidence that most cases of autism nowadays are being caused by mercury vapor poisoning from dental amalgams. In such cases, something has indeed "gone wrong", namely they have got mercury poisoning, and they do indeed "have" something, namely excessive mercury. But it remains the case that the excessive mercury is not the autism. And some cases of autism could be entirely due to very high levels of the antiinnatia genes, especially where two ultra-high-IQ ultra-classy parents are involved. In such cases the child simply IS autistic and does not "have" anything other than too much of a good thing genetically. I don't know for sure whether there is or can be any cure or treatment for such a condition; maybe yes maybe no. I hope to have more to say on the matter at a future date.

(By the way, and this is a most important point here, as most autism is now caused by mercury poisoning, researchers who think they are studying autism are as often as not actually unwittingly studying mercury poisoning instead. And in consequence they become even more convinced of their false notion that autism must be some disorder of the body. There's even a book titled "Autism: Oxidative Stress, Inflammation, and Immune Abnormalities." (Chauhan et al., 2009), which expertly overlooks that that's three major consequences of mercury listed in its title!)

In addition to the parents' preference of terminology, there is the researchers' preference. Saying that your research is about a terrible "disorder" sounds a lot more important and prestigious than saying you are just studying some atypicalities of behavior. And the false "disorder" language gives your research career a free pass to the medical charities funding world. And why bother with mere scientific truthfulness when you can get promotion so much easierly by means of false propaganda drivel-words?

Oh, but!.....surely the researchers are merely using the terminology officially established in the DSM (Diagnostic and Statistical Manual), as they should? But this notion is incorrect. The researchers are supposed to be the leading edge of understanding. It is the DSM that is supposed to be following the researchers rather than the other way round. And furthermore, the DSM is very far from being the uncontroversial, evidence-based tome of accumulated competence which it tends to be assumed to be. The book *Cracked* by James Davies (2013) does a good job of discussing the not-so-impressive reality underlying the DSM. And even the chairman of DSM-3, Allen Frances, came out of retirement to publish a similarly scathing condemnation of DSM-5.

The DSM is profoundly misconceived in another respect. It is trying to serve three distinct purposes and ends up serving none properly. We need:

(a) A ("scientific") answer to the everyday question of "what is (the proper definition of) autistic"? (or "how does autism manifest itself?");

(b) A working criterion for researchers to use to sort people into "autistic" and "control" in their studies, for instance studying whether autistic people have longer fingers than controls;

(c) A working criterion for clinicians and administrators to decide who should qualify for disability services and support.

And there is no reason why those three things should be anything like identical. Indeed the latter criterion would properly take major account of the practical impact of any disabilities, which is certainly not any proper part of the other two. What a ridiculous muddle. (Though at least it was written by graduates.)

Update: Unlike most academics Professor Casanova has a quite good blog on the public internet, titled "Cortical Chauvinism". Subsequent to my sending him an early draft of this chapter and now having finished writing the rest of this book, I notice that he has meanwhile put up a blogpost defending the standard notion that autism is a disorder and not an aspect of normal variation (as the antiinnatia theory entails). I guess he's waiting for me to reply to it!

Anyway, it appears to me that his most cogent (/least uncogent) new point is that a high proportion of autistics have seizures (epilepsy). To which I have two points of rejoinder. Firstly, most autism nowadays is caused by mercury, and seizures are known to be one of the symptoms which mercury can cause. The brain processes causing seizures appear to be poorly understood anyway, but a websearch of { mercury seizures } shows up numerous people identifying mercury as a cause of seizures, including a report titled "Effects of continuous low-dose exposure to organic and inorganic mercury during development on epileptogenicity in rats" (Szasz et al., 2002; Klinghardt, 1998). This is of course *yet more* evidence in support of my claim that perinatal mercury has caused the autism increase – while also causing that epilepsy as well.

Secondly, an outright "disorder"-like symptom can still be the result of pure "normal" variation. This is exemplified by variation in height of humans and indeed of other creatures. Above a certain height, the gravity forces on the bones become excessive such that they tend to break or have joint failures. Of course in practice that causes natural selection to disfavour people being too tall, such that such problems in practice are rare. (I can think of other examples of the same principle but they would take too much space to explain here, especially as one such suffices anyway.)

Finally here, I have not yet explained my point about autism not being a characteristic of just the brain or even just of the body. It would be better if I leave that explanation until after you have read the presentation of the antiinnatia theory first so I can take it from there. Meanwhile here are some examples of de-irrationalised language for you to practice with.

Autistics with childness
Persons with degrees (usually incurable, sadly)
Women with Blackness
Men with Muslimness
Persons with Professorships
Persons with Doctorates
Researchers with Academism Spectrum Disorder

"And now please let me introduce our speaker with distinguish-edness Irva Hertz-Etc, who is a Person with Doctorate and Person with Professorship, and may soon also be awarded a diagnosis as a Researcher with Academism Spectrum Disorder...."

Yet more abusive language from academics

A further word which many researchers have become routinely accustomed to misusing is *hypothesis* (or in plural, *hypotheses*).

In later chapters here I will be presenting one or more theories. In the first chapter here I have already explained the evidence of how the medical science bureaucracy's research has become grossly perverted by a hostility to new theories to such an extent that it barely merits recognition as genuine science any more. A symptom of that perverted hostile attitude is misuse of the word "hypotheses" to refer to what are actually theories.

It is impossible for a theory to be a hypothesis and impossible for a hypothesis to be a theory, because they are categorically different things.

The "fuzzy" sciences such as psychology, sociology, and clinical and epidemiological medicine use what is known as "inferential statistics" to ascertain whether a "statistically significant" effect or relationship has been observed in a study. Every student of those fields learns about testing the *"null hypothesis"*, which is.... well please let me explain from the beginning.....

You can generally tell a hypothesis from a theory by the fact that a hypothesis can't have the word *"because"* or *"causes"* incorporated into it. For instance:

"Autistics look cuter" = hypothesis.

"Autistics look cuter <u>because</u> the antiinnatia suppresses the gene-expression of idiosycracies of their appearance" = theory.

"There is a higher prevalence of autism in Las Vegas" = hypothesis.

"There is a higher prevalence of autism in Las Vegas <u>because</u> it has been invaded by Martians recently." = (somewhat daft) theory.

"Banging a hammer on your finger is followed by more pain" = hypothesis.

"Banging a hammer on your finger is followed by more pain because the pressure causes injury to the finger, which activates pain receptors which then send impulses down nerves to your brain where the impulses are interpreted as pain." = theory.

"Higher mercury intake <u>is associated with</u> higher autism scores" = hypothesis.

"Mercury <u>causes</u> autism" = barest-bones basic theory.

"Mercury causes autism by (/because of its) selectively suppressing gene-expression" = slightly more developed theory.

"Mercury causes autism because [process a; process b; process c...] as is evidenced by [observation a; observation b; observation c...] which are logically related to those processes by [reason a; reason b; reason c...]" = highly developed theory but which *still might be a load of rubbish.* <u>But can never be a "hypothesis" just as a sandwich can never be a lunchbreak.</u>

Another useful way of understanding it is that a hypothesis is a putative answer to a "What is the fact of the matter?" question, whereas a theory is a putative answer to a "Why is it so?" question.

Now back to the students studying inferential statistics, which is a very important part of your own education here. Most research studies are investigations of whether more of x is associated with more (or less) of y, such as "Is there more autism in areas where more of the cars are red?" Or something similar. The *null hypothesis* is the (alternative) hypothesis that there is no such association or difference. So from the examples above we can see null hypotheses to test such as:

"Autistics DON'T look cuter."

"There is NOT a higher prevalence of autism in Las Vegas."
"Banging a hammer on your finger is NOT followed by more pain."
"Higher mercury intake is NOT associated with higher autism scores."

At this point I shall hypothesise that I have sufficiently explained to you the categorical difference between a hypothesis and a theory. Pending evidential confirmation of that hypothesis, I shall now move on to the way the word is regularly abused by academics.

Things vary in quality and worth. A brand new Ferrari is a car but a rusted bashed 20-year old Ford with broken windows and clattering engine and worn tyres is likewise a car, and not some sort of "carpothesis".

Likewise theories vary greatly in their quality and worth. But it gets more complicated. You will often encounter the phrase "The theory that ......" (usually followed a bit further on by "has been disproven by numerous studies"). This is where you can get confused. Consider for instance "the theory that mercury causes autism". This is not the same as "the theory that mercury causes *all* autism" or "the theory that mercury causes *some but not all* autism", or even the same as "the theory that mercury is one of the factors in the causation of autism". Such distinctions are important, because these are simply not the same theories even in basic outline.

But I have made a mistake in the preceding paragraph. Did you notice it? It's this. There is not one single "theory that mercury causes autism". Rather there can be many. Including a sub-collection of "theories that mercury kills braincells and thereby causes autism". Those ones I don't personally rate very highly. Then there is the theory that "mercury randomly binds to DNA and thereby acts as an antiinnatia factor and thereby causes autism". Which is one which I argue for in later chapters here.

A theory such as "Autism is being caused by visiting Martians because Martians are yellow-striped and the yellow stripes are very relaxing and that relaxation causes people to learn foreign languages which is the main symptom of autism." is a load of rubbish. And yet it is a theory none the less, just a very rubbishy theory. Likewise "Autism is now being caused by the absence of mercury from most modern vaccines" is a theory of very low credibility. But it still cannot be a hypothesis.

And here's a crucial point. Even a very decent theory well-supported by evidence and argument, if it is nevertheless new and thus has not yet undergone some process of bureaucratic herd endorsement (baah!), tends to be treated with the greatest of hostility as evidenced in the preceding chapter. And as part of the process of contempt, it is belittled as supposedly not even being a theory anyway, but as something supposedly categorically different, namely a mere "hypothesis", just as a Person with Professorship or Person with Doctorate is somehow categorically different in their very essence from a mere unqualified "person". In the status-obsessed mindset of academics, a theory can only be an outstanding great discovery by a Darwin or Einstein, whereas Simon Baron-Cohen's disputed theory that high fetal testosterone is a major cause of autism can only be a piddling "hypothesis" (not that I rate it much myself either).

Wikipedia declares that "A theory is a well-substantiated explanation...", and "Theories are the single highest level of scientific achievement". Meanwhile some famous journals such as the Lancet and Nature have a category of articles they call *"Hypothesis"*, and yet they clearly must be having in mind would-be theoretical explanations given that they are required to have not yet been "tested" and yet take up up to 1500 words whereas just about any genuine hypothesis can be stated in a single sentence such as the examples above. It is impossible to take a whole article to propose the hypothesis that "Vitamin C intake below 2 mg is associated with autism a year later (but *no-one has tested it yet!*)". I've just done it fully in that sentence there. But it could take an article to propose the theory that "Vitamin C intake below 2mg causes autism because [process a; process b] as supported by [reasoning c; reasoning d]".

And that position of Wikipedia and the academic parrotting is arguably a very harmful terminology, because just about every great theory starts its life as a mere rough idea to which only later is there attached more and more evidence and reasoning. And the last thing we need for the advancement of science is such a false pseudo-categorising barrier blocking even more the way to recognition of new and better understandings.

And the other last thing we need is such sloppy abusive use of the terminology which makes it all the harder for readers to accurately understand what writers are talking about.

And no, the fact that x million people have sloppily abused some language for decades does not make it acceptable or valid via some rationale that "words only mean what people mean them to mean anyway". Which people, when, where, why? Certainly not myself. I have higher standards and will not be lowering them for any number of superior experts.

The autism increase controversy

The following Chapter 3 contains a discussion of the notion that there has not really been an increase of autism in recent decades. That notion is also revisited in Chapter 12. But it would be useful add some further prefatory content here for unpicking the false reasonings of those denying the increase.

Firstly it might be useful to be clear about some motivations. Such motivations do not necessarily cause any bias, but being aware of them can enable due scepticism in one's reading of the debate.

A first motivated group are those of the medical establishment, who have a very heavily-developed reflex which could be well-characterised as a perversion of the Hippocratic Oath: "First do not admit to doing any harm". This reflex is particularly liable to be excited whenever the word "mercury" is in the air (for reasons that might have something to do with Chapter 3 here). These establishment people are strongly motivated to deny there has been an increase because that helps towards denying that themselves the medics have caused the catastrophe revealed by the increase.

A second motivated group consists of the more fanatical of the "Neurodiversity" or "autism pride" people, according to whose viewpoint autism is never a problem or disability and certainly not a disorder or illness, and "therefore" it cannot have been caused by some adverse factor, and "therefore" an increase cannot have been caused. (This is an example of a very common phenomenon of human mentation, namely adjusting the "facts" to fit the prior theory (chosen for emotional reasons) rather than correcting the theory to fit the actual facts.)

A third motivated group is some parents of autistic children, who are somewhat motivated to find someone to blame and to seek compensation from (though many parents are more motivated to just find out the truth of what caused and what could un-cause the autism). It is only some of this third group who might be motivated to falsely perceive an increase rather than deny one.

The idea that there had indeed been an increase originated with facts noted by researchers in the field. There were the direct observations of people who had been in the field for decades, such as Bernard Rimland, Sally J Rogers, and Lisa Blakemore-Brown, who insisted that there had been a real increase of behaviours. And there were the statistics from surveys of autism prevalence, which showed sharp increases of numbers (and continued to do so).

In reaction against these reports, speculations were put forward by some observers, basically three in number: the increase could be due to (1) widening of the diagnostic criteria; (2) increased awareness; (3) diagnostic substitution (from "mental retardation" to "autism" or "ASD"). Or a combination.

The notion of substitution from mental retardation was argued for in a study by Croen et al., but subsequently Dr Croen ended up agreeing that substitution could not explain the increase of numbers. A decade later the substitution concept was revived in a paper by Polyak et al., whose graph features in Chapter 6 here along with my explanation of its gross incompetence and unsoundness. And autism is very unlike ordinary mental retardation, which is usually characterised by high empathy and sociability and low "cuteness".

The dismissal of the increase in terms of widening of diagnostic criteria is also unsound. A wider category of "autism spectrum disorder" does indeed now exist, but the increases have also been observed in respect of the two diagnostic concepts separately (Blaxill 2004) and with care taken to keep the criteria constant.

The remaining ground for doubting the increase, namely in terms of increased awareness, seems very credible at first glance for anyone who has not actually been involved in the field for more than a few years.

And yet on only slightly more reflection, that attempted explain-away in terms of mere increased awareness is laid bare as the most utterly absurd one, as shown in Chapter 12 here. That some prominent "experts" have resorted to such claptrap and are still doing so, is symptomatic of the forcefulness of the malign motivation of "do not admit to doing any harm", which was the first on my list above here.

In support of the official increase-denialism quackery there has been created a whole mythology of a fictional "lost generation" of older autistics, as discussed in Chapter 12. Under this crackpot pseudo-science, we are asked to believe that huge numbers of severely disabled children were somehow never noticed before and that all preceding generations of parents and pediatricians were grossly incompetent in failing to notice them. And that thousands of these non-verbal head-banging incontinents somehow managed to sneak successfully through the normal school systems and on into normal employment. Autism is very different from ordinary low IQ.

Meanwhile a number of studies have confirmed the reality of the increase. These include Nevison (2014) and three of the studies she cites (namely Hertz-Picciotto et al. 2009, Mind 2002, and California 2002). And to all this evidence we can add the further observations I make in Chapter 3. There isn't really a scientific debate here, but something more like a corporate agenda in alliance with the fanatical ideology held by some very vocal "neurodiversity" advocates. A severely-flawed "award-winning" "best-seller" book, *Neurotribes* (featuring a promotional plug for Janssen's Risperdal®), has been heavily promoted recently. Its over-arching theme is a grossly one-sided mis-portrayal of the supposed non-increase. On the internet you can read some damning crtitiques from Professor Manuel Casanova.

Appendix to Chapter 2:
More advanced understanding of how the processes of mutation are subject to natural selection

> "When you put English text into [the code], it generates very frequent stop codons in the genetic code and won't produce big proteins .... *It's designed to be biologically neutral.*"
> – Nobel Laureate microbiologist Hamilton Smith

After I was mercury-poisoned by distinguished experts I became severely mentally disabled, and in subsequent decades other people then prevented me from continuing via the usual social means my education and research efforts. So I generally had to resort to working things out for myself, alone. This tended to involve the application of logic to facts. And oftentimes my personal conclusions turned out to be already confirmed findings of professional specialists. This can be seen in at least two instances in the theory paper presented in Chapter 7 here. Firstly, I perceived in autism the re-emergence of characteristics lost millions of years earlier, and this turned out to be a well-established phenomenon which biologists called atavisms. Secondly, I reasoned to the conclusion that there would be greater reliability of expression of more advantageous characteristics. And now, here in respect of my thoughts of those "evolving" Bechstein pianos we have a further example of such concurrence of my own naive inferences with specialist experts.

In my reasoning-obsessed worldview, it simply stands to reason that the cellular processes affecting mutation would themselves be subject to evolutionary pressure of "survival of the fittest"; and that this evolution of mutational processes would be such as to make deleterious mutations less easy to occur and advantageous mutations relatively more likely to occur; and that such evolution of the mutational processes would be expected to occur in practice rather than just theory; and therefore most mutations would not be harmful, even though the grand evolutionary process overall would be like a randomly-driven "blind watchmaker" with no teleological guidance towards purposive ends.

With these ideas I enter into a hotly "controversial" area, because a great many people have learnt "the facts" in their university courses (as per an earlier chapter here), and don't see any merit in learning something which conflicts with them and so "therefore can't be true". (And those minds have been made even more rigidified due to their confrontation against creationist would-be-science.) But in recent years the field of study of genomes and evolution has become rather turbulent, because of the arrival of so many new facts enabled by the development of technologies for genome-sequencing and genome engineering. And I remind you of that quote from Max Planck:

> ".... A new scientific truth does not triumph by convincing its opponents and making them see the light, but rather because its opponents eventually die, and a new generation grows up that is familiar with it."

And in this case a lot of those funerals will be required. Because as a cheeky guy called Ron Maimon says (Maimon, 2013): "All these things are things that biologists got wrong, because they were going by stupid dogma." And: "The RNA "brain" is also making "knowing" modifications in the DNA through the action of reverse transcriptase."

Keynes famously said that politicians were the slaves of defunct economists. Likewise, most authors of medical research papers are slaves of defunct, superceded, genomics theorists. Not least with the simplistic theoretical notion that just about all mutations are nasty evil things creeping up to make you ill.

The understanding of DNA and mutations is currently undergoing a substantial revolutionary paradigm shift, from a simplistic flawed 20th-century model to a more complex more accurate 21st-century model. As is usual with these changes, those holding the outdated views continue to hold on to them and tend to be dismissive of those presenting the new understanding. So rest assured that some "leading" people will tell you that the following is just rubbish!

DNA and mutations are matters which just about every medical scientist has to learn about, even if they are not reckoning to be a cutting-edge genetic theorist themselves. It's hardly surprising that most scientists even including those working in genetics fields tend to be stuck with the outdated 20th-century model they learnt at school, rather than having the most modern under-standing.

Meanwhile some more words from Nobel laureate Werner Arber (2011) on the matter:

"....evolution genes. Some of their gene products act as variation generators, others as modulators of the rates of spontaneous genetic variation. ...." " .....increasing evidence .... indicates that principally the same natural strategies of genetic variation, local sequence changes, intragenomic DNA rearrangements, and DNA acquisition, are also in action in higher multicellular organisms. ...... one can postulate that all kinds of organisms living today on our planet earth dispose of a set of evolution genes that had become fine-tuned in the course of long periods of past evolution...." So you see that a Nobel prizewinner thinks alike with this Nobody no-prizes-winner.

This field is currently very much in flux due to new data coming from the improving technologies. But the newer thinkers are tending to reckoning like myself that the mutation profile of a species evolves to a steady state of *"balanced mutation"* with "a balance between slightly deleterious and slightly advantageous" (Razeto-Barry et al., 2012; Ohta & Gillespie, 1996). Like those Bechstein pianos.

Another analogy might be useful here. It is well-known (at least to experts in these things) that the southern end of the island called Great Britain is gradually sinking into the sea, at a rate of about five millimetres per decade. Plus the sea is gradually rising due to the melting ice caps. Meanwhile the tide goes in and out daily. And furthermore there are waves coming up the beaches, typically about 20 cm high and moving at walking speed. Now, aware of claims that England is progressively sinking below the waves, an ignorant amateur geologist might check by doing some measurements on a beach. He measures the rise of the water as a wave comes in. And wow!, the water rises 20 cm in less than a second. At that rate the whole of Norfolk and Kent will be drowned by tea-time!

People looking at data about mutations of DNA could be likewise assuming they are observing a whole picture of relentless long-term negativity of mutation when in reality all they are noticing is some more transient change, analogous to those waves coming up on a beach, without grim longer-term trend implications.

A fundamental problem with this mutation and parental ages research is that it is analogous to that silly geologist measuring the rising side of the wave but ignoring its falling side. Likewise these mutation researchers look at only one side of the matter, namely the negative effects (profitable for the drugs industry of course!). But suppose (for mere sake of argument....) that I am a person who is exceptionally reasonable and patient, exceptionally slow to anger or take offense, exceptionally resistant to losing my head in traumatic circumstances, exceptionally capable of enduring and coping with decades of stressful adversity and sneering demeanment, and then reacting only with creative positivity and ingenious sense of humour.... (indeed a person such as described in Chapter 8 here?).... Perhaps thus we could say that Robin P Clarke has "mental superiority syndrome"** ("MSS"). Which might have been caused by some of those balancing advantageous mutations mentioned by Razeto-Barry a few paragraphs back. But who's doing any studies of the mutational or parental age correlates of my MSS? Precisely no-one. And such abnormally positive people are potentially of huge value to society (at least if it is capable of letting them be).

(** Or at least "mental conceit syndrome".)

And there is another way the researchers are only looking at one side of the matter, as follows. They look for de novo mutations occurring when a non-autistic parent has an autistic child. But they don't look to see whether there could be exactly as many de novo mutations occurring in the opposite event, when an autistic parent has a non-autistic child. Which is precisely what would be happening under the balanced mutation situation reckoned to be the reality by the new thinkers.

At this point it could be useful to recall that a key concept of the unfaulted and unrivalled antiinnatia theory of autism is that the genetic (and other) antiinnatia factors which contribute to "risk" of autism are basically the same ones that also contribute to "risk" of high IQ.

From that point of view, any de novo mutations which "cause" autism would also be causative of higher IQ (and genius) in other individuals. (An exception to this might be if there were some mutations with extra-large antiinnatia effect, just as while most potatoes are a sensible size for eating, a potato as big as a cow would be quite harmful to eat in one meal.)

Now here is where this subject gets quite amusing, at least for my own perverted sense of humour. At the same time as some researchers are reckoning to confirm that those nasty paternal mutations cause increased risk of autism (which I say is caused by *high* level of antiinnatia factors), concurrently some other researchers are reckoning to confirm that the nasty paternal mutations are also causing increased risk of .... lowered IQ (which I say is causally the exact opposite of the autism, caused by *low* antiinnatia instead). But "strangely" these researchers' research isn't going to plan! As follows.

   Arslan et al. (2014) have recently done a study in this field which is particularly superior because it controls for the IQs of the fathers of the children (to rule out that as a possible confounder). Their report includes a good discussion of the theoretical issues, of which I will give a reasonably unmangled summary here.

   They observe that intelligence is regarded as an attractive trait in mates across cultures, and also that it has had survival value in recent times. This leads to a question of why low intelligence has not become extinct, and why high intelligence has not become "fixated", by which they mean everyone now having the genes for maximal IQ.

   On this question they point to the (mistaken) ideas of an earlier paper. Which (mistakenly) suggests that the reason why high IQ has not become fixated is that there is a substantial stream of unhelpful new mutations keeping the IQ low. And that there is consequently a *"mutation-selection balance"*, with new nasty mutations tending to make the population's IQ go down while *"directional selection"* tends to make it go up. (But all this is mistaken!)

   I think what people are overlooking here is that the output of a human brain is subject to the quirks of a stupendous number of neuronal connections and those quirks are in turn dependent on a huge number of individual genes in each neuron and their varying expression under a huge number of varying conditions inside those neurons. Scientists who ought to know better assume the brain is some sort of amazing super-computer, whereas it should more reasonably be thought of as a would-be computer rather randomly emerging from lumps of not-entirely-organised meat. Computer chips are carefully designed by expert engineers, and formed of highly stable solids such as copper and silicon. By contrast brains are not designed but rather emergent from random mutations and blind selection, and are made from very unstable living cells. Information input to a computer does not change the hardware. But information input to a brain *does* change the brain's "hardware", in terms of new or altered synapses and so on (more than actually known at present). Computers are designed to be boringly logical. Brains are evolved to be seriously prejudiced.

   Now here's the crucial problem for evolution. You can't evolve your way out of all that quirkyness of the brain functioning, because there are vastly too many genes and non-genetic factors involved. Even if you could de-select them from the cells of the inherited germline, there would still be many "somatic" de novo mutations among the billions of individual cells forming the brain.

There is a lot of potential for quirky error in the outputs of those neurons, or in other words in the gene-expressions of those neurons, and there needs to be some means for editing down their contributions to reduce the unhelpful rubbishy noise output. In the published autism theory paper I argued that antiinnatia factors (including antiinnatia genes) would have their main function in suppressing such unhelpful error-causing expressions (which I called a class of "innatons" namely "IQ impairers"), and thereby tending to raise IQ. But these same antiinnatia factors would have the downside of also tending to suppress the advantageous innatons and making people a bit autistic-y. And that "but" is where these mutation researchers go wrong.

Sure, high IQ is an important quality in human affairs. But so have been "Sense and Sensibility", not to mention "Pride and Prejudice" and "Persuasion". Consequently these antiinnatia genes which these researchers are unwittingly studying are under evolutionary pressure from two directions. For any given environmental situation, there is an optimum level of antiinnatia: between being too retarded on the one hand and being too geeky on the other. And so the genes for IQ are not under that "directional selection" leading to "mutation-selection balance", but instead under something more like "stabilising selection".

Arslan et al. (2014) say of this stabilising selection that it: "leads to a buffering against both deleterious and beneficial changes (robustness)" and that "higher robustness would imply smaller effects of new mutations".

Which brings us back to the concept of "balanced mutation", which I mentioned earlier is becoming the new main paradigm of mutational change. And back to my thoughts about the Bechstein pianos.

Meanwhile, poor old Prof Arslan and colleagues were still thinking along the old lines, so they were expecting their results to confirm the "mutation-selection balance" assumptions instead. Quite often, when scientists get "wrong" results they are very embarrassed about it, and fearful that they will be laughed at and even demoted for their "incompetence". So they tend to squirm about with their study, briefly mention the "wrong" thing only on page 7, or hide it away altogether. But to their credit the Arslan team didn't, but instead just stated their surprise at their result:

> "We did not find support for our hypothesis that higher paternal age at offspring conception, as an indicator of more new, harmful mutations, would predict lower offspring intelligence."

Which is exactly what you would expect if those mutations are analogous to those waves going both up *and down*, rather than to a one-way trend threatening to drown the entire populations of Canterbury and Cambridge before the end of the day.

In summary about the Arslan et al. study, they ended up confirming my own theory of the genetics of IQ even though they didn't even know it existed and they were expecting to prove the opposite anyway. Thus so much more becomes clear once you dump the evidence-defying parrotting of "autism is a disorder".

Meanwhile, those older parents are also survivors of many more years of natural selection, to the extent that the positive selection from that surviving could entirely cancel out any deleteriousness from some of the added mutations. If older paternity really was very disadvantageous one would expect that it would have been naturally selected away millennia ago, with human paternity starting and ending at the same age as for horses and dogs.

We should also bear in mind the fallacy of averages. It is a standard dogma of corporatised medical propaganda that large studies of thousands of people are the best form of evidence, while the wonderful experience of Fred after taking some herbal tablets bought by his mom is supposedly no evidence at all. These studies of increasing parental age fall into this same fallacy of averages. Sure, as Mr Average gets older he is more likely to need a walking stick and to get cirrhosis of the liver. But those persons who don't drink alcohol and who take (expert, haha) care of their bone nutrition are not Mr Averages and those results will have no relevance to them. Many older people have not so much spent x years alive as having spent x years living self-abusively in various unhealthy ways almost guaranteed to damage their children, but nothing to do with age per se.

And the list of other conditions most asserted to be associated with parental age is notable. Schizophrenia commonly begins around the time of becoming adult, and hence can prevent a young man from becoming registered as a young husband. But thereafter a proportion recover or become more stable, so the former schizophrenic may then become one of those "older fathers" which the researchers are finding. And again, in respect of manic-depressive illness, that condition has been notably associated with valuable creativity and higher social class, which again is associated with older parenthood, with no need for adverse mutations to be involved.

If later paternity were really genetically harmful, as per my silly mutilations of the Mona Lisa, then we would expect the resulting children to be weak, sickly, stupid and cancer-ridden. But they aren't. A review by Tournaye (2009) concluded that the absolute risk of genetic anomalies from older paternity is low, and that "there is no clear association between adverse health outcome and paternal age".

And finally, any genetics which ignores the context of changing environmental factors is half-baked. A hugely important factor is dental mercury. In Chapter 3 here I show how just about all of this autism, schizophrenia, manic depressive, and more, can be accounted for as the consequence of the introduction of dental amalgam in the 19th century followed by its "improvement" from the 1970s with the even worse non-gamma-2 amalgams. Get rid of that dental mercury and just about all this disability caused thereby disappears, nothing whatsoever to do with genes being harmful per se, but merely genes conceivably making a person vulnerable to an abnormal environment which would not be there anyway if fewer "distinguished experts" were liars.

The bottom line here is that the proper understanding of the genome and mutations does not at all correspond with the still-predominant assumptions of the outdated simplistic model. And too many people in autism genetics research are assuming that it does.

[P.S.: Ruben Arslan has commented: "You refer to me as "poor old Prof Arslan". I'm neither a Prof nor a Dr, I'm still a PhD student. The "poor" is quite right though." However, the very next month I noticed some other research of his reported in the *New Scientist*. Some "student".

He also informed me that that Arslan et al. 2014 "wrong" result has since been confirmed by "a much bigger study (D'Onofrio et al., 2014)...."]

(The main text of this chapter continues back at page 60.)

~~~~~~~

3

A suppressed report of
millions of (non-autistic) victims

*"Academic journals and societies show an auto-immune response
to information that should be the life-blood of medicine."*
– Prof. David Healy, author of *Pharmageddon*

"Your paper is important"
– mercury expert Dr med. Joachim Mutter

Before reading this chapter I recommend that you read the first two
chapters of this book. Otherwise you may come to it with considerable misconceptions which could make for difficult and unproductive reading here.

The main content of this chapter is a scientific paper. I wrote it
with the intention of it being accepted in a scientific journal, and so
you might find it rather turgid reading and with too many of those
citations such as (Authorname, 2012) intruding into my florid prose.
On the other hand one journal editor condemned it for (supposedly)
appearing to be written like a newspaper article, so maybe there's
hope for non-academic readers nevertheless.

You may be wondering whether you can have the competence to
make any useful judgement of the soundness or credibility of this
article. Wouldn't the experts perhaps point out all manner of hidden
things wrong with it? But I am providing you with a special
resource here. In the next two chapters, you can see the world's top
experts telling me (off the record) the reasons why this article is
such rubbish that you shouldn't even be informed of its existence
anyway. I suggest that you study those critiques and my rejoinders
to them, and (as is always necessary eventually) then decide for
yourself who if anyone has the more credibility. I can't print the re-
rejoinders from these experts because none have replied back.
Perhaps you could write to these journals yourself to ask them why
you shouldn't be persuaded by what I said in my own replies.

Scientific papers normally end with a list of the references
cited. In this book I will transfer this paper's reference list into the
list at the end of the book. But this article is unusual in that it
contains an appendix which itself contains three further lists of

references. I will leave those in place just as they were present in the original documents contained in that appendix. Other than that, what follows after this paragraph is the most updated version of the manuscript I have sent to now eighteen journals. It is usual for scientific papers to begin with a summary called an "abstract". This gives an overview for those who don't already have the full text, but may be hard as a non-specialist to follow until you have read that full text, and you shouldn't let yourself get bogged down by this one here. Also this chapter contains some graphs of disability epidemiology. If you are not already a wizard with such graphs, you may find it useful to jump forward to the section of Chapter 6 which discusses some misuses and abuses of similar sorts of graphs. Lastly, the "p<" values stated herein indicate the probability of obtaining that result due to random chance.

(NOTE: AT NO POINT HAVE I EVER SAID THAT *ALL* AUTISM IS CAUSED BY MERCURY OR AMALGAMS – See Chapter 7!)

Autism, adult disability, and 'workshy': Major epidemics being caused by non-gamma-2 dental amalgams

Robin P Clarke

Abstract: It is unknown to most people that the dental amalgams which have been used as standard in recent decades, namely non-gamma-2 dental amalgams, have been substantially unlike those used before the 1970s, in that they constantly emit 20 to 50 times more mercury vapor than the older types. This is the first-ever study of health consequences of non-gamma-2. Following the changeover to non-gamma-2 amalgams, there promptly began a tenfoldish increase of autism, a tenfoldish change of ratio between late onset and early onset, a change from mainly genetic to mainly environmental, and a change from lifelong incurable to sometimes clearly recoverable. Exactly simultaneously there occurred a fourfoldish increase of claims for adult disability in the UK, with disabilities all or mostly of the nature that would be expected from chronic mercury poisoning (including mental disabilities and neurological disabilities). And similarly in the US. These timings cannot be dismissed as coincidence because there are no credible alternative explanations for the increases. Data strongly suggests that non-gamma-2 amalgams are currently by far the main cause of chronic disability in the UK, US, and other such countries, with about 10% of the UK working-age population disabled thereby.

An experiment on millions of dis-informed subjects

Dental amalgams in patients' teeth constantly emit mercury vapor, and that vapor is easily measureable. This has been known for decades as indicated in at least 18 published studies (Berglund, 1993; Berglund et al., 1988, Boyer, 1988; Brune et al., 1983; Clarkson et al., 1988; Ferracane et al., 1995; Mackert, 1987; Mahler et al., 1994; Moberg, 1985a, 1985b; Olsson et al., 1989; Olsson and Bergman, 1987; Patterson et al., 1985; Psarras et al., 1994; Svare et al., 1981; Vimy and Lorscheider, 1985a, 1985b, 1990).

And yet in stark contradiction of all this clearly established basic science, the UK's Chief Dental Officer (2009) has publicly asserted, as some supposed fact, that dental amalgams do *not* constantly emit any mercury vapor (or in his second thoughts on being challenged, at least "not measureably").

Such mercury vapor has been recognised for centuries as one of the most toxic of substances, causing various mental, neurological and physical disabilities. For more than a hundred years prior to the 1970s, strong condemnations were regularly issued against the use of amalgam in dentistry. These warnings were consistently ignored by health authorities, and dismissed with claims that there was no real evidence of harmfulness.

Much further evidence of harmfulness of dental amalgam has come to light in recent decades (Mutter, 2011; Hanson, 2004; Homme et al., 2014), not least in thousands of cases of improvement following amalgam removal which cannot be dismissed as merely anecdotal or placebo. Some relatively large-scale trials have been asserted to show amalgam safety, but they have been substantially flawed and in at least one case in reality showed harmfulness rather than safety (as explained by Mutter, 2011 and Homme et al., 2014).

In the 1970s a new type of dental amalgam was introduced as the new standard, partly on the basis that it was very much more durable, with far less tendency to corroding and crumbling. This new type was called non-gamma-2.

These non-gamma-2 dental amalgams constantly emit 20 to 50 times more of the toxic mercury vapor than the older types (Berglund, 1993; Boyer, 1988; Brune et al., 1983; Ferracane et al., 1995; Mahler et al., 1994; Moberg, 1985a, 1985b; Psarras et al., 1994). The amalgam constantly emitting this neurotoxic mercury vapor is located in a person's mouth, less than two inches from their brain, and in the pathway to the lungs (where 80% is absorbed at each inhalation). Any notion that the levels of mercury vapor caused by amalgams are very low has to be put in the context of the general outdoor levels being many times lower still at around 0.002 mcg/m3.

No safety testing was undertaken before or after it was introduced. Patients and the public in general have still not been informed of the change, let alone of the increased levels of mercury involved. No informed consent has been sought, and no warnings have been given of any possible harmfulness. Indeed, throughout the US it was actually made illegal for dentists to issue such warnings, and Hal Huggins and other dentists were struck off the register of practitioners for doing so.

In the UK, a number of untruths were adopted by the NHS and DH such as to prevent people being diagnosed with mercury toxicity and to thereby further reduce any concern about risk. The following untruths have been identified by the author, but it is unlikely that they have been the only ones.

1. Untrue assertion that "Chronic mercury poisoning is highly unlikely to present in a psychiatric setting".
2. Use of proven useless urine tests for supposed (dis-) diagnosis of chronic mercury poisoning.
3. Use of proven useless blood tests for supposed (dis-) diagnosis of chronic mercury poisoning.
4. Chief Dental Officer's untrue assertion that "no mercury vapor" emits from amalgams, or alternatively "not measureably".
5. Chief Dental Officer's untrue denial that amalgams are the main source of mercury in the body.
6. NHS Chief Executive's re-insistence on the untruth that dentists have capability for mercury diagnosis whereas doctors do not.

The existence of these untruths is authenticated via my Freedom of Information requests as documented partly in an Appendix hereto and more fully via http://tinyurl.com/dentmerc

Dates of introduction and usage

Non-gamma-2 amalgams are very much more durable than the previous types. Consequently, declining rates of amalgam install-ation would conceal an increase of prevalence of the amalgams in patients' mouths. And it is here expected that the key variable would be that rising prevalence rather than the declining rate of installations and replacements.

A number of US patents for non-gamma-2 were granted in the mid-1970s. The famous US dentist Hal Huggins states that the changeover to "high copper", i.e. non-gamma-2, occurred in 1976. In 1986 the ISO standard was changed retrospectively to incorporate them. The non-gamma-2 amalgams took over in the period 1975-79 in Denmark (Hansen et al., 1993). In Germany the use of the earlier types was banned in 1992, making the non-gamma-2 the only option. And according to the manufacturer's product sheet,

Dispersalloy is the most widely used amalgam with over 25 years of proven performance, i.e., since before 1979, but perhaps after their 1974 patent no. 3841860.

I have been unable to obtain any numerical data on usage or total prevalence of non-gamma-2 in people's mouths. The DH have told me they have no such records. And NHS dental records have not recorded the types of amalgam used. It is unlikely that any better information is available in other countries. But we can very reasonably assume that the overall prevalence of non-gamma-2 will have gradually, progressively increased in the decades following its introduction.

My epidemiological investigations

Having become aware of the changeover to non-gamma-2 amalgams, I decided to look to see if there might be epidemiological evidence of any consequences. It appears that no-one has ever done this before.

In respect of the following accounts it is important to understand that I have not cherry-picked selected data to prove any point, but instead have used all the best data readily available to me.

To avoid undue length here, the reader is referred to consult prior reviews of substantial important other data pointing to similar conclusions as those here, including Hanson (2004), Mutter (2011), Geier et al. (2010), Homme et al. (2014), and others not specifically cited.

Is mercury involved in causation of autism?

Before presenting the epidemiological findings it will be useful to first show the context of existing evidence from clinical studies on this question.

A number of reviews have suggested there is persuasive evidence that mercury is importantly involved in causing of autism (Geier et al., 2010; Bernard et al., 2001; DeSoto and Hitlan, 2010; Kern et al., 2012). And yet the evidence can be shown to be far more decisive than any of these suggest, and indeed beyond all reasonable doubt.

In any combinatory review of studies it is necessary firstly to rule out those which lack a sound rationale. A number of studies have used blood mercury or urine mercury as criterion measures, and yet it has been known for decades that these lack merit as indicators of chronic mercury toxicity. Indeed, the most prominent such study, Hertz-Picciotto et al. (2010), stated in its second-last sentence that: "This report did not address the role of prenatal or early-life Hg exposure in the etiology of autism" [i.e., the study could not provide any evidence against causation by mercury].

Another danger in meta-reviewing of studies is the merging together of data which should be kept separate. In respect of mercury in autistics' hair, the most enlightening study is that of Majewska et al. (2010). They found that in younger children autism was associated with markedly decreased hair mercury ($p<0.01$), whereas in older children autism was associated with markedly increased hair mercury ($p<0.01$). If they had just lumped all their results together they would have got an entirely unwarranted "no difference" non-result instead. Viewed in the light of Majewska et al, all or most of the other hair mercury studies fall into a coherent pattern. There are several which have smudged together the different ages and therefrom invalidly declared non-results. Meanwhile others strongly reinforce the notion that there are real effects.

Holmes et al. (2003) obtained an eightfold difference of mercury in hair, with significance level of 1 in 250,000 ($p<0.000004$). Some commenters dismiss that study on a basis that it was done by opponents of mercury, and "therefore" their results may have been biased or fraudulent. But one would have expected any bias or fraud to result in a finding that hair mercury was increased in autistics, as that would have been in accordance with the standard rationale for diagnosing toxin exposure from increased hair measurements. They found instead 8-fold reduced levels, which strongly suggests that they were instead acting competently and honestly. Their rationalising notion of paradoxical reductions of measurements in mercury toxic subjects has since been supported by much other evidence that mercury sometimes impairs its own excretion.

A study in India (Lakhshmi Priya and Geetha, 2010) found 8-fold increased hair mercury ($p<0.001$). Another in Kuwait (Fido and Al-Saad, 2005) found 15-fold increased hair mercury ($p<0.001$).

Bradstreet et al. (2003) found that a challenge test with the chelating agent DMSA caused a release of mercury 3.15 times greater in autistic cases than in controls ($p<0.0002$). That is a 1 in 5000 probability that that excess mercury was just a fluke.

The probability of just these results listed above being all due to mere chance is 1/5000 x 1/250000 x 1/100 x 1/100 x 1/1000 x 1/1000, that is one in 12,500,000,000,000,000,000, vastly beyond the standard of proof ever required in any criminal prosecution.

And far more than one negative result is required to call into question one significantly positive result. There are far more ways of making a "negative" car that does not move than of making a "positive" one that does. I and thousands of others have lived in the UK for many years and never seen the Queen in all that time, and yet that does not constitute significant grounds for dismissing the testimony of those who claim she has existed.   If there were in reality no mercury-autism connection there should be a huge pile of "no-difference-found" results among which these high-significance results would be a small minority. But there is no such pile of null results to speak against the mercury-autism connection.

One could seek to interpret all those results with a notion that there could be an unknown factor which both causes autism and also harmlessly causes mercury to vary in hair and other tissues. But that notion is brought into question by the extensive commonalities between autism and mercury toxification (Kern et al., 2012). And it is completely demolished by the observations of the Autism Research Institute which has for decades been surveying the effectiveness of many potential treatments for autism. Of more than 80 treatments tested, the ARI has found that one of the most effective has been removal of mercury by careful chelation.   And Blaucok-Busch* et al. (2012) obtained highly-significant behavioral improvements even with the rather poor Hg chelator DMSA ($p<0.001$; $p<0.001$; $p<0.001$). [*incorrect spelling of Blaurock-Busch]

Meanwhile, three studies have been promoted as supposedly disproving any mercury-autism thesis. The study by Ip et al. (2004) was shown to be riddled with arithmetical errors, and in reality indicated that there was indeed a mercury connection (DeSoto and Hitlan, 2010).   Likewise Soden et al. (2007) actually proved the opposite (DeSoto and Hitlan, 2010).   And Hertz-Picciotto et al. (2010) stated in their own second-last sentence that their study did not address causation of autism by prenatal or early-life mercury exposure. Such falsely proclaimed studies are all that stands in supposed defiance of that astronomically large number calculated above. There is even more evidence that merits mention here but it would be superfluous. We can resolutely conclude that mercury is now a major cause of autism.   [Updates: Autism association with prenatal SSRI use (Harrington et al., 2014) = amalgam causes both depression of mother and autism of baby. Widespread reports of seizures in 1/3 of autistics = perinatal mercury causes both autism and seizures (Szasz et al., 2002; Klinghardt, 1998).]

Increased autism?

In academic papers and elsewhere, certain myths about autism are constantly portrayed as self-evident truths, so they must be addressed here. Firstly, the human race does not divide into those "with" autism and those "without" it, or those "on the spectrum" and those "not on the spectrum". Rather, there is a continuum of variation in the extent to which individuals are more or less autistic (in varying ways). Secondly, there is no scientific basis for a distinction between autism and Asperger's. It was merely a historical accident that Kanner and Asperger made simultaneous rediscoveries of the syndrome described by JL Down in 1887. Thirdly, there is no scientific basis for the routine references to autism as a "disorder". Autism can be severely disabling, is often terribly distressing, and may often be *a consequence of* a disorder (such as maternal infection), but rather than a disorder it is properly considered to be just atypicality (as is genius). [This is now more fully discussed in Chapter 2.]

Some researchers with decades of direct experience, such as Bernard Rimland and Lisa Blakemore-Brown, have been of the view that there has been a substantial increase of autistic behaviors, and not just increase of diagnoses.

[Update for this book: Significant further discussion of the increase "controversy" is contained in Chapter 2 in the section "The autism increase controversy" (page 68), just before the appendix to that chapter, and also majorly in Chapter 12 and pages 188-189.]

The NHS has published a report claiming to show that there has not been any increase, by supposedly showing the prevalence of autism among older adults to be the same as in children (Brugha, 2011). The report detailed the elaborate measures taken to ensure reliability of the autism assessments. And yet it gave no details at all of any measures taken to ensure the validity, that is the (infinitely more important) comparability of the diagnostic procedures as applied to adults relative to applied to children. The reason there were no such details is because there was no way of establishing such validity. And in absence thereof, such a study proves nothing about changing prevalence of autism. I myself have direct knowledge of two older persons given baseless diagnoses of autism by this same NHS that proclaims as expertise the untruths listed on a preceding page here.

The Autism Research Institute has a uniquely extensive historical database of cases. Figure 1 [here 3.1] is my re-plot of a graph published by the Autism Research Institute of its own records. Figure 2 shows my extraction from Figure 1 of the time-series of case ratios between late and early onset. Before 1980, onset at birth was twice as frequent as onset in the second year (i.e. regressive autism), whereas after 1990 the later onset rose to become five times more frequent than the onset at birth. The switch-over began at the end of the 1970s and was well under way by 1990. It closely related with the apparent increase of autism illustrated in Figure 3 and elsewhere. Figure 3 shows the data from the California DDS 2003 report (2003), with the earlier 1999 report (1999) (1998 data) recalculated to the same basis. [Note added to book chapter version:

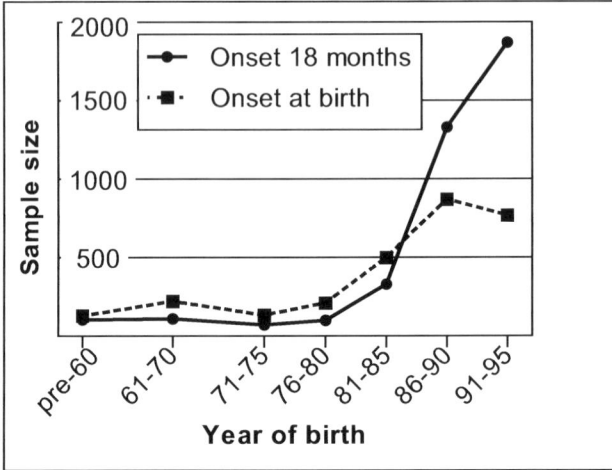

Fig. 3.1. "U.S. Cases: Autistic children who behaved normally before 18 months vs. those with no normal period." From Rimland (2000) (replotted)

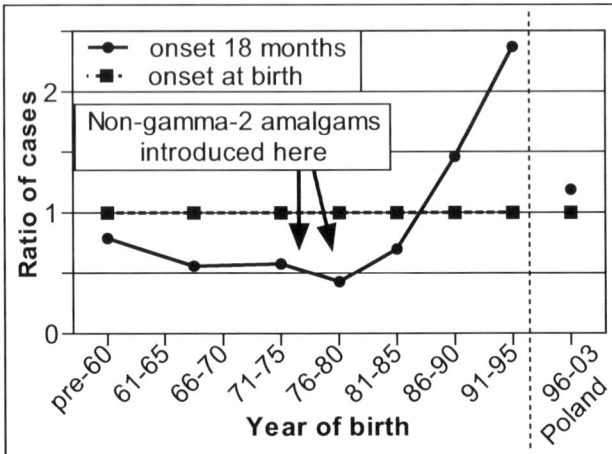

Fig. 3.2. Data from Figure 1 here used to show the changing ratio of cases in respect of age-of-onset. A further datum is from Mrozek-Budzyn et al. (2009) p.109.

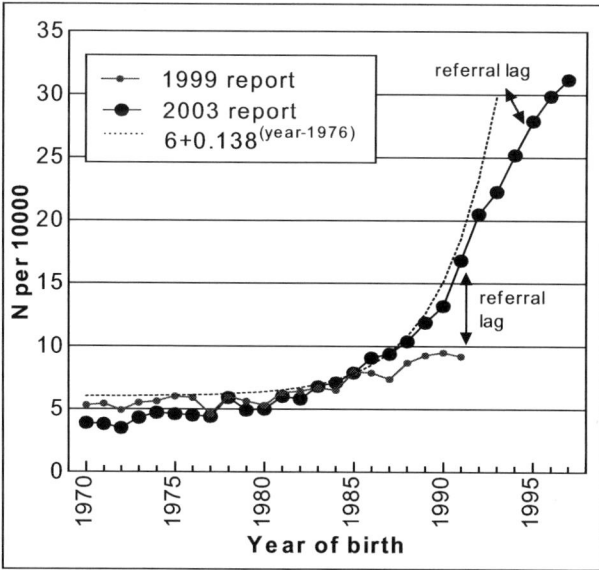

Fig. 3.3. Autism enrolment in California.

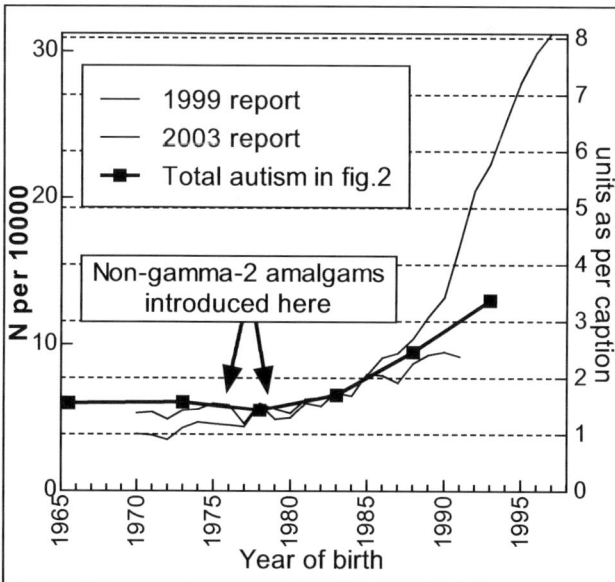

Fig. 3.4. Concurrence of California data of Figure 3.3 with total autism implied in Figure 3.2 if onset at birth is assumed to have constant incidence of one unit.

Figure 3 also shows what mathematicians call an *exponential increase* curve; basically it gets increasingly steeper exactly in proportion to the higher it gets.]

In Figure 4 I have added together the two series of Figure 2 such as to give a nominal "total autism" curve based on an assumption that onset at birth has had constant prevalence during those years, and that early onset cases plus late onset cases equals total autism. Figure 4 shows that the increase curves of Figure 3 peculiarly coincided in time with the ratio-change curve of Figure 2. This enables substantial confidence that the conceptually independent Figures 2 and 3 are tracking exactly the same causal phenomenon.

The late-onset, regressive autism is much more difficult to overlook than the at-birth autism, as parents are baffled by the regression of their children. Any under-awareness would not have been concentrated on those late-onset cases. And yet it is those which have increased about tenfold, not the more overlookable early-onset. So this data argues against interpretation in terms of mere changing of awareness or diagnostic thresholds. And it cannot be dismissed as due to demise of the diagnosis of "childhood schizophrenia", because ARI's survey questionnaire asked about age of onset rather than presumed about it, and indeed the ARI was neutrally called the "Institute for Child Behavior Research" until 1991.

These curves strongly suggest that the autism increase was caused by something that started having an effect on children around the end of the 1970s and also caused a tenfold change of ratio of late-onset cases relative to early onset.

An overview of autism trends in the US and UK found essentially the same trends of increase in both areas and in respect of both autism and "autism spectrum disorders" (Blaxill, 2004). Information about other capitalist countries has been less systematic, but generally similar trends appear to prevail. In respect of Sweden, Gillberg's three prevalence studies in Gothenburg (Stehr-Green et al., 2003) could have been plotted into Figure 3, but they would have collided impressively with the California data. The data of Denmark is rich in potential for confusion but the careful analysis by Goldman and Yazbak (2004) shows an increase from at least about 1987 onwards. Likewise, the general observation in the other countries is that there has been an increase in recent decades. And the age-of-onset data in Figure 2 follows the same pattern too. (The notion of Bernard (2003) that autism decreased in Denmark after removal of mercury from vaccines is misfounded for various reasons partly explained by Hviid (2004).)

So there is here a simple thing to be explained, seemingly beginning around the end of the 1970s.

Some years ago there was published "A theory of general impairment of gene-expression manifesting as autism" (the antiinnatia theory). It remains unchallenged in reasoning and evidence, and unrivalled as the only comprehensive fully satisfactory explanation of the supposed mystery of autism. Martha Herbert has recently been arguing that autism is not a brain/behavior condition but rather "whole body", and also not essentially genetic or developmental and fixed. But the antiinnatia theory already embodied all those notions decades ago.

The theory also specified circumstances in which autism would change from a mainly genetic condition to a mainly environmental one. Autism has now indeed markedly changed to a mainly environmental causation (Hallmayer et al., 2011).

That antiinnatia theory paper made no mention of mercury or an increase of autism (which was only vaguely becoming apparent at the time of writing it). But it did explicitly explain why molecules which randomly, dose-dependently bind to DNA and thereby reduce gene-expression would thereby cause autism. Mercury is now known to do exactly that binding and reducing at levels far below those producing other toxic effects (Ariza et al., 1994; Goyer, 1991; Rodgers et al., 2001; Walter and Luck, 1977).

A preceding section here has shown the decisive recent evidence of major involvement of mercury in many autistic cases. And thimerosal in vaccines cannot have been a main source of that mercury, for reasons explained in [Chapter 6]. So the question arises of:

where else is the source of the mercury that is now so strongly associated with most autism.

An update review of the antiinnatia theory was subsequently written, and showed confirmation of various peculiar predictions [Update: including Clarke (2015)], and explained the amalgam-autism causation more fully. But almost all medical researchers have a false presumption about theories, whereby "skepticism" (in reality a prejudice against new ideas) is supposedly a characteristic of intellectual superiority (Eysenck, 1995). And "peer review" systems block from effective publication any ideas that are more than routinely original (Eysenck and Eysenck, 1992).

Because readers are deprived of that update review I will outline here just a few of its important points. (1) Many mothers keep their infants close by at all times, and many people keep their homes very unventilated, even installing draught-proofing. The new prediction that autism would be associated with lack of ventilation (of the mercury vapor breathed out by parents or carers then inhaled by infants) has already found significant accidental confirmation (Waldman et al., 2008).   (2) The antiinnatia theory points to causation not so much like an overdose "hammer-blow" but rather more like a sustained suppression of genetic data, and thus the every-day inhalation of mercury would be much more impactful than occasional large injections. (3) The tenfold change to predominantly later onset is explained by gradual accumulation when infants regularly inhale the vapor.   (4) Any persons who dismiss the antiinnatia theory must logically be supporting one of a handful of utterly absurd alternatives, and this author requests that such "skeptics" kindly state which ones they find so credible: (i) "anti-innatia factors don't tend to produce biological advantageousness"; (ii) "they don't exist anyway despite their experimental demon-stration" (genuine flat-earthers will prefer that one); (iii) "they would not tend to become excessive"; (iv) "excess would not manifest as autism".

Some studies have found positive associations between maternal dental amalgams and autism (Holmes et al., 2003; Geier et al., 2009).   There have also been some seemingly conflicting findings, such as Adams et al. (2008) compared to Holmes et al. (2003).   But rather than concluding from these that the whole mercury or amalgam theories are unsound, or that there has been falsification or error, we may better understand them as reflecting a fact that autism is far from being simply "a novel form of mercury poisoning", and instead other factors impact in ways not yet known. Even the causation of autism by amalgam vapor alone would be complicated by variables of ventilation, parental habits, galvanic contacts in the mouth, genetics and epigenetics, intake of protective selenium, and other intakes and exposures. That complexity could explain why small cross-sectional studies have given inconsistent results. And meanwhile the time-series data shown in the charts here reflects varying levels of non-gamma-2 applied to whole populations, such that all those confounding variables are evened out, which explains why they show a clear association with the growing prevalence of the non-gamma-2 in adults' mouths.

Increased adult disability?

In 2010 I heard on BBC Radio a claim by a government minister that "There certainly hasn't been a threefold increase of disability". This suggested to me that perhaps there had indeed been an increase of adult disabilities, threefold or even greater.

On investigating this possibility, the most extensive data I could obtain was a chart on page 9 of pathways-presentation.pdf,

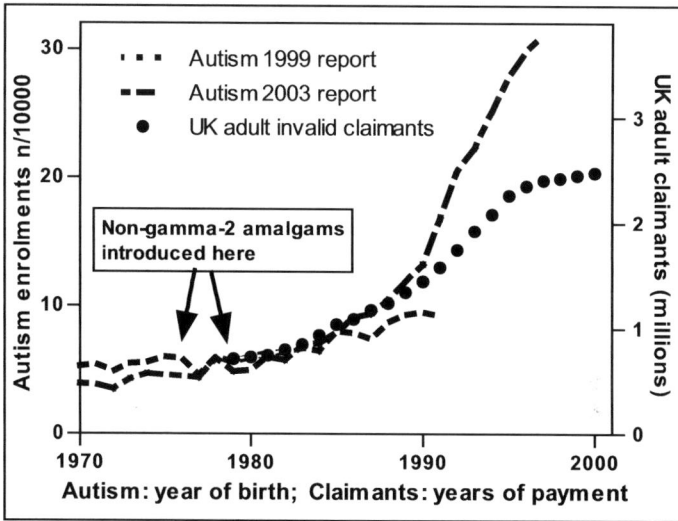

Figure 3.5. Autism enrolments (DDS) in California compared with UK adult invalidity benefits claims granted (excluding short-term lower-rate cases and excluding claims denied for policy reasons of "caseload growth now controlled")

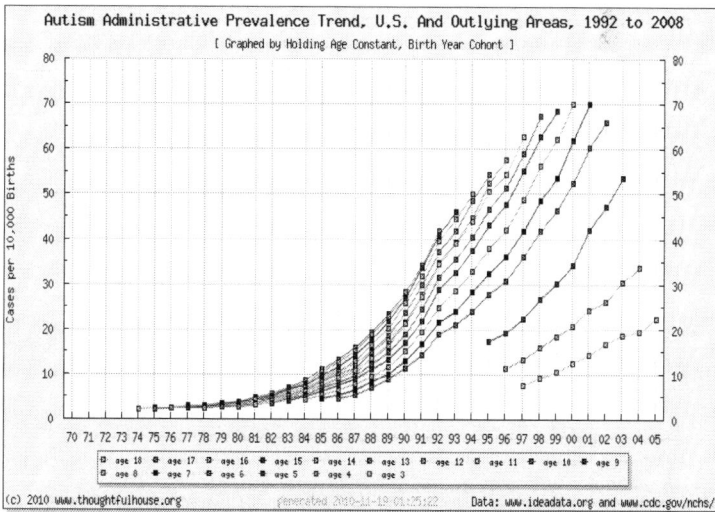

Figure 3.6. Autism enrolments under the
Individuals with Disabilities Education Act (IDEA)

(DWP, no date a) and online data timeseries (DWP, no date b) from the DWP's website.

I then took the Figure 4 chart from my (long-obstructed) autism theory update review draft, and removed my data-series derived from age-of-onset ratio-change, leaving only the two data-series of autism enrolment in California. I then added in the data of granted invalidity benefits from the DWP's chart. I used only zero-baselines, so as to not to misuse the statistics to create artificial alignments. All I did was set the righthand scale such that the first datum of the invalidity benefits data was level with the autism data at that same year, 1979.

This showed a close relationship of timing between the two, as shown in Figure 5 here.

At this point it will be useful to show you a second chart of the autism increase, this time a different administrative database (IDEA rather than DDS) and covering the whole US, namely Figure 6. This is a more complex graph, with each data-series representing a different age at recording of the cases.

With the increasing of age, fewer children from any particular birth-year cohort remain undiagnosed. So in respect of each year on Figure 6, the highest datum is the most accurate estimate to date of the real underlying level. And the falling off at the top of the latest years is due to diagnoses not yet being made.

The first important thing that this chart of IDEA data shows is that the increase has been a remarkably uniform exponential sort of curve, with just a moderate decrease of slope after 1992. The other curves, from the California DDS data, can be understood as showing what would be a similarly uniform exponential, but distorted by noticeable "noise" due to smaller samples or mislaid records.

Another important thing to understand about all these curves is that we are not here counting clear distinct things like apples or oranges. The number of people granted invalidity benefits in a particular year is a precisely-known integer, but the underlying number of people who were more or less "disabled" is necessarily a debatable, fuzzy one. Likewise with the autism numbers, and this goes some way to explaining why these two autism databases (DDS and IDEA) show significant discrepancies, most obviously in the starting levels before the increase. So we must understand that none of these curves document validly exact measurements of the underlying pathologies in their vertical scales. And therefore we should not be looking for particularly close alignments in the vertical scales; and if we do find such precision it should be considered largely a fluke. Also there is a lack of numerical data on usage or total prevalence of non-gamma-2 in people's mouths.

But these charts nevertheless do give an accurate documentation on the horizontal scale, of the timing of the increases and of
the form of the increases (i.e. not one big jump over a couple of
years). And the four series (DDS, IDEA, onset ratio, and invalidity
claims) show closely similar timing, of an increase that was gently
starting off just before 1980, and then accelerating rapidly through
the 1980s and well into the 1990s.

Meanwhile, there is also a weight of other facts attesting to the
reality of an increase of invalidity.

The symptoms of chronic mercury vapor poisoning have been
known for centuries, and include most especially all manner of
mental and neurological disturbances, but also a variety of other
symptoms. The wide variability of the presentation is easily understood in terms of the effects of mercury as a general anti-anti-
oxidant, and as an antagonist to zinc thereby disrupting hundreds of
enzymes, and also binding to the body's own proteins thereby
causing the immune system to identify them as alien and thereby
producing auto-immune reactions.

Page 14 of pathways-presentation.pdf gives an analysis of
diagnoses of the claimants. It shows that 83% of cases are
accounted for by those categories especially readily attributable to
amalgam illness:

Mental disorder	35%
Nervous system	10%
Musculo-skeletal*	22%
Others**	16%

(* Which could be mostly fibromyalgia, a modern "mystery" illness
commonly sharing features of typical amalgam illness and often
cured by amalgam removal.)
(** An all-too-likely official label for cases of the amalgam illness
which officially does not exist.)

[Book update: In David Brownstein's book *Overcoming thyroid
disorders*, he quotes Dr Derry saying: *"Chronic fatigue and fibromyalgia were non-existent before 1980. So where did these two new
diseases come from?"* Errm.... no idea, please tell me, folks.]

Further evidence supports the reality of the increase. I web-
searched for the minister's words "been a three-fold increase in
disability" and found instead that in Finland 1987-1994 there was a
threefold increase of disability pensions granted in respect of
affective disorders (mainly depression) (Salminen et al., 1997),
which is one of the most common effects of amalgam illness.

And the disability claimants are now being regularly characterised by ministers and propagandists as "workshy", "bogus", or
merely making a "lifestyle choice" of fraudulent leisure.

In 2010, the government minister Mark Harper declared on BBC Any Questions that "There are definitely some people in this country—and everyone in every community knows who they are—who are perfectly able to work, and don't." and then reiterated with "Everybody knows them, able-bodied people with no barriers to work who choose not to."

Another government minister, George Osborne, asserted that there were a sizeable number for whom claiming disability was a "lifestyle choice".

Meanwhile we are also being told that immigrants are subst-antially more hardworking than the natives of the UK, who appear by contrast to be "workshy". And indeed employers confirm such a difference.

In the real world of disability, the effects of adult mercury vapor poisoning can be far from obvious to "everyone in every community". As stated in the book *Amalgam Illness* by Andrew Hall Cutler, at page 78, "Extremely poisoned patients do not look as sick as they are .... they make adequate adrenaline during the stressful time and perform. Then they collapse for a long time while nobody is around." And at page 13, "One very important note: the patient looks a lot healthier than he is.....It is important to keep in mind that the patient may look well during appointments and yet be unable to conduct day-to-day activities, as well as be experiencing great discomfort on an ongoing basis."

And note also the following 1926 account by the famous chemist Alfred Stock of his own mercury vapor poisoning. Note how easily it could be "known" to be "workshy" were it not that the author was a notable professor.

"Mental weariness and exhaustion, lack of inclination and ability to perform any, particularly mental, work, and increased need for sleep. .... My memory, which had previously been excellent, left more and more to be desired and became worse and worse until, two years ago, I suffered from nearly complete memory loss..... I forgot the content of the book or theater play I had just read or seen as well as my own work, which had been published. ..... Obstacles, which formerly I would have overlooked smilingly (and am overlooking again today), seemed insurmountable. Scientific work caused great effort. I forced myself to go to the laboratory without being able to get anything useful accomplished in spite of all efforts. Thought came laboriously and pedantically. I had to deny myself working on solutions to questions beyond the nearest tasks at hand. The lecture that used to be a pleasure became a torture. The preparations for a lecture, the writing of a dissertation, or merely a simple letter caused unending effort in styling the material and wrestling with the language." (translated by Birgit Calhoun)(Stock, 1926)

You can see from all the above that the characteristics ascribed to the allegedly bogus claimants are characteristics of mercury poisoning. With this understanding we can even account for the peculiar observations that workers from Eastern Europe and from more distant countries are found to be more "hardworking" than the native British, who by contrast are accused of being "workshy". In fact a whole peculiar myth about normal human nature has been deployed here. Any normal healthy person, yourself for instance, would positively want to go out and do things rather than just lie in bed or slump in front of the tv all day every day. The normal healthy person would experience the latter prospect as more like a form of imprisonment than as an agreeable "lifestyle choice".

[[Update for this book: Here are the words of Frank Field MP speaking on BBC Any Questions (Field, 2012):

"London's got the second highest youth unemployment, and yet it is the mecca for immigrants to come in and work. Now why is it that our schools produce people who cannot work or don't work, as opposed to other people who at the very same time have work as part of their dna and the best thing in the world they want to do is to actually work? (loud applause)." [He then answers in terms of lazy racist white people, presumably with inferior dna, before continuing....]

"It doesn't take much money to get the kids to school on time, washed, clothed, breakfasted, and to school on time, and it is worrying that something is happening here..." [Indeed, and my own inability to get to the grammar school on time had nothing to do with my family's shortage of money either.]

And here are words about chronic fatigue syndrome from the book *Plague* (Heckenlively & Mikovits, 2014):

"If this had been going on in the fifties and sixties, even if we had discarded it as psychiatric, it would have been written about, and [yet] it's not in the literature." ..... "How could we have possibly missed this disease for all these years?". ....

"....by the mid-1980s, distressed doctors and desperate patients had turned the disease into the top category of inquiry at both the CDC and public health departments ...."

"Aided by a passive lay press, government scientists have sought to dismiss the disease by labeling sufferers with all manner of deficiencies and malevolent motives. That list has included malingering and cheating welfare systems, ... or people who [had] read about the disease and "wanted to have it".

"By 2009.... patients were denied not merely medical care, payouts on disability claims, and the emotional support that might have been forthcoming from family and friends had they suffered from a "real" disease,..... If they were children, they were denied educations ...." [like don't I know myself, and see Chapter 8 here]]]

And furthermore, in reality almost all people are desperate to avoid becoming categorised as disabled, going to near-psychotic lengths of denial in the opposite direction. Few people would be pleased to be in any social context, with no better answer to a common question than: "I've been chronically disabled for the past five years (mentally rather than physically of course)." Virtually no-one in any society treats mentally disabled people as even near to being social or intellectual equals of themselves (in terms of marriage or educational opportunities for instance) (notwithstanding their pretentions to otherwise).

An even greater catastrophe?

Notably in line with the UK data, recipients of disability benefits in the US (SSI/SSDI) also increased more than twofold between 1987 and 2007.

Here are some further facts. Figure 5 indicates a levelling off at 2.5 million claimants from 1995 onwards. But this must be put in the context of the words of the DWP document those figures came from. It was an internal discussion document about the "Personal Capability Assessment", and its page 11 was headed "Caseload growth now controlled". Translating those words from Officialese, they mean that there has been political resistance to the growth of disability claims, and that many thousands of persons genuinely disabled by DH recklessness have been denied the disability benefits they needed for survival, and that if the graph had reflected the real increase of disability it would not have levelled off, but instead would probably have surpassed more like 4 million by 2000 (which is about 10% of the UK's working-age population). [Update August 2015: "Statistics [reluctantly] released by the DWP on Thursday revealed that 2,380 people died between December 2011 and February 2014 within 14 days of being taken off Employment and Support Allowance because a Work Capability Assessment had concluded they were able to work." (Butler, 2015).][Update November 2015: 590 additional suicides linked to WCA reassessments (Barr et al., 2015; Benefits and Work, 2015).]

And yet more. Four of the most characteristic symptoms of chronic mercury vapor poisoning are fatigue, depression, sleep disturbances, and poor memory. And surveys in recent years have found that now a gigantic proportion of the NON-claimant population have these very symptoms, as follows.

Depression:

A survey of 2000 women and girls in England and Wales found 63% had been affected by mental health problems, having "a devastating impact on their lives", and "48% experiencing mental health problems had stayed in bed or not left the house for a long period as a result" (Platform 51, 2011). Meanwhile, Colin Walker of Mind said his organisation's research showed men and women experienced mental health problems such as depression and anxiety in roughly equal numbers (Hill, 2011).

Insomnia:

A report from the Mental Health Foundation (2011) states: "Only 38% of survey respondents (2522 people) were classified as 'good sleepers', whilst 36% were classified as possibly having chronic insomnia (2414 people). .... Other estimates of insomnia have put the total figure at around 30% of adults, ... although rates depend upon the criteria used to define it. Of the people reporting insomnia in the survey, over 30% have had insomnia for 2–5 years, and over 25% for over 11 years (figure 4)."

The figure 4 in question then shows a distinctly bimodal distribution, in which the larger, longer-term, mode can be reasonably attributed to the effects of the dental amalgam toxicity.

Fatigue:

In a survey by Pharmaton (2010) in the UK, 24% said they are mentally or physically exhausted every day, 45% say they miss socialising due to tiredness, and 60% of the young are too tired to socialise, compared to 40% in 2002. And that is in line with the widespread experience that immigrants from less-developed countries are substantially more "hardworking" than those who have grown up in the UK, who are conversely "workshy" as discussed on a preceding page here.

Memory:

Almost everyone nowadays wishes they had "better" memory, by which they mean more remembering rather than less. And yet contrary to the common assumption, memory is not something which natural selection would always be pressuring for more of (such as health or beauty). On the contrary, some persons (e.g. Solomon Shereschevsky) have had more memory than was actually useful for them. And history attests to the powerful memorising abilities of our ancestors.

(This chapter continues on the next page.)

Update 1

All the preceding evidence here was suggesting to me an obvious further question, namely whether the original introduction of amalgams in the 19th century had caused an earlier increase of mental disabilities to the baselines shown here. Subsequent to my writing all the preceding, I learnt of the detailed historical review by Torrey & Miller (2002) of what was then called "insanity", and the time-series graphs therein (at pages 94, 152, 188, 271, and frontispiece). In Figure 7 here I have re-plotted their data along with dates relating to the introduction of amalgam. Their book makes no mention of amalgam, or dentistry, nor of mercury as a possible cause of that increased morbidity. And yet their graphs show that rates of mental disability steadily increased from the original introduction of amalgams till a century later, by <u>fourteenfold</u> in Ireland and Canada, <u>elevenfold</u> in the US, and <u>fivefold</u> in the UK. These increases occurred in the context of vociferous contemporary condemnations of the use of amalgam due to its causing of mercury toxicity disabilities. The ASDS disbanded and the ADA replaced it because too many dentists preferred making quick profits from poisoning their patients with fillings deceitfully referred to as "silver".

Two curious observations on Figure 7. Firstly, the starting level being much higher in England/Wales, which could be because England was the first industrialised country, and with the main fuel both in houses and factories being mercury-emitting coal, besides which mercury was used for other purposes (such as hat-making). And indeed there is much reference in Torrey & Miller to insanity having been considered "the English disease".

Secondly, the ending level being much higher in Ireland, which could be because Ireland gets high rainfall from the Gulf Stream and consequently people are much more indoors and hence breathing in the amalgam mercury (as per my citation of Waldman et al earlier here). These two reality-harmonious observations suggest that these statistics reflect real increases rather than what some might construe as just some speculated mysterious spontaneous increase of awareness of what was then called insanity.

And the Preface of their book states: "It has now been almost thirty years since one of us—E. Fuller Torrey—submitted a paper for publication suggesting that epidemic insanity was a recent phenomenon. .... The paper was summarily rejected by all journals .... and it was never published.... ".

And then even my own copy of their extraordinary book had come from being dismissed from a library in Illinois.

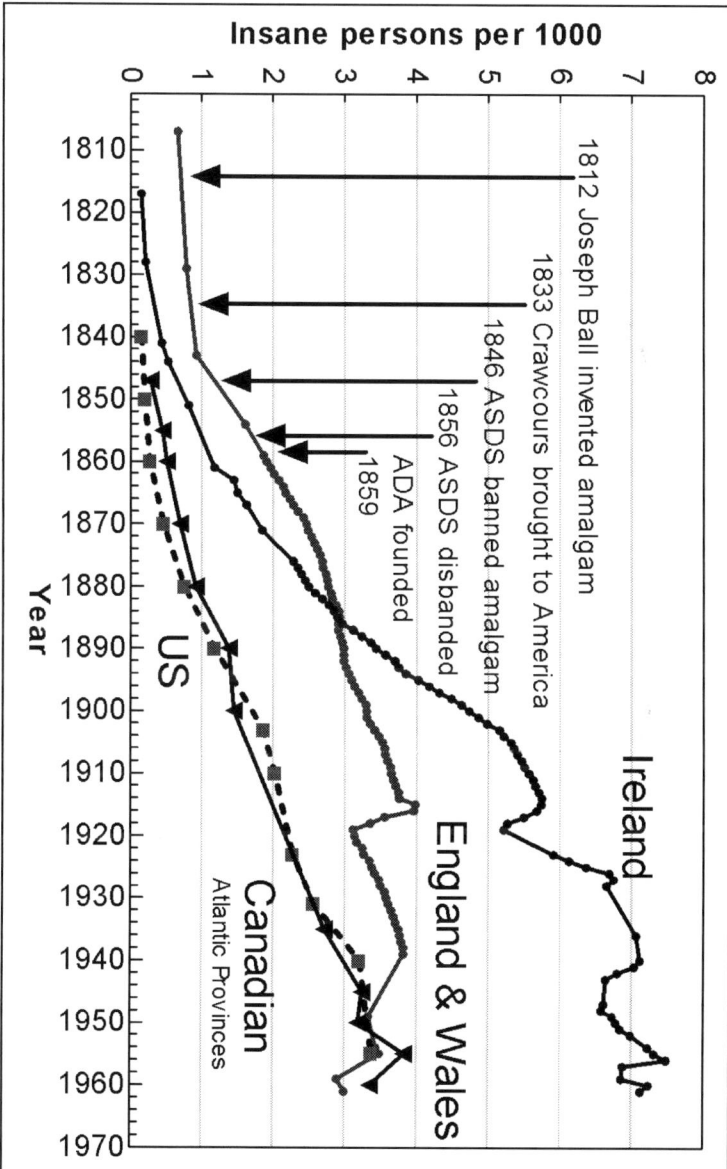

Figure 3.7. Insane persons in relation to the history of amalgams

[Update 2

Since about 2012 there has been a very peculiar and "mysterious" change to the appointments systems used in the UK by the clinics of NHS GPs. The new systems require the patients to phone in at 8.15–8.30 am or else wait to phone in next day at 8.15–8.30. If a patient missing the deadline asks to be listed for the next day, they just get a blank reasonless reply that "We can't do that", as if the ability to write down a note on a piece of paper has somehow been lost by receptionists.

On the NHS Choices website you can see countless people complaining about this appointments system and how it was so much better for many years before it was thus "improved". So why make this weird change which no one asked for and many have been complaining bitterly about? Why "fix" something that wasn't broken anyway, and then only with a hugely inconvenient and annoying disimprovement rather than an improvement?

Well here's the answer to this mystery. Basically the new systems are designed to get rid of the mercury-poisoned people who (speaking from *far* too much personal experience) (a) cannot wake up in the morning, (b) even if they are awake, still cannot remember to phone at just that time, (c) are too exhausted to keep dialling and likely phone-phobic as well. So the system successfully disappears all the mercury-poisoned would-be patients who would be complaining of Tired All The Time (TATT, the most frequent complaint received by GPs which of course they can do nothing honest about anyway as the MHRA has decreed that "amalgams are harmless"). Thereby are got rid of those who raise tedious questions about mercury poisoning (as I did) or who get angry at the constant shifty nonsense they encounter from the medical professionals. And furthermore, because they fail to get registered for an appointment, their reports of illness do not even exist in legal terms. Thereby is the epidemic detailed in this book pretended into non-existence by this new appointment system perfectly designed for exactly that purpose.

Chapters 8 and 9 will show you more on the huge deceitfulness shown against a severely disabled person very obviously poisoned by amalgams, and despite years of informative efforts about the matter.]

Conclusions and Predictions

It is important to bear in mind here the further supporting data reviewed by Mutter (2011), Hanson (2004), Geier et al (2010), Homme et al (2014), and others.

There are roughly two alternative viewpoints which may be reached from the data presented here. On the one hand there is a notion which entails that:

(1) The heavy involvement of mercury in modern autism has nothing to do with the largest source of mercury input but instead is due to some other mysterious source or process.

(2) And these graphs and other observations are mere coincidences in time.

(3a) And either some mysterious unknown substance caused all these disabilities just so as to resemble the mercury symptoms that Mutter, Hanson, Geier, etc., have long been predicting anyway *on entirely different evidence*, and just happened to coincide at the right time to neatly confuse the author.

(3b) Or there has been either a huge moral degeneration into "workshy" or else millions of people have enthusiastically embraced a "lifestyle choice" of living like a prisoner combined with the social leper dis-status of being mentally disabled, and furthermore these shirkers by some fluke just happened to be getting diagnosed with mercury symptoms even though they knew nothing about mercury toxicity, and by further impressive fluke so closely coincided with the increases of autism diagnoses and non-gamma-2 prevalence. And these "workshy" millions are somehow descendants of the people who hand-built the huge medieval cathedrals in a cold wet small island and then went on to create the largest empire (of hardworking foreigners) in history.

(4) And a many-fold increase of mercury burden has not had any harmful effects on the millions thus burdened.

(5) And the change of autism from life-long genetic to environmental and recoverable is just another of these mysteries.

(6) And those gross untruths from the NHS just happened by fluke to all relate to preventing people getting diagnosed with mercury poisoning (two evidence-defying pseudo-tests, the "birds are highly unlikely to have wings" nonsense, the "see a dentist instead" - "see a doctor instead" nonsense, the review of my non-dental problems complaint exclusively by a dental panel with no toxicological or neurological expertise, the NHS's own pseudo-study to pretend away the autism increase, and the Chief Dental Officer's evidence-defying insistence that no mercury vapor comes off anyway).

(7) And merely by yet another fluke Torrey's graphs confirmed my suspicion that there would have been a previous increase of mental disabilities following the original introduction of amalgam 150 years earlier.

(8) And merely by yet another fluke there is that observation that most mental disorders start in the 12-25 age-range.

Alternatively there is a notion that non-gamma-2 amalgam has been the main cause of a tenfoldish increase of autism and a fourfoldish increase of adult disability including so-called "workshy". It is the view of this author that this latter interpretation of the data strains credibility very much less than the former. It is hardly a surprising discovery given what Mutter, Hanson, and others have previously predicted on entirely different evidence already.

And likewise the data of an increase in the 19th century cannot be lightly dismissed as "merely" coincidence. Some such increase was to be suspected by inference from the later non-gamma-2 data; it is scientifically explainable in terms of known mercury toxicity; and indeed it was very much pre-warned of already by ASDS members 170 years ago. And the ADA then adopted the propaganda language of "silver amalgams" by way of the ongoing cover-up. And I obtained that data from a very detailed review book which did not even mention dental or amalgam, so can hardly be dismissed as some sort of cherry-picking.

Editors of putatively scientific medical journals have a duty to ensure that the public is not being kept unaware of evidence of possible serious harm from standard medical practices. It is a serious breach of ethics for such evidence as contained here to be refused publication other than for rigorously justified reasons. If there really are any serious faults in the case presented here, they should be openly published in the scientific literature rather than used as mere excuses to prevent the evidence being raised in the first place.

It is here predicted that these increases will tend to correlate together in comparisons between different nations, due to the common causality. It is predicted that these epidemics will only be reversed by reduction of prevalence of non-gamma-2 in victims' mouths. And meanwhile the risk of autistic disability can be reduced by ensuring adequate ventilation (in practice with a through draught at breathing-level).

[[**Update 3**

Subsequent to all the preceding I have noticed the words of Professor Stephen Wood, as follows:

"My research aims to understand the health paradox of adolescence – the years between 12 and 25 are a time of great physical fitness, yet this is the period during which 75% of all mental disorders have their onset. Why should this be the case? Clearly changes in the brain are likely culprits, but how they interact with genetic and environmental factors to produce illness is unclear." (Wood, 2015)

But I suggest that there is not really much paradox or unclarity here (in the context of the graphs on the preceding pages). It could be simply that medical experts start installing those great lumps of harmlessly neurotoxic mercury into the mouths of people two inches from their brains shortly before that age.

In 2012 Professor Wood got a grant of £818,000 from the MRC for this research on adolescent mental problems. The entirety of *all* my own research to date has been funded to the tune of £0.]]

Additional Files

Additional File 1.htm: Four Freedom of Information requests (outlined in the Appendix). [www.tinyurl.com/dentmerc]
Additional File 2.pdf: Mercury in vaccines as alleged cause of autism increase. [see Chapter 6]
Additional File 3.pdf: Prior responses from journals.
[Chapter 5]
Additional File 4.pdf: Prior responses from Neurotoxicology journal.
[Chapter 4]

[Update: One in six American adults taking psychiatric drugs (Moore and Mattison, 2016).]

[Update: "About 300,000 [UK] people with a long-term mental health problem lose their jobs each year, a review commissioned by Theresa May has found." (Siddique, 2017)]

Appendix: Four Freedom of Information requests

(more fully documented via Additional File 1.htm) or
http://tinyurl.com/dentmerc

Why "Chronic mercury poisoning is highly unlikely to present in a psychiatric setting."?

Mr Clarke made this Freedom of Information request to
Birmingham and Solihull Mental Health NHS Foundation Trust
RESPONSE TO THIS REQUEST IS LONG OVERDUE
6 September 2011

Dear Birmingham and Solihull Mental Health NHS Foundation
Trust,

1. Given that it has been well-known for years, decades, and even
centuries, that among the most characteristic symptoms of chronic
mercury poisoning are nervousness, shyness, depression, agitation,
fatigue, impaired memory, lack of concentration, and indecision (as
per abundant documentation indicated below):
Why did the BSMHFT (Birmingham and Solihull Mental Health
Foundation Trust) state this year in a FOI reply that "Chronic
mercury poisoning is highly unlikely to present in a psychiatric
setting."?
2. What scientific or evidential basis existed to justify such a
statement?
3. Who in the BSMHFT gave that answer, and from where did they
derive that conclusion? Where did the notion originate?

Yours faithfully,
Mr Clarke

DOCUMENTATION:

Numerous studies and reports exist, for example:
Alfred Stock 1926:   "Mental weariness and exhaustion, lack of
inclination and ability to perform any, particularly mental, work,
and increased need for sleep..... nearly complete memory loss.....
Obstacles, which formerly I would have overlooked smilingly,
seemed insurmountable.... merely writing a simple letter caused
unending effort...."
BMJ 287:1961 (1983) Did the Mad Hatter have mercury poisoning?
HA Waldron: "The principal features of erethism were excessive

timidity, diffidence, increasing shyness, loss of self confidence, anxiety, and a desire to remain unobserved and unobtrusive. The victim also had a pathological fear of ridicule and often reacted with an explosive loss of temper when criticised."
1899 Tuthill: "makes a mental wreck of its victim".
1974 J Am Dent Soc 98(4),904: "symptoms include ....
self-consciousness, embarrassment without justification, disproportionate anxiety, indecision, poor concentration, depression, irrational resentment of criticism, and irritability."

TOXICOLOGICAL PROFILE FOR MERCURY. U.S. DEPARTMENT OF HEALTH AND HUMAN SERVICES
Public Health Service Agency for Toxic Substances and Disease Registry March 1999 Page 276:
Neurological Effects. The nervous system is the primary target organ for elemental and methylmercury-induced toxicity. Neurological and behavioral disorders in humans have been observed following inhalation of metallic mercury vapor and organic mercury compounds, ingestion or dermal application of inorganic mercury-containing medicinal products (e.g., teething powders, ointments, and laxatives), and ingestion or dermal exposure to organic mercury-containing pesticides or ingestion of contaminated seafood. A broad range of symptoms has been reported, and these symptoms are qualitatively similar, irrespective of the mercury compound to which one is exposed. Specific neurotoxic symptoms include tremors (initially affecting the hands and sometimes spreading to other parts of the body), emotional lability (characterized by irritability, excessive shyness, confidence loss, and nervousness), insomnia, memory loss, neuromuscular changes (weakness, muscle atrophy, and muscle twitching), headaches, polyneuropathy (paresthesias, stocking-glove sensory loss, hyperactive tendon reflexes, slowed sensory and motor nerve conduction velocities), and performance deficits in tests of cognitive and motor function (Adams et al. 1983; Albers et al. 1982, 1988; Aronow et al. 1990; Bakir et al. 1973; Barber 1978; Bidstrup et al. 1951; Bluhm et al. 1992a; Bourgeois et al. 1986; Chaffin et al. 1973; Chapman et al. 1990; Choi et al. 1978; Cinca et al. 1979; Davis et al. 1974; DeBont et al. 1986; Discalzi et al. 1993; Dyall-Smith and Scurry 1990; Ehrenberg et al. 1991; Fagala and Wigg 1992; Fawer et al. 1983; Foulds et al. 1987; Friberg et al. 1953; Hallee 1969; Harada 1978; Hook et al. 1954; Hunter et al. 1940; Iyer et al. 1976; Jaffe et al. 1983; Jalili and Abbasi 1961; Kang-Yum and Oransky 1992; Karpathios et al. 1991; Kutsuna 1968; Langauer-Lewowicka and Kazibutowska 1989; Kutsuna 1968; Langolf et al. 1978; Langworth

et al. 1992a; Levine et al. 1982; Lilis et al. 1985; Lundgren and Swensson 1949; Matsumoto et al. 1965; McFarland and Reigel 1978; Melkonian and Baker 1988; Miyakawa et al. 1976; Ngim et al. 1992; Piikivi and Hanninen 1989; Piikivi and Tolonen 1989; Piikivi et al. 1984; Roels et al. 1982; Sexton et al. 1976; Shapiro et al. 1982; Snodgrass et al. 1981; Smith et al. 1970; Tamashiro et al. 1984; Taueg et al. 1992; Tsubaki and Takahashi 1986; Verberk et al. 1986; Vroom and Greer 1972; Warkany and Hubbard 1953; Williamson et al. 1982). Some individuals have also noted hearing loss, visual disturbances (visual field defects), and/or hallucinations (Bluhm et al. 1992a; Cinca et al. 1979; Fagala and Wigg 1992; Jalili and Abbasi 1961; Locket and Nazroo 1952; McFarland and Reigel 1978; Taueg et al. 1992). Although improvement has often been observed upon removal of persons from the source of exposure, it is possible that some changes may be irreversible. Autopsy findings of degenerative changes in the brains of poisoned patients exposed to mercury support the functional changes observed (Al-Saleem and the Clinical Committee on Mercury Poisoning 1976; Cinca et al. 1979; Davis et al. 1974; Miyakawa et al. 1976).

The characteristic symptoms of chronic mercury vapour are also documented in innumerable other studies and sources and case histories:

a) "References documenting symptoms to mercury exposure" published by the International Academy of Oral Medicine and Toxicology, www.iaomt.org ; the first seven in their list are all very familiar as major symptoms of this inquirer, namely irritability, anxiety/nervousness, loss of memory, inability to concentrate, lethargy/drowsiness, insomnia, mental depression/ despondency/ withdrawal; plus also very familiar, 9: muscle weakness, 11: tremors of hands, legs, eyelids, 12: decline of intellect, 13: loss of self-confidence, 16: bleeding gums, 18: loosening of teeth, etc.

b) Mats Hanson "Effects of Amalgam Removal on Health; 25 studies comprising 5821 patients" lists the main removal findings as "fatigue, anxiety/depression, muscle pains, headache, concentration problems, joint problems, metal taste, mouth symptoms, vertigo/dizziness, gastrointestinal problems, memory disturbances, problems with sight, irritability, sleep disturbances, heart problems, skin problems, allergies, problems with hearing, numbness, infection-prone (bold added here to indicate this inquirer's most notable symptoms in that list).

c) Extensive further documentation of causation of these same symptoms can be seen in excerpts here appended from www.flcv.com/depress.html and www.flcv.com/amalg6.html.

Excerpt from http://www.flcv.com/amalg6.html

Bernard Windham compilation of references re amalgam removal cases

[....]

VI. Results of Removal of Amalgam Fillings

[...] There are extensive documented cases (many thousands) where removal of amalgam fillings led to cure or significant improvement of serious health problems such as: [excerpts here:]

epilepsy (5,35,309,229,386e,557),

dizzyness/vertigo (8,40,95,212,222,229,233bcdgh,271,322,376,453,525c,551,552), 523,525c,538,551, 552,556,557,583),

insomnia (35,62,94,212,222,233ag,271,317,322, 376,525c,583),

MS 2,94,95,102,163,170,212,222,229,271,291,302,322,369, 469,485,34,35c,229,523, 532),

ALS (97,246,423,405,469,470,485,535,35),

Alzheimer's (62,204,251c,386e,535,35),

Parkinson's/ muscle tremor (222,248,228a,229,233f, 271,322, 469,557,212,62,94,98,35),

Chronic Fatigue Syndrome (8,35,47f,60,62,88,185,212,293,229,222,232,233abcdfgh,271, 313, 317, 322,323,342, 346, 369,376,386de, 440, 469, 470,523,532,537,538, 551,552,556,557,595),

nausea (525c),

neuropathy/paresthesia (8,35,62,94,163,212,222,322,556,557),

memory disorders (8,35,94,212,222,322,437,440,453,552,557,595),

depression (62,94,107,163,185,212,222,229,233bcfh,271,294,285e,317,322,376,3 86de,437,453, 465,485,523, 525c,532,538,551,556,557,583,595,35,40),

anxiety & mental confusion (62,94,212,222,229,233abcfgh,271,317,322,440,453,525c, 532,551, 557,583,35,57),

neuropathy/paresthesia (8,35,62,94,163,212,222,322,556,557),

Why SWBHNHST uses well-known useless quack tests of dental amalgam mercury poisoning?

Mr Clarke made this Freedom of Information request to Sandwell and West Birmingham Hospitals NHS Trust

RESPONSE TO THIS REQUEST IS LONG OVERDUE

23 September 2011

Dear Sandwell and West Birmingham Hospitals NHS Trust,

1. Given that it has been well-established and well-known for decades that blood mercury level and urine mercury level are useless as indicators of chronic mercury toxification (as documented below)....

Why did the toxicologists of the SWBHNHST / the City Hospital in Birmingham propose in 2010/11 these well-known useless tests in respect of a patient presenting substantial evidence of being disabled by dental amalgams?

2. What scientific or evidential basis existed to justify such proposals?

3. From where did the SWBHNHST toxicologists get that notion of usefulness of those blood and urine tests? Where did that notion originate?

4. What worthwhile purpose could be served by those tests given that the patient already had reported extraordinarily high mercury vapour measurements of 460 mcg/m3 (unprovoked, open mouth) (a world record level, about 100x higher than typical levels)?

DOCUMENTATION:

Goldwater et al. (1964) stated:

> "Those investigators who have studied the subject are in almost unanimous agreement that there is a poor correlation between the urinary excretion of mercury and the occurrence of demonstrable evidence of poisoning."

and a joint statement of the National Institute of Dental Health and the American Dental Association (NIDH/ADA, 1984) stated in 1984 that: "The distribution of mercury into the body tissues is highly variable and there appears to be little correlation between levels in urine, blood or hair and toxic effects." And later studies have further confirmed that conclusion. Even with normal or low mercury levels in blood, hair and urine, high mercury levels are found in critical organs such as brain and kidney (Danscher et al., 1990; Drasch, 1997; Hahn et al. 1989, 1990, Hargeaves et al., 1988; Lorscheider et al., 1995; Opitz et al., 1996; Vimy et al., 1990; Weiner & Nylander, 1993). Drasch et al. (2001, 2002, 2004) found that 64% of individuals occupationally exposed to mercury vapor and having typical clinical signs of mercury intoxication had low mercury levels in blood. A more recent autopsy study again confirmed the lack of correlation between inorganic (e.g. dental) mercury levels in urine or blood and mercury levels in brain (Björkman et al. 2007).

Bjorkman L, Lundekvam BF, Laegreid T, Bertelsen BI, Morild I, Lilleng P. 2007. Mercury in human brain, blood, muscle and toenails in relation to exposure: an autopsy study. Environ Health 6:30.

Danscher G, Hørsted-Bindsley P, Rungby J. 1990. Traces of mercury in organs from primates with amalgam fillings. Exp Mol Pathol 52:291-299.

Drasch G, Wanghofer E, Roider G. 1997. Are blood, urine, hair, and muscle valid bio-monitoring parameters for the internal burden of men with the heavy metals mercury, lead and cadmium? Trace Elem Electrolyt 14:116-123.

Drasch G, Böse-O'Reilly S, Beinhoff C, Roider G, Maydl S. 2001. The Mt. Diwata study on the Philippines 1999 - assessing mercury intoxication of the population by small scale gold mining. Sci Total Environ 267:151-168.

Drasch G, Böse-O'Reilly S, Maydl S, Roider G. 2002. Scientific comment on the German human biological monitoring values (HBM values) for mercury. Int J Hyg Environ Health 205:509-512.

Drasch G, Böse-O'Reilly S, Maydl S, Roider G. 2004. Response to the letter of the Human Biomonitoring Commission. Int J Hyg Environ Health 207:83-184.

Goldwater, L.J. Ladd, A.C. and Jacobs, M.B. 1964. Absorption and Excretion of Mercury in Man; VII Significance of mercury in Blood. Arch Envir Health. 9:735-741.

Hahn LJ, Kloiber R, Vimy MJ, Takahashi Y, Lorscheider FL. 1989. Dental "silver" tooth fillings: a source of mercury exposure revealed by whole-body image scan and tissue analysis. FASEB Journal 3:2641-2646.

Hahn LJ, Kloiber R, Leininger RW, Vimy MJ, Lorscheider FL. 1990. Whole-body imaging of the distribution of mercury released from dental fillings into monkey tissues. FASEB Journal 4:3256-3260.

Hargreaves RJ, Evans JG, Janota I, Magos L, Cavanagh JB. 1988. Persistant mercury in nerve cells 16 years after metallic mercury poisoning. Neuropath Appl Neurobiol 14:443-452.

Lorscheider FL, Vimy MJ, Summers AO. 1995. Mercury exposure from "silver" tooth fillings: emerging evidence questions a traditional dental paradigm. FASEB Journal 9:504-508.

NIDH/ADA Workshop on Biocompatibility of Metals. 1984. J Am Dent Assoc 109, September 1984.

Opitz H, Schweinsberg F, Grossmann T, Wendt-Gallitelli MF, Meyermann R. 1996. Demonstration of mercury in the human brain and other organs 17 years after metallic mercury exposure. Clin Neuropath 15:139-144.

Vimy MJ, Takahashi Y, Lorscheider FL. 1990. Maternal-fetal distribution of mercury (203 Hg) released from dental amalgam fillings. Am J Physiol 258:939-945.

Weiner JA, Nylander M. 1993. The relationship between mercury concentration in human organs and different predictor variables. Sci Tot Environ 138:101-115.

Yours faithfully,
Mr Clarke

Seriously misleading falsehoods about dental amalgam by Chief Dental Officer Barry Cockcroft

Mr Clarke made this Freedom of Information request to Department of Health

RESPONSE TO THIS REQUEST IS LONG OVERDUE

1 November 2011

Dear Department of Health,

The Chief Dental Officer Barry Cockcroft declared (on ITV, see link below) that no mercury vapour is emitted from dental amalgams, or --on second thoughts-- at least "not measureably". Yet this is violently at odds with the real bleedingly obvious long-established facts of the matter, as per documentation below.

He further queried the point that dental amalgam is the main source of mercury exposure in humans. Again this flies in the face of the known evidence. As per documentation below.

In the context of the above, would you please tell me:

1. On what scientific basis did Barry Cockcroft assert that no measurable mercury is emitted from amalgams?

2. On what scientific basis did Barry Cockcroft assert that dental amalgam is not the main source of mercury exposure?
3. In the absence of such a scientific basis, why did Barry Cockcroft make these very seriously misleading assertions on the major ITV Tonight program?
4. Do you appoint utter incompetents/liars/idiots to your most senior positions as a matter of deliberate policy or did you make some mistake in the case of Barry Cockcroft?
5. Why is Barry Cockcroft still the Chief Dental Officer more than two years later?
6. Why do you everywhere keep the public in the dark about those two very important most basic points of amalgam toxicity (that measureable amounts of mercury are constantly emitted and that that is the main source of mercury exposure)?

Yours faithfully,
Mr Clarke

DOCUMENTATION:
This video:
http://www.youtube.com/watch?v=mMI_em8UPo4
shows at 5-7 minutes: (a) three measurements (9.93, 2.58, 1.66); (b) CDO Barry Cockcroft declaring that the measurements are impossible; (c) a further measurement (2.44).

Here are TEN studies from twenty years earlier, of the measurements that Chief Dental Officer Barry Cockcroft says are impossible.

Svare, C.W., Peterson, L.C., Reinihardt, J.W., et al. (1981): The effect of dental amalgams on mercury levels in expired air. J Dent Res 60:1668-1671.
Patterson, J.E., Weissberg, B.G., Dennison, PJ. (1985): Mercury in human breath from dental amalgams. Bull Environ Contam Topical 34:459-468.
Vimy, M.J., Lorscheider, F.L. (1985): Serial measurements of intra oral air mercury: estimation of daily dose from dental amalgam. J Dent Res 64:1072-1075.
Berglund, A., Pohl, L., Olsson, S., Bergman M. (1988): Determination of the rate of release of intra-oral mercury vapor from amalgam. J Dent Res 67: 1235-1242.
Vimy, MJ., Lorscheider, FL. (1985): Intraoral air mercury released from dental amalgam. J Dent Res 64:1069-1071.

Clarkson, TW., Friberg, L., Hursh, JB., Nylander, M. (1988): The prediction of intake of mercury vapor from amalgams. In: Clarkson, TW., Friberg, L., Nordberg, GF., Sager, P.R. editors. Biological Monitoring of Toxic Metals, New York. Plenum Press: 247-260. ·

Vimy, M.J., Lorscheider, F.L. (1990): Dental amalgam mercury daily dose estimated from intra oral vapor measurements: a predictor of mercury accumulation in human tissues. J Trace Elem Exp Med 3:111-123.

Mackert, J.R., Jr. (1987): Factors affecting estimation of dental amalgam mercury exposure from measurements of mercury vapor levels in intra oral and expired air. J Dent Res 66:1775-1780.

Olsson,, S., Berglund, A., Pohl, L., Bergman, M. (1989): Model of mercury vapor transport from amalgam restorations in the oral cavity. J Dent Res 68:50~508.

Olsson, S., Bergman, M. (1987): Intraoral air and calculated inspired dose of mercury [Letter]. J Dent Res 66:1288-1289.

And here are EIGHT more studies from more than fifteen years ago, comparing these impossible measurements for differing types of amalgam:

Mahler DB, Adey JD, Fleming MA: Hg emission from dental amalgam as related to the amount of Sn in the Ag-Hg (g1) phase. J Dent Res 1994, 73:1663-1668.

Berglund A: An in vitro and in vivo study of the release of mercury vapor from different types of amalgam alloys. J Dent Res 1993, 72:939-946.

Boyer DB: Mercury vaporization from corroded dental amalgam. Dent Mater 1988, 4:89-93.;

Psarras V, Derand T, Nilner K: Effect of selenium on mercury vapor released from dental amalgams: An in vitro study. Swed Dent J 1994, 18:15-23.

Ferracane JL, Adey JD, Nakajima H, Okabe T: Mercury vaporization from amalgams with varied alloy composition. J Dent Res 1995, 74:1414-1417.

Moberg LE: Long-term corrosion studies in vitro of amalgams and casting alloys in contact. Acta Odontol Scand 1985, 43:163-177.

Moberg LE: Corrosion products from dental alloys and effects of mercuric and cupric ions on a neuroeffector system [dissertation]. Stockholm; 1985.

Brune D, Gjerdet N, Paulsen G: Gastrointestinal and in vitro release of copper, cadmium, indium, mercury and zinc from conventional and copper-rich amalgams. Scand J Dent Res 1983 Feb, 91(1):66-71.

Finally, references for amalgam being the main source of mercury:
-Criteria 118 WHO 1991 states that amalgam is up to 6x the other sources combined;
-Aposhian HV, Environ Health Perspect 1998: – 2/3 comes from amalgam.
-Richardson GM. Assessment of mercury exposure and risks from dental amalgam. Health Canada 1995. Tolerable Daily Intake is exceeded in adults with 4 or more amalgams.

Dentist training in diagnosis of mental/physical symptoms of mercury

Mr Clarke made this Freedom of Information request to University of Birmingham
The request was **successful**.
26 October 2011

Dear University of Birmingham,

I have been informed by an NHS Chief Executive that dentists have the capability to diagnose chronic systemic mercury poisoning whereas GPs do not (and thus the GP was correct in telling me to instead see a dentist about my fatigue and mental and other problems).

In that connection, could you please tell me the following.

1) What training in this diagnosis do your dental students receive?
2) What methods do they use in this diagnosis?
3) Why have all the dentists I have consulted invariably insisted that they do not have any capability of making such diagnosis and insist that I have to seek it from a doctor instead?

Yours faithfully,
Mr Clarke

1) What training in this diagnosis do your dental students receive?
    Undergraduate dental students at the University of Birmingham are **not** taught to diagnose chronic systemic mercury poisoning.

2) What methods do they use in this diagnosis?

Undergraduate dental students at the University of Birmingham are not taught to diagnose chronic systemic mercury poisoning and therefore the question is not relevant.

3) Why have all the dentists I have consulted invariably insisted that they do not have any capability of making such diagnosis and insist that I have to seek it from a doctor instead?

Under the Freedom of Information Act 2000 the University of Birmingham is only required to provide information that it holds rather than to express an opinion; therefore the University can provide only limited information in respect of this part of your request

The diagnosis of systemic poisoning clearly falls into the area of clinical toxicology and therefore would require a diagnosis from a medically qualified specialist. A general dental practitioner would not have the knowledge or skills to exclude all other systemic possible causes of the symptoms an individual was suffering without considerable postgraduate training. Therefore only a limited number of dentists would have this capability.

References

The references cited in this paper would normally be listed at the end here in a scientific paper but as this is incorporated in a book chapter they have here been merged with the list at the end of the book instead.

"the most insidious myth, increasingly pervasive, is that the poor are workshy, scrounging"

 – Labour former UK Prime Minister Gordon Brown, November 2015

"Everyone in receipt of benefits is not a scrounger."

 – Conservative former UK Prime Minister John Major, November 2015

~~~~~~~

4

Expert excuses from "Neurotoxicology" journal

"Academic journals and societies show an auto-immune response to information that should be the life-blood of medicine."
– Prof. David Healy, author of *Pharmageddon*

This chapter consists of just the reviewer reports from this "scientific" journal, with my replies interpolated. The reviewers' words are in **bold** and mine are non-bold. It is presented here in the same order the reviewers made their comments, and so what you see at the beginning here is not the most important or exciting points first.

Reviewer reports from Neurotoxicology journal, with author's replies
Ref.: Ms. No. NEUTOX-D-13-00253 Robin P Clarke
Autism, adult disability, and 'workshy': Major epidemics being caused by non-gamma-2 dental amalgams

Reviewer #1:

1. The Abstract is misleading as to what information this manuscript provides, stating that, "This is the first-ever study of health consequences of non-gamma-2." This is not a "study," as usually defined, as no measurements of non-gamma-2 were made, nor were any health consequences assessed except population-level statistics about prevalence of disability.

Three baseless pseudo-points in one sentence there – I will chop it up for my replies.

> no measurements of non-gamma-2 were made,

As my review stated, indeed, no-one has ever bothered to keep records of the usage or prevalence of non-gamma-2.

That lack of data is not a fault of this work but rather of those authorities who didn't bother to even keep records. However, an indisputable inference can still be made that the overall amount of non-gamma-2 in people's mouths would have progressively increased as more and more of their teeth were fitted with the new materials. This review thus provides the absolute best quantitative information currently (and almost certainly ever) available.

> nor were any health consequences assessed except population-level statistics about prevalence of disability.

Again, that lack of data is not a fault of this work but rather of those authorities who didn't bother to even seek reports on possible adverse events from amalgam, but instead implemented the cover-up measures documented in the paper. Which means those population-level statistics are about as good as it can get. It does not follow that they are worthless, else quite a number of other "not-really-studies" in very prestigious journals would also have to be dismissed.

> This is not a "study", as usually defined, as no measurements of non-gamma-2 were made, nor were any health consequences assessed except population-level statistics about prevalence of disability.

Really? In that case there are numerous other papers which were "not really a study", despite being published in the most prestigious journals and highly promoted as indeed being important "studies". Their authors likewise didn't do any measurements or diagnoses but instead presented existing data as I have. These include for instance:

o **JAMA**. 2003 Oct 1;290(13):1763-6. Association between thimerosal-containing vaccine and autism. Hviid A, Stellfeld M, Wohlfahrt J, Melbye M.

o **Pediatrics**. 2003 Nov;112(5):1039-48. Safety of thimerosal-containing vaccines: a two-phased **study** of computerized health maintenance organization databases. Verstraeten T, Davis RL, DeStefano F, Lieu TA, Rhodes PH, Black SB, Shinefield H, Chen RT; Vaccine Safety Datalink Team.

o **N Engl J Med**. 2002 Nov 7;347(19):1477-82. A population-based **study** of measles, mumps, and rubella vaccination and autism. Madsen KM, Hviid A, Vestergaard M, Schendel D, Wohlfahrt J, Thorsen P, Olsen J, Melbye M.

o **Pediatrics**. 2003 Sep;112(3 Pt 1):604-6.Thimerosal and the occurrence of autism: negative ecological evidence from Danish population-based data. Madsen KM, Lauritsen MB, Pedersen CB, Thorsen P, Plesner AM, Andersen PH, Mortensen PB.

o **J Child Psychol Psychiatry**. 2005 Jun;46(6):572-9. No effect of MMR withdrawal on the incidence of autism: a total population **study.** Honda H, Shimizu Y, Rutter M.

o **Pediatrics**. 2004 Sep;114(3):584-91. Thimerosal exposure in infants and developmental disorders: a retrospective cohort **study** in the United kingdom does not support a causal association. Andrews N, Miller E, Grant A, Stowe J, Osborne V, Taylor B.

o **Pediatrics**. 2006 Jul;118(1):e139-50. Pervasive developmental disorders in Montreal, Quebec, Canada: prevalence and links with immunizations. Fombonne E, Zakarian R, Bennett A, Meng L, McLean-Heywood D.

No-one has ever proposed that any of those were not really studies. And that's just a few I've come up with this minute. A more reasonable consideration of the matter is as follows. Journals categorise papers as either "reviews", or "studies", or something else such as commentaries. But that categorisation is rather crude, like categorising people as either "black" or "white". In reality there is a fudging between two notional ideal types, namely "proper reviews", of which the input data consists entirely of pre-existing published studies (of for instance whether walking causes autism), and "proper studies", in which the investigators do some measuring either in a laboratory or out in the wider world. Those seven famous papers listed above fit into neither of those ideal categories, just like this present one. But so what. There has never before been ANY scientific paper about the health consequences of non-gamma-2 amalgams. And no-one has ever compiled any measurements into a published study. It follows that it cannot be either of those ideal types, but it does not follow that it cannot be an excellent scientific paper any more than those seven above are not. In reality it is properly described as both the first ever study of the known data, and as the first ever review of the evidence.

2. P.4: Evidence needs to be provided for the statement that "...Hal Huggings and other dentists were struck off the register of practitioners." for issuing warnings about the

amount of mercury released from non-gamma-2 amalgams.

Firstly, that point is far from a key foundation for any conclusions of this review.   I doubt whether it warrants taking up additional space on documentation merely on the basis that some people might wish to not believe it.   Secondly here are some evidential details of the matter which I have quickly dragged from the web:

Hal Huggins de-licenced for challenging amalgam:

http://www.quackwatch.org/01QuackeryRelatedTopics/huggins.html

http://connection.ebscohost.com/c/articles/9608142846/huggins-vows-fight-after-license-revocation

"Judges Block Dental Board Gagging Dentists Who Discuss Risks of Mercury Fillings":

http://www.cdchealth.com/judgeblocks.html

"California's compliance with dental amalgam disclosure policies";

"The American Dental Association has a gag rule – yes, a gag rule telling dentists not to give warnings about the toxic effects mercury might have":

http://www.gpo.gov/fdsys/pkg/CHRG-108hhrg93640/html/CHRG-108hhrg93640.htm

Details of several more dentists struck off, and it only takes a handful to scare all the rest into never telling their victims that "silver" fillings are actually mainly mercury:

http://www.mercurypoisoned.com/dentists_disciplined/dentists_gagged.html

3. P.5: The statement that, "Consequently, declining rates of amalgam installation would conceal an increase of prevalence of the amalgams in patients' mouths" is a non-sequitur. If fewer amalgams are being placed, how could their prevalence increase? It might mean that this trend would conceal an ongoing release of mercury vapor in the mouths of individuals with such amalgams, but not the number of individuals with them.

Dear Reader, please go to your kitchen sink, put the plug in firmly and water-tight, and then turn on the tap to flow fairly fast, till an inch or two of water accumulates. Then turn the tap down so there's only a little more coming out per second. And now you can see that the water level in the sink stops rising but instead quickly goes down, as it must because the rate of additional input of the water has decreased, so obviously the total amount in the sink must decrease correspondingly. Or at least that is presumably what happens in the kitchen of someone with enough scientific expertise to judge such things.

For the educationally-deprived among us I'll go through that paragraph again, with tutorial hints added:

Dear Reader, please go to your kitchen sink [analogous to patients' mouths], put the plug in firmly and water-tight [analogous to the fact that non-gamma-2s stay in those mouths for whole lifetimes], and then turn on the tap [analogous to dentists installing non-gamma-2s] to flow fairly fast, till an inch or two of water accumulates. Then turn the tap down so there's only a little more coming out per second [analogous to "declining rates of amalgam installation"]. And now you can see that the water level [analogous to the prevalence of the amalgams in the mouths] in the sink stops rising [contrary to silly me's expectations] but instead quickly goes DOWN [well, highly-qualified expert Reviewer #1 apparently thinks so, so there], as it must because the rate of additional input of the water has decreased, so ["]obviously["] the total amount in the sink must decrease correspondingly. Or at least that is presumably what happens in the kitchen of someone with enough scientific expertise to judge such things.

I did emphasise in my review that the whole point of non-gamma-2 was that they are <u>far more</u> durable (indeed can easily last a whole lifetime). Just like that water which doesn't suddenly start to rush out of the sink just because you turned the tap down.

4. P.5: The author states that information is not available on "usage or total prevalence of non-gamma-2 in people's mouths." Given this, any statements made about the health consequences must remain purely conjecture.

Firstly Reviewer #1 here misrepresents what I wrote. I did not state that "information is not available...". My words were:

"I have been unable to obtain any **numerical data** on usage or total prevalence of non-gamma-2 in people's mouths. The DH have told me they have no such records. And NHS dental records have not recorded the types of amalgam used. It is unlikely that any better information is available in other countries. But we can very reasonably assume that the overall prevalence of non-gamma-2 will have gradually, progressively increased in the decades following its introduction."

And you can see there that I had already pre-answered this half-baked objection. It is in the nature of reality that the prevalence of something *must* inevitably increase for some period after its introduction as the new standard product. And it is common knowledge that people usually have their further tooth fillings put in in dribs and drabs over the years so their prevalence will correspondingly increase over a period of years rather than of minutes or millennia. Which is very much in line with those increase curves of autism, adult disability, and later age of onset, which also occur over years following the change to non-gamma-2.

5. P.6: The author states that he or she did not "cherry-pick.. selected data to prove any point," yet that is done in the last paragraph on this page, when reviews supporting the hypothesis that mercury is etiologically involved in autism are cited, but reviews that conclude that it is not are not cited.

But again, Reviewer #1's assertions are multiply untrue. Firstly, reviews are not data. Secondly, *in that very section supposedly at fault here, I did indeed explicitly cite the entire (supposed) counter-data*, namely the three studies which have been claimed to disprove the mercury-autism link, namely Ip et al, Soden et al, and Hertz-Picciotto et al. So that instance asserted by Reviewer #1 shows the exact opposite of what Reviewer #1 asserts. And thirdly, my statement about not cherry-picking was only in my section headed "My epidemiological investigations", and specifically a comment about my own presentation of data of the time-trends of autism, adult disability, and amalgams. What great contrary data have I omitted there? In reality there has been not the slightest cherry-picking and this is merely yet more nonsense from this so-called peer reviewer.

6. P.7: The fact that mercury excretion is increased following administration of DMSA in individuals with autism does not prove much, as the action of DMSA is nonspecific. Excretion of other metals (lead, antimony) is also increased.

Yet more cheap muddle from Reviewer #1. The finding in Bradstreet et al was not "The fact that mercury excretion is increased following administration of DMSA in individuals with autism". Rather it was the finding of a major difference between autistics and non-autistics, with the autistics outputting three times as much mercury as the non-autistics (with fluke probability of 1 in 5000). AS ALREADY CLEARLY STATED RIGHT THERE.

7. P.7: The conclusions of the Holmes et al. (2003) study are weak, not because of whatever biases the investigators might or might not have but because the findings are not credible. In this study, the mean mercury level in the hair of controls was 3.63 ppm, which is much higher than would be expected in a representative sample of infants. By comparison, measurements of mercury in children's hair in an NHANES survey conducted about the same time (1999-2000) (McDowell et al., Environ Health Perspect 2004;112(11):1165-1171) reported a mean of 0.12 ppm (and 0.16 among fish-consuming children). This suggests that the controls included in the Holmes et al. study were biased with regard to their mercury status and that an 8-fold reduction reported in the hair mercury level of "autistic cases" is likely an artifact.

Here Reviewer #1 shows a bit less incompetence, and stumbles only in terms of a rather more subtle fallacy. We could call it "the fallacy of the assumed all other things being equal". A good other example of it is found in various comments about the Hallmayer et al 2011 twin study finding of autism being mainly environmental. Commenters on Hallmayer et al have concluded that it shows that the earlier twin studies were "wrong". But well, they "must be wrong" mustn't they?, because Hallmayer et al is a big powerful new study and so it must trump those little old ones into the wastebin of "wrong" results.

The fallacy here is the unfounded assumption that all other things are equal (constant). In respect of those twin studies, please have a look at my still-unchallenged paper "A theory of general impairment of gene-expression manifesting as autism", which appeared in print years ago and is still essential reading for anyone who wants to have a clue about the subject. Therein I specified the conditions under which autism would change from a mainly genetic condition to mainly environmental: *"If a rare perinatal adversity were to become somewhat more common, then obviously, autism of the environmental category would become more prevalent."* And now with the huge impact of non-gamma-2 in parents' and carers' mouths, exactly such a condition has indeed occurred, and so hardly surprisingly the causation of autism has indeed CHANGED from mainly genetic to mainly environmental. There is no real conflict between Hallmayer and the earlier twin studies, merely differences of the underlying and unexamined variables. Likewise, in respect of mercury and autism we know that there is a lot we do not know. You can see in my own review section there how the various studies of autistic hair give divergent results and that there is nevertheless good reason to find them all valid and true. Likewise, to dismiss the Holmes et al result as "not credible" just because of those non-standard levels entails an unwarranted gross presumption that there are no important unknowns going on between the different studies. And so the finding of Holmes et al should not be dismissed unless there is a more substantial basis for doing so. And on the contrary, later studies have supported their 'perverse' data of lower hair mercury levels in autism. This Reviewer #1 is here categorising the careful work of Holmes et al as {either grossly incompetent or grossly fraudulent}, on a basis of no real evidence but merely because he/she does not find their results in accordance with the required commercially/professionally-convenient dogma.

> I don't think it is appropriate to state that a pattern of findings provides any evidence as to whether an investigator was "acting competently and honestly."

Whereas I do think it appropriate. And that is because fraudsters or incompetents are extremely unlikely to come out with a whopping strong result that is:

(1) markedly contrary to what they would have expected;

(2) markedly contrary to what they would have found convenient to report; and

(3) only subsequently supported by the collection of results of later other-people's studies of autistic hair mercury.

And in the context that many have presumed to shallowly discredit Holmes et al as either incompetent or fraudulent (as Reviewer #1 here does him/herself), that consideration is outstandingly eminently appropriate to be stated.

8. P.7: The author multiplies the P-values from 6 studies to calculate the probability that the findings are due to chance. This is a meaningless calculation. First, the studies included reached different conclusions about the hair mercury levels of children with and without autism (although the author argues that age needs to be taken into account). Second, given that all P-values are less than 1, multiplying them necessarily results in a smaller and smaller number the more studies one includes. If each of the 6 studies yielded a P-value of 0.5 (indicating no statistically significant relationship), then using the author's method, the combined P-value would be 0.0156, which would suggest that, in aggregate, the studies provide significant evidence of an association. Third, even if the author's method was valid, it

would be necessary to include in the calculation all of the studies ever conducted of a particular hypothesis, not just those selected because they purport to show an association (just as it is necessary, in a meta-analysis, to include all available evidence).

Again I shall have to chop the above into shorter bits for reply, as follows.

> The author multiplies the P-values from 6 studies to calculate the probability that the findings are due to chance. This is a meaningless calculation.

(It is absolutely standard probability maths to multiply together probabilities to get the compound probability of them all happening merely by fluke, as any betting shop can confirm, but we must continue here with Reviewer #1's further exposition on this point......)

> Firstly, the studies included reached different conclusions about the hair mercury levels of children with and without autism (although the author argues that age needs to be taken into account).

This misrepresents the situation. I don't "argue" that age needs to be taken into account, rather I *observe* that age needs to be taken into account, in that the earlier ages always give lower mercury in autistics, while the later ages always give higher mercury. Thus none of those studies are in any conflict with the reasonable hypothesis mentioned by Majewska et al that the adrenarche plays a role in the hair mercury levels. There is therefore not any real conflict between these studies but rather voices declaring in common that mercury is involved in autism in some way. (And Reviewer #1 is here again employing that fallacy of the presumed all other things being equal – age in this case.) And so there is no valid ground there for not multiplying together those probabilities.

> Secondly, given that all P-values are less than 1, multiplying them necessarily results in a smaller and smaller number the more studies one includes.

That is of course true. [Note for non-expert readers: smaller P-values indicate the results are less likely to be mere flukes and so are more "significant".]

> If each of the 6 studies yielded a P-value of 0.5 (indicating no statistically significant relationship), then using the author's method, the combined P-value would be 0.0156, which would suggest that, in aggregate, the studies provide significant evidence of an association.

And that is also indeed true. But so what. It is indeed the reality that several bits of weak evidence can add up to strong evidence. Indeed that is the whole point of making a (for instance clinical) study large enough to give a significant result. Any such study can be conceived of as being a combining together of lots of smaller sub-studies, any one of which could give non-significant results, but when all put together would enable a highly significant result. And that high significance is not some specious false result, rather it is the entirely sound statistical inference. And that's what I've done there, **except that my p values were all highly significant already**. And the fact that the evidence there is of diverse types adds all the more to its methodological robustness, as it is not wholly founded on any one premise.

> Thirdly, even if the author's method were valid, it would be necessary to include in the calculation all of the studies ever conducted of a particular hypothesis, not just those selected because they purport to show an association (just as it is necessary, in a meta-analysis, to include all available evidence).

Again, not so. Firstly, there IS no contrary evidence on the mercury-autism question such as could make any meaningful reduction of my combined calculation. I've pointed out that even the three supposedly counter results were actually pro in reality. Secondly, I made the point that that is the probability only from those few studies combined. It logically follows that if there were more studies, and continuing on the same 100% positive connection trend, then that would simply make my big fluke number even bigger (smaller). So there is still no sound objection to my probability calculation.

9. **P.8: The argument about the evidentiary value of never having seen the Queen is a little ridiculous and, in my view, has things completely backwards. It is by means of the falsification of hypotheses that science advances. A single negative result is enough to call into question a positive result that has repeatedly been observed and might be the**

result of bias (all it takes is the observation of one black swan to refute the statement that, "all swans are white"), but no number of positive observations is sufficient to demonstrate the universality of a statement.

Again I will need to chop this up for my replies.

> **9. P.8: The argument about the evidentiary value of never having seen the Queen is a little ridiculous and, in my view, has things completely backwards.**

As we'll see in the next few lines...(?)

> **It is by means of the falsification of hypotheses that science advances.**

Partly so, but also there cannot be any advance at all if hypotheses are prevented from being properly raised in the first place. And Reviewer #1 is doing a great job of preventing some very important hypotheses being raised, via these unflattering would-be-critiques right here.

> **A single negative result is enough to call into question a positive result that has repeatedly been observed and might be the result of bias (all it takes is the observation of one black swan to refute the statement that, "all swans are white"), but no number of positive observations is sufficient to demonstrate the universality of a statement.**

Reviewer #1 here uses some extremely incompetent language to confuse the matter. Namely the notion of a "negative result". For example an investigation of whether or not the Queen actually exists could come up with two very different types of results, both of which Reviewer #1 would have us class as "negative results". On the one hand, there could be a failure to see the Queen on peeping over the palace wall; on the other hand there could be a finding of the absence of the Queen anywhere in the UK following an insanely detailed mega-search from South to North and back. The difference between a "negative" failure to find something and a (positive) finding that that something is actually absent, is complete and absolute, and not to be confused by conflating into a false notion of "negative results".

> **A single negative result is enough to call into question a positive result that has repeatedly been observed and might be the result of bias**

I shall here now correct Reviewer #1's grossly incompetent language.

"A single FINDING OF POSITIVELY CONTRARY evidence is enough to call into question THE UNIVERSALITY OF [an earlier] result that has repeatedly been observed and might be the result of bias."

"A billion mere FAILURE-TO-FIND results CAN BE STILL NOT enough to call into question [an earlier] result that has repeatedly been observed and might be the result of bias."

When I used the words "negative results" it was self-evident from the context that I could only mean the latter, more common meaning of the term, and not the "positively contrary" meaning. But Reviewer #1 still managed to muddle it as ever.

> **a little ridiculous and, in my view, has things completely backwards.**

Indeed.

10. P.8: The discussion of the validity of the three studies sometimes described as refuting an autism-mercury link requires fleshing out. It is necessary to tell the reader the arithmetic error Ip et al. made and to demonstrate the extent to which it altered the study conclusions. The reader is told that DeSoto and Hitlan (2010) concluded that Soden's study "actually proved the opposite," but no information is provided that would enable the reader to evaluate this statement. The conclusions of Hertz-Piccioto et al. are misstated. The second-to-last sentence of this paper actually states, "This report did not address the role of prenatal or early-life Hg exposure in the etiology of autism." The major finding was that total Hg in blood was not elevated or reduced in preschool children with autism/ASD compared with unaffected controls and resembled those of a nationally representative sample. The reason for the authors' qualification is that only concurrent measures of blood Hg were available, meaning that they could draw no conclusions from their data about the role of prenatal or early-life mercury exposure. To say that the authors concluded that their data, ".constituted no evidence whatsoever against causation of autism by mercury" is simply wrong.

Again, I need to chop this up for my replies.

> 10. P.8: The discussion of the validity of the three studies sometimes described as refuting an autism-mercury link requires fleshing out.

....because.....

> It is necessary to tell the reader the arithmetic error Ip et al. made and to demonstrate the extent to which it altered the study conclusions.

Really? I cited the conclusion of DeSoto and Hitlan (2010) that the study actually proved the opposite. (Ip et al was retracted due to their major but elementary errors.) On this question this reviewer should either <u>explain why D&H were wrong</u> or else shut up. Here's what they said:

"The author of record has publicly acknowledged that these numbers and the statistical calculation were in error in an erratum (Ip et al. 2007) and the journal editor notes the reason given was a series of typographical errors (Brumback 2007). Furthermore, a careful and correct analysis of the full data set results in a statistically significant difference (Brumback 2007, DeSoto and Hitlan 2007, DeSoto 2008) with autistic children having higher mean levels of mercury. As can be seen by comparing the erratum to the original article, the standard deviations were wrong for both groups, the stated statistical significance in 2004 was not even close: their original stated level of statistical probability was off by almost 10 fold."

> The reader is told that DeSoto and Hitlan (2010) concluded that Soden's study "actually proved the opposite," but no information is provided that would enable the reader to evaluate this statement.

Not so. I provided the citation of D&H along with the citation of the original Soden, which is all the information that is needed for that evaluation. If Reviewer #1 reckons there is something wrong with D&H's conclusions then he/she should state what it is, or else shut up. Here's what D&H said:

"In the end, the statistical test conducted by Soden and coworkers is meaningless and distracting from the essentials of what was done. The authors measured metal levels, then (based on the lab definition of toxicity) all values were defined as zero, then – they tested this actual zero statistically and found that one could not rule out zero. "

"But let readers be clear about this central point: if one is willing to consider the actual numbers reported and test those numbers, the results are clear - a larger proportion of autistics had heavy metals excreted as the result of chelation."

It is not the business of authors of papers to have to recite the details of all the prior papers they cite in support; if they did there would be even more that everyone had to read. Any half-proper peer reviewer would check out the background references themselves (where required), and indeed in this case ought to be an expert familiar with these important key papers (on **_Neurotoxicology_** of autism) already anyway. What a timewasting pseudo-expert charlatan.

>The conclusions of Hertz-Piccioto et al. are misstated.

Not so. They are not in the slightest mis-stated in my report.

> The second-to-last sentence of [their] paper actually states, "This report did not address the role of prenatal or early-life Hg exposure in the etiology of autism."

Indeed that is the case. But so what? That is exactly my point about it. [Note to non-expert readers: "Hg" means mercury and "etiology" means causation.]

> The major finding was that total Hg in blood was not elevated or reduced in preschool children with autism/ASD compared with unaffected controls and resembled those of a nationally representative sample.

Indeed that is the case. But so what? I never said otherwise.

> The reason for the authors' qualification is that only concurrent measures of blood Hg were available, meaning that they could draw no conclusions from their data about the role of prenatal or early-life mercury exposure.

Indeed that is the case. But so what? That is exactly my point about it.

> **To say that the authors concluded that their data, ".constituted no evidence whatsoever against causation of autism by mercury" is simply wrong.**

No it isn't. Their words quoted above indicate PRECISELY that. As Reviewer #1 appears to be having some peculiar difficulty with either language or logic I will try to parse this for them as follows. (I apologise that I have to assume the reader is an idiot here.)

We begin with their paper's second-last sentence that:
"This report did not address the role of prenatal or early-life Hg exposure in the etiology of autism."

That means effectively the same as:
"This report *was not capable of providing any information about* the role of prenatal or early-life Hg exposure in the etiology of autism."

Which means that it is also the case that:
"This report *did not provide* any information about the role of prenatal or early-life Hg exposure in the etiology of autism."

And hence:
"This report did not provide any *evidence* about the role of prenatal or early-life Hg exposure in the etiology of autism."

And hence:
"This report did not provide any evidence about the role of prenatal or early-life Hg exposure in the *causation* of autism."

And hence:
"This report did not provide any evidence about the role of prenatal or early-life *mercury* exposure in the causation of autism."

And hence:
"This report did not provide any evidence about the causation of autism by prenatal or early-life mercury exposure."

And hence:
"This report did not provide any evidence *against* the causation of autism by prenatal or early-life mercury exposure."

And hence:
"This report *constituted no* evidence against the causation of autism by prenatal or early-life mercury exposure."

And hence on merely removing a redundant word:
"This report constituted no evidence against [~~the~~] causation of autism by prenatal or early-life mercury."

....which would be identical to my own statement except that there is that extra bit about "prenatal or early-life".

So I was wrong there. I overlooked that autism could still be <u>not</u> caused by exposure to mercury later in life, after that person has already become autistic. So we'd best not publish my non-gamma-2 rubbish after all.

And whatever it takes to become a reviewer for *Neurotoxicology*, it's all too clear I don't have it myself.

Reviewer #2:

Dental amalgams are a continual source of controversy. The current review attempts to survey the adverse health consequences of the amalgam formulation known as non-gamma-2. It asserts that these restorations "are currently by far the main cause of chronic disability in the UK, US, and other such countries, with about 10% of the UK working-age population disabled thereby." It also claims that its introduction led to a 10-fold increase in the incidence of autism.

Indeed. But no faults are there to provide basis for non-publication so far.

As a contribution to this specialized journal, the manuscript lacks any clear connection. It offers no neuro-mechanistic foundation for such a correlation, especially for autism, which is a product of disordered early development.

Not so. In respect of autism, my review(/study/rant/) ties in the newer mercury factual data with the prior unchallenged theory and the related fact of how the mercury binds with DNA to reduce gene-expression and hence [as my antiinnatia theory had predicted] cause autism. And meanwhile in respect of adult mercury poisoning there is quite a developed understanding of how the symptoms are caused. The details of that causality are in the cited literature or secondarily-cited.

It doesn't attempt to demonstrate any kind of dose-response relationship.

No data is available that would enable that. But it doesn't follow that there is no other useful evidence presented.

Its definition of autism lacks specificity.

It doesn't need to have any "specificity". It just uses the definitions that are used as standard by others. As is usual practice.

In addition, the claim that this amalgam formulation accounts for 10% of chronic disability requires advanced statistical modeling of exposure-consequence relationships in which other kinds of exposures are concurrently evaluated.

Firstly, I did not claim that it accounts for 10% of chronic disability. I reckoned from the data of Figures 5 and 7 that it now actually accounts for MOST chronic disability (something like 70-95%). That 10% figure was my estimate that wholly 10% of the UK workforce has been disabled by non-gamma-2 (about 4 million victims out of a 40 million workforce).

That 10% is not a "claim" but rather was expressly only a rough estimate, from looking at figure 5 (plus the further context of Figure 7). You can see that it shows an increase of about 2 million accepted claimants, easily all attributable to non-gamma-2. And you can see that it peculiarly levels off about year 2000 as would be expected from the stated political agenda of "claimant count now controlled". And you can see that otherwise it would most likely have continued upward to something like 4 million – hence 10% of the working-age population.

And no fancy statistical modelling is required to understand what these graphs are showing us. Of course they are not absolute proof, but neither are they any lack of evidence, else we'd have to retract an amazing lot of highly-acclaimed "studies" from the most prestigious journals.

In the absence of these kinds of information, it is difficult to see how this manuscript is compatible with the aims and audience of this journal. Perhaps the author should consider another kind of journal and audience.

Or perhaps instead the so-called *Neurotoxicology* journal should consider changing those aims and audience, or change its name to reflect its restricted nature, for instance to *Pedantic Neurotoxicology* or *Pseudoneurotoxicology*.

Reviewer #3: This is an opinion piece on the possible role of mercury exposure in the causation of autism.

Not so. It is not "an opinion piece". Like all scientific papers it does include proposed conclusions which are necessarily of an opinion nature. But for the most part it consists of presentation of data and reasoning thereon, which is entirely in line with any normal scientific paper and not "an opinion piece".

The author makes a very impassioned case for non-gamma-2 amalgam fillings being the major cause for the rise in incidence of autism using ecological data from UK, US and few other countries.

Not so. It is not at all "very impassioned" but rather "very filled with as much useful factual evidence as can be found".

No primary research has been undertaken by the author to test this hypothesis.

So what. Exactly the same could be said about all those seven highly-rated studies listed on the first page here. Has anyone ever called for their retraction yet?

My main concern with this work is that it is not an objective assessment of the evidence available at present.

....because / for instance.....

Key statements that form the basis for the author's argument are unsupported by high-quality evidence.

...such as....

For example, the exposure of children to mercury from their parents' amalgam restorations needs to be confirmed before the author can make such a far-reaching conclusion.

Indeed, no one has bothered to do any measurement studies of this question to date. But that is not the fault of this author or this review. Rather it highlights the urgent need to make a start by publishing this first study of the subject, which can be then followed up by testing studies. But I did already explain why we can be confident that there is enhanced exposure. That is because there is very low background atmospheric mercury vapor, and it is known to constantly emit from parents' and carers' amalgams, and they commonly spend much time together with babies in enclosed spaces, even talking at them through their amalgam-filled mouths, and so it logically follows that many babies are going to breathe in an increased amount of mercury vapor at least on average. [Studies have also shown prenatal transmission.]

Randomized clinical trials of dental amalgam (Bellinger et al 2006; DeRouen et al. 2006) showed no significant neurodevelopmental deficits in the children receiving amalgam restorations compared to non-mercury fillings.

Those two studies have already been solidly debunked as evidence, as I pointed out via my first page citation of Mutter 2010 (and others). Not least they started too old to relate to causation of autism, and they stopped too young to relate to causation of adult disability. In fact (as in my earlier journal replies) if I myself had been in those studies I would have been recorded as evidence of *harmlessness*, because I only became chronically disabled (by the amalgam scam) *after* the age at which those studies stopped. And an editorial in the very same issue of the journal stated that those two studies did not constitute evidence of amalgam safety. Why didn't Reviewer #3 mention that counter-point in their "unbiased" commentary here?

[Update: The Bellinger, DeRouen and Maserejian studies have now been further demolished by Homme et al. (2014). See also IAOMT (2008).]

In fact, Maserejian et al. 2012 have reported that compared to amalgam restorations, children receiving composite (non-mercury) fillings showed impaired psychosocial function. There are several other such instances in the manuscript where important data have been ignored.

Maserejian et al had not been published when I first sent this review to a journal in July 2012, else I might have mentioned it. But exactly the same methodological problems arise as with the two others cited above. I myself was doing fantastically well at school before the effects of the amalgam scam imposed themselves so heavily on my life. And perhaps bisphenol-A might well have injurious effects but that is a separate matter out of the range of my own documents.

In my opinion, this manuscript does not add unbiased scientific knowledge to the topic of mercury and autism, and I cannot support it being published.

But rather it is this Reviewer who is biased, and has raised only bogus reasons for suppressing the publication of this outstandingly important cautionary information.

IN CONCLUSION:

These three reviewers have failed to raise even a single sound reason for preventing the publication of this very important information. And they have meanwhile deployed a whole load of shallow pseudo-objections, which raises considerable questions about both their competence and their honesty.

And that comes in the context of ten previous journals likewise raising only specious excuses for refusing publication.

~~~~~~

Further reply from "Neurotoxicology" (23rd October 2013):

".... Thank you for your email. I forwarded it to the editor of the journal. After review it was concluded that your manuscript was handled appropriately and the original decision stands....."

Notably there was an absence of any rebuttal of any of my rejoinders.

~~~~~~~

5

Expert excuses from other "scientific" journals

"Academic journals and societies show an auto-immune response to information that should be the life-blood of medicine."
– Prof. David Healy, author of Pharmageddon

This chapter consists mainly of just the "peer reviewer" replies from 18 journals with my rejoinders added in between. I sent the lengthening compilation to each successive journal in turn. You can see that not a single real fault of evidence nor reasoning (nor presentation) has been shown by any of these "scientific" journals.

1. BMC Medicine

In an email reply sent 21 August 2012, Claire Tree-Booker declared on behalf of the editors of *BMC Medicine* that their refusal to consider this present manuscript was because:

> " we did not feel that it was sufficiently different from the 2011 article published in *Journal of Occupational Medicine and Toxicology* (Mutter J. Is dental amalgam safe for humans? ".

And yet only one of Mutter's 160 references overlapped with the 50 cited here. There is no other overlap of evidential basis between Mutter's review and this one. And this one concludes with evidence-based estimates of the huge scale of morbidity being caused, whereas Mutter's makes no such estimates. And this one contains six (highly-original) graphs of data whereas Mutter's contains no graphs nor tables. Plus my predictions and preventive advice none of which are contained in Mutter's review. Above all, my review is explicitly of consequences of *the change to non-gamma-2 amalgams* whereas Mutter's makes no mention whatsoever of non-gamma-2 or any change. *BMC Medicine's* sole ground for rejecting is thus shown to be wholly false.

2. Journal of Occupational Medicine and Toxicology

The *Journal of Occupational Medicine and Toxicology* then took 14 weeks to refuse the paper without giving any reason at all.

3. Environmental Health

The paper was then sent to *Environmental Health* on 4th December 2012. On 10th December, David Ozonoff sent a reply whose least unsubstantive content consisted of the following:

> "Our journal requires prior approval for review articles. In this case the Editors feel that having a plausible hypothesis is not sufficient. There is an abundance of speculation on what is causing the increase in autism or even if that increase is real and not an artifact. Over the time period at issue many things have changed, not just dental amalgams. Whether any of them, including your hypothesis, are credible or not will require a more fine grained and targeted analysis."

But there is not even one genuine scientific objection shown by those comments, as is explained in the following.

>"Our journal requires prior approval for review articles."

The only proper criterion for a journal that validly claims to be scientific is to publish the best possible (or potentially best) content in whatever form it has to take. The very essence of science is that it is an exploration of the <u>unknown</u>. It follows that unless an editor is content to confine their mind to some pseudic form of "prophetically anticipated science" they must be open to publishing whatever form and origin of content happens to present itself, especially when a very important catastrophic situation is carefully presented with clear practical implications as here. Of all the duties of a medical research community, there can be none greater than facilitating the publication of substantial warnings of harm being done by medical practices themselves.

>**"In this case the editors feel that having a plausible hypothesis is not sufficient."**

But the paper does not present merely a "plausible hypothesis". If so I wouldn't have bothered writing it let alone sending it to the journal. Instead (even as stated in the abstract) it presents extremely substantial evidence and reasons for ruling out all other possibilities. Furthermore it is very far from mere hypothesis but instead a causal theory. A journal editor ought to know and understand the important fundamental difference between the concepts of theory and hypothesis. [*Hypothesis:* "Sugar tastes sweet".; *Theory:* "Putting sugar on your tongue induces a chemical reaction in the taste-buds (which have evolved to detect nutrients), and this in turn induces action potentials in neurons which thereby transmit signals to other neurons in the brain which register a sensation generally reported to be sweetness; Blaggg (1987) showed pictures of the taste-bud receptors in which the blue dots are the etc....; Freddd (1997) showed that the increased action potentials only occurred when sugar was present etc...."]

>**"There is an abundance of speculation on what is causing the increase in autism or even if that increase is real and not an artifact."**

Indeed an abundance of *speculation*. By contrast, I present strong *evidence* and *reasoning*. What this editor should be doing is explaining what specific errors or gaps there are in it, not just adding his own rather facile speculations of what errors he reckons he would find in it if he bothered to check.

And indeed, the huge abundance of mere speculation about these matters should properly be recognised as showing that this is an extraordinarily important subject and one in which there is indeed too much mere speculation and not enough actual evidence-based and reason-based coherent theory such as presented by this paper. So he got it exactly the wrong way round there - it's all the more reason that they *should* be publishing it (or at least not casually dismissing it).

And as for the alleged non-increase, please explain to me how anyone credibly accounts for those charts figs 1-4 other than by a real increase (let alone the peculiarly close parallel increase in Fig. 5).

>**"Over the time period at issue many things have changed, not just dental amalgams."**

That is a statement of the idiotically obvious – as if it would never have occurred to myself to ask if anything else might have changed, before I wasted months producing that review of the possibilities. But this editor's cheap words fail to address the fact that not even one of those other things can account for the clear involvement of mercury in the increase of autism (let alone also account for the timing and other details). I made that point clearly in the paper, but it seems we have here the reply of someone who is so clever that he doesn't need to actually read something before having yet more prophetic revelations of what it will "obviously" have failed to say.

>**"Whether any of them, including your hypothesis, are credible or not will require a more fine grained and targeted analysis."**

But I challenge anyone to suggest even <u>one</u> alternative to "my" "hypothesis" which I have not already ruled out in that manuscript. You can't. And that's the <u>whole point</u> of it. And there exists no alternative review of the subject – this is the best now and likely best there ever can be (in consequence of the failure to keep records).

Editors of *Environmental Health* failed to respond to these rebuttals, so I proceeded to send to a further journal.

4. BMC Public Health

It was next sent to *BMC Public Health*, on 13th December 2012. On 20th December Natalie Pafitis replied that:

"We have now looked over your submission and are sorry to inform you that the journals in the BMC series do not generally consider narrative reviews for publication. We are therefore unable to consider your manuscript for peer review and are closing your file."

Again there is no sound ground for non-consideration offered there. Even if it is in some aspects a "narrative review", so what? It still remains the <u>only ever</u> review to date of non-gamma-2 amalgam consequences. It must therefore at this date be the best available science on this most important question (and probably best-ever given the institutional failures to record data), and the fact that editors can speculate some notional "proper" sort of review as a hypothetical substitute is entirely irrelevant. As already pointed out at top of page 2 here, any journal having pretences to being scientific should be definition be open to the unknown nature of new discoveries and becomes merely pseudoscientific to the extent that it insists on confining itself to its prior presumptions of what the best science should look like, a false "prophetically anticipated science".

5. Health Research Policy and Systems

On 20ᵗʰ December it was sent to *Health Research Policy and Systems*. On 24ᵗʰ December the HARPS Editorial Team replied that:

> "Pre-peer review of your manuscript is now complete and I am sorry to say that we cannot consider the manuscript for publication given that your article is out of scope for our journal."

And yet that notion that it was "out of scope" for that journal is difficult to square with the following evidence copied from the Covering Letter I had sent to them:

"

Why this is suitable for *Health Research Policy and Systems*? Please note all the relevant bits of your journal statement which I have **bolded herebelow**:

> *"Health Research Policy and Systems* aims to provide a platform for the global research community to share their findings, insights and views about all aspects of the organisation of health research systems including **agenda setting, building health research capacity**, and **how research as a whole benefits decision makers and practitioners in health and related fields and society at large**."
>
> *"Health Research Policy and Systems* considers **manuscripts that investigate the role of evidence-based health policy and health research systems in ensuring the efficient utilization and application of knowledge to improve health and health equity**, especially in developing countries. Research is the foundation for improvements in public health. The problem is that **people** involved in different areas of research,

together with managers and administrators in charge of research entities, **do not communicate sufficiently with each other. How well informed is the public of the results of their research? How do they make sure that what they do will actually improve health? Do they have good links with the decision makers who can actually influence how their research findings are used? Is the money used to sponsor their activities spent wisely, fairly and efficiently? Are there means to assess the impact and utility of their work? How many of them are leaving the country for greener pastures? How can they be enticed to stay?"**

And this is indeed an article which presents proof of the **agenda setting** avoidance of having dental amalgam toxicity on the agenda, with avoidance of **building research capacity**, and **how research as a whole** is prevented from **benefiting decision makers and practitioners in health and related fields and society at large**.

It is a **manuscript that investigates the** prevention of a **role of evidence-based health policy and health research systems in ensuring the efficient utilization and application of knowledge to improve health and health equity**, about **people** who deliberately set out to prevent others to **communicate sufficiently with each other**.

How well informed is the public of the results of their research?: They are kept in deliberate ignorance by systematic censorship and deceit as documented both in the review and in its shallow blocking by editors of four pretendedly scientific journals.

How do they make sure that what they do will actually improve health?: The review shows how they go out of their way with deceits to prevent such improvement. **Do they have good links with the decision makers who can actually influence how their research findings are used?** Yes, evilly-"good" links as indicated in the review.

Is the money used to sponsor their activities spent wisely, fairly and efficiently? No, it is used criminally in support of cover-up of a gigantic crime. **Are there means to assess the impact and DISutility of their work?** Yes, this review. **How many of them are leaving the country for greener pastures?** This review documents the reasons why just about all the honest researchers have been driven out by a Lysenkoist regime of pseudo-science and persecution of those who try to do honest study of the subjects.

How can they be enticed to ~~stay~~ <u>come back</u>?" <u>By publishing this review</u>.

It should be clear from the above that this review fits very much with your statement of what would be relevant.

6. Emerging Themes in Epidemiology (*Permitted Themes in Epidemiology?*)

It was next sent to *Emerging Themes in Epidemiology* on 25th December 2012.

An email reply from the ETE Editorial Team dated 8th February 2013 stated the following two paragraphs of rationales for not accepting. These rationales have at least an appearance of being much more substantive than those received in earlier responses, but they do fall apart on proper examination as I will now show.

"1. The aim of the paper is to present evidence of a causal relationship between exposure to dental amalgams and autism, as well as other disabilities. We found no evidence to support such a claim in this article. The article presents time trends demonstrating secular increases in autism diagnoses and disability claims. There is, however, no data presented regarding the population level exposure to non-gamma-2 dental amalgams over this period."

Firstly, as regards data of the population exposure to non-gamma-2: In response to my FoI request the UK Department of "Health" stated that they have kept no records of usage or prevalence. And indeed I can myself confirm that my own dental notes from many years under the "care" of a leading Dental Hospital and School give no indication of which types of amalgams were installed or present, even though I was well aware that in earlier decades I frequently had amalgams crumbling in my mouth (indicating they were the crumbly earlier types), whereas I later had a large number of amalgams which never degraded even over decades (indicating they were the non-gamma-2 types). And in the UK more generally, dental notes are only kept for ten years. And with the substantially more complex and fragmented medical system in the USA it is highly unlikely that there would be any better records there. However, despite that callous neglect of documentation, we can still reasonably infer that the prevalence of the highly-durable non-gamma-2 progressively increased from the time of its introduction in 1975-6 onwards. At first there would be mostly just ones and twos in a few patients, while later there would be many patients accumulating more and more high numbers. The review thus presents about the best evidence as we can ever hope to obtain and yet it is still indicative enough of close relationships to increases of both autism and adult disability such that the precautionary principle should be strongly evoked thereby.

"There is also no evidence presented that those exposed to these products have higher rates of these conditions compared with those not exposed to them, nor that those with these conditions are more likely to have been exposed to these products."

Not so. In respect of autism I cited Holmes et al 2003 and Geier et al 2009, and could have added Majewska et al 2010. In respect of adult disabilities I cited the separate reviews by Mutter 2011 and Hanson 2004, which reached similar causality conclusions to my own via almost entirely different data. And that is despite the gross avoidance of carrying out any studies of these sorts, in line with the pseudo-scientific denialism documented in the Appendix of the paper.

Besides which, this is specifically a review of such evidence as exists of an epidemiological nature. It would take an even much longer paper to re-review all the other data which has already been adequately covered in the cited Hanson 2004 and Mutter 2011 (in respect of adult disability) and Geier et al 2010 (in respect of the clear involvement of mercury in much autism).

"2. There have been at least two large-scale randomised clinical trials with long-term follow-up that have invest-igated whether use of dental amalgams has adverse neurological or psychosocial effects. Neither has shown evidence of an effect, yet these studies are not mentioned in the manuscript."

Not so. Firstly, the paper's second paragraph stated: "Some relatively large-scale trials have been asserted to show amalgam safety, but they have been substantially flawed and in at least one case in reality showed harmfulness rather than safety (as explained by Mutter [19])."

And on the contrary the Childrens' Amalgam Trials showed significantly decreasing urine mercury despite increasing intake, which is evidence of developing toxicity. And there were severe limitations in those studies, such that an <u>accompanying editorial</u> stated they were not capable of showing amalgam to be safe. And they certainly did not have "long-term follow-up", indeed, if I myself had been included in those studies I would have been registered as evidence of harmlessness because I became chronically disabled only after the age at which the trials ceased. By remarkable fluke of PhD-qualified professional design and peer-review those studies started too late to detect autism and ended too early to properly detect adult pathology. (And despite their very poor quality they had no difficulty getting promptly published (and in prominent journals) in contrast to this present paper)

And again, these defective studies were not mentioned because they had already been demolished in the cited Mutter 2011 (and by others such as Boyd Haley) and it is not reasonably to be demanded that this present review should completely re-review every defective propaganda study anew, else it would need to be even longer.

Finally, even if the editors of ETE indeed did not find the presented evidence compelling, their proper response should still have been to act in accordance with the precautionary principle, publishing the review while stating alongside it their notions about the unsoundness of inferring causality from it.

Annals of General Psychiatry (not fully submitted to)

It was next sent to *Annals of General Psychiatry* on 15th February 2013. But they were unwilling to allow a waiver to below their discounted fee of £1,180 / $1,880 / €1,480. That would be beyond my means as a chronically mercury-disabled benefits-dependent with no earning prospects, so I decided to seek another journal which would provide open-access without a high publishing fee. [I haven't added this journal to the counting here.]

7. Chinese Medical Journal

It was next sent to *Chinese Medical Journal* on 2nd March 2013 (CMJ20130601). The editor replied on 25th March, stating as follow:

> We provide a list of the most common reasons why we reject your article instead of a detailed description of comments about the article from our reviewers.
> **First reviewer's comments:**
> To the Author
> In this long review article, the author described in

detail the potential toxic effects of non gamma-2 dental amalgam, a most commonly used dental filling material used in the last decades world wide. The consequences including autism, adult disability, and 'workshy' seem astonishing, but dental amalgam is seldom used in dentistry nowadays, and the data the author cited was mostly from online with lower grade and published years ago.

Conclusion: Reject

Second reviewer's comments:

汞合金作为补牙材料已经完全被树脂材料所替代，尽管汞合金作为重金属可能对中枢神经系统造成影响，但作者应用综述的方式来作出相关的论述已有较多文献发表，而本文并无相关的实证数据，故论文缺乏现实性、科学性。

不建议在本刊发表。

Conclusion: Reject

My rough translation of the above: "Amalgam as a dental filling material has been completely replaced by resin material, the amalgam's heavy metals may affect the central nervous system. But reviews of health effects of amalgam have already been widely published in the literature. In this article there is no empirical data, so the paper is not realistic or scientific."

On 31st March I sent a reply which included the following replies to quoted points.

>"The consequences including autism, adult disability, and 'workshy' seem astonishing,"

But huge increases in these outcomes are evidenced in reality as shown in various references cited in the article (and shown in the graphs). And they are not so astonishing given that mercury is well-known to have various such neurotoxic effects and a huge increase of mercury was introduced with no attempt at monitoring.

>"but dental amalgam is seldom used in dentistry nowadays,"

Maybe that is true in China (of which it is difficult for me to get information from due to my limited language capability). But certainly not elsewhere.

Indeed on the contrary, in the UK (and US and many other countries too) amalgam use is still being taught to the dental students (as entirely harmless)(I just now phoned 0121 466 5000 to obtain confirmation of this), and it is the only treatment approved for molar teeth in the UK's NHS and in the various health insurance schemes in the USA.

"Immediate phase-down of dental amalgam use in the UK unlikely":
http://www.dental-tribune.com/articles/news/europe/7333_immediate_phase-down_of_dental_amalgam_use_in_the_uk_unlikely.html
There continues to be a huge international industry of installation of new amalgams. That is the reason why there has just this year been a call from the UN for worldwide "phase-down" of amalgam usage as detailed at
http://www.prnewswire.com/news-releases/scientific-dental-academy-to-aid-un-global-phase-down-of-mercury-fillings-188091681.html
[....]

And also of crucial importance, as my review states, the causal factor is not the amount of new installation, but rather the amount already existing in people's mouths, and that is with these non-gamma-2 amalgams being extremely long-lasting.

>"and the data the author cited was mostly from online with lower grade and published years ago."

But as the article states, that data is the best that is available on the matter and none of the opponents of this article have shown any proper scientific objection to that data.
(The second reviewer wrote in Chinese which I will try to translate here to English.)

>汞合金作为补牙材料已经完全被树脂材料所替代，
>"Amalgam as a dental filling material has been completely substituted by resin material,"

Not so (outside China), as detailed above in reply to the first reviewer.

>但作者应用综述的方式来作出相关的论述已有较多文献发表，
>"But review of applications to make the exposition has been widely published in the literature,"
(I guess a correct translation here is more like:
>"But reviews of health effects of amalgam have already been widely published in the literature,")

But again, the article explains that the other reviews have never examined any epidemiological data, and there have never before been any reviews of the change to non-gamma-2 (which is the whole point of the article).

>而本文并无相关的实证数据，故论文缺乏现实性、科学性。
>"this article there is no empirical data, so the papers to the lack of realistic, scientific."
(Again, I guess a more correct translation would be:
>"In this article there is no empirical data, so the paper is not realistic or scientific.")

But again that is not true. The article presents all the empirical data that is available on the subject. Most of its content is such presentation. There are many references, almost none of them previously cited by for instance J Mutter, and which include the various graphical data.

8. Journal of Psychiatry and Neuroscience

There was no response to the above replies and so after some revision (minor improvements plus rearranging to produce a new section titled "Is mercury involved in causation of autism") it was next sent to Journal of Psychiatry and Neuroscience on 14th May 2013.

The Co-Editor in Chief, Dr Joober, replied on 27th May, saying that it was *"not suitable for publication in the journal. Because of increasing space constraints, we have to be extremely selective about the manuscripts that we ultimately publish."* And yet no faults or inadequacies or other evidence were adduced to support that assertion.

9. Iranian Biomedical Journal

Then after some adjustment between the different journal formatting requirements, it was sent to Iranian Biomedical Journal on 30th May.

The Executive Manager replied on 17th June that:

"Our referees have carefully reviewed your manuscript and suggested that this paper is more suitable for other journals than Iranian Biomedical Journal. We hope that you can publish this valuable manuscript in the above mentioned journals."

10. Acta Medica Iranica

After some further adjustment for journal formatting requirements, it was sent to Acta Medica Iranica on 22nd June 2013. On 17th September a reply stated that it "has been evaluated by referee(s) and I am sorry to inform you that we have therefore decided that this manuscript cannot be accepted for publication."

Again these two Iranian journals did not raise any actual criticisms of the paper.

11. Neurotoxicology

At this point I became aware that the publishers of *Neurotoxicology* had introduced a possibility of a waiver of the fee (for not only designated countries), which had not previously been the case. It might otherwise have been my first choice of journal before all those listed above.

After further adjustment for journal formatting requirements, it was received by Neurotoxicology on 24th September 2013.

On 12 October a reply from assigned editor Pamela Lein stated it had been declined on a basis of three reviewers' reports. And yet, just as with the previous responses documented above here, those three reports contained no reasonable basis for refusing publication. More importantly, they contained a spectacular compilation of half-baked pseudo-expert pseudo-faults, as is made clear in my rejoinders which I have put in a separate document.

12. Molecular Autism

Following a further reasonless reply from Ms Lein, and further adjustment for differing journal formatting requirements, it was sent to *Molecular Autism* on 7th November 2013 with a request for a waiver (which was granted on 8th November. The editors replied on 29th November 2013 as follows:

> Dear Mr Clarke,
>
> We very much appreciated reading your manuscript on dental amalgams as an autism risk factor. We think you have done a good job reviewing the literature and the question is of considerable interest.
>
> The advice we have received is that the methodology would not get through critical peer review from our journal, so we think that it is better for you if you submit this to the

other journal that has expressed an interest in this. This will also save you time.

  We wish you success with your research and thank you for considering our journal.

Best wishes,

Profs Joseph Buxbaum and Simon Baron-Cohen.

The references in that reply to "the other journal" mis-characterise the general-readership magazine I had mentioned (What Doctors Don't Tell You) as a (perfectly reasonable alternative) "journal" when that would incorrectly suggest it functions as a primary science journal publishing scientific papers (indexed in for instance Index Copernicus, DOAJ, or PubMed), which is of course far from the case – WDDTY has to date only published popular journalism articles reviewing or commenting on the primary journals' papers. That reply furthermore notably fails to specify any actual *reasons* why my paper would "not get through the critical peer review". And that is in the context of all those previous "peer review" critiques being shown to be vacuous as above.

Indeed it is those journals' own "peer reviews" that glaringly fail any honest test of "critical" examination, not my own work.

And this reply appears to be outrightly deceitful, because it is the editors themselves who decide whether or not it does indeed "get through critical peer review from our journal". (That's exactly what being a journal editor is about.) This reply is thus very much like an executioner saying "I really wish you the best in your hopes of staying alive, but I'm terribly sorry that my arm isn't pulling hard enough to prevent this axe falling on your neck. Anyway, I wish you survive in future executions". Note that Chapter 12 here contains further discussion of whether Dr Baron-Cohen tells the truth or not.

Before [, in the event, not] finally sending to WDDTY I decided to first send to just two more journals, namely the *Russian Open Medical Journal*, and the new journal *eLife*.

13. Russian Open Medical Journal.

After further re-formatting it was sent to ROMJ on 9th December 2013. The editor sent an email reply on 19th March 2014, of which the here-relevant content was as follows:

"....We received several conflicting reviews on your article. Editorial board members carefully studied and reviewed the text of article. The views of members were different. In sum of debates, all members concluded unanimously that style of presented article not suited to the format and scope of our journal and our readers. ....

We recommend you submit your article to another journal (mass media), specializing in the acute medico-social problems and not having narrowly specialized readership...."

So yet again, no actual faults of the paper were identified. As for the notion that there might be some unsuitability of style, this is evidently not a real problem given that no such comments on style were made by any of the other journals, including the abundant false criticisms from Neurotoxicology journal.

14. eLife

I then noticed there was the journal eLife recently founded by the 2003 Nobel laureate, which claims to have a novel approach to publishing and does not cause much delay in its decisionmaking anyway. So I sent it to eLife on 24th March 2014.

The next day the editors of eLife sent the following reply.

Dear Dr. Clarke,

Thank you for choosing to send your work entitled "Autism, adult disability, and 'workshy': Major epidemics being caused by non-gamma-2 dental amalgams" for consideration at eLife. Your initial submission has been assessed by Prabhat Jha in consultation with a member of the Board of Reviewing Editors. Although the work is of interest, we are not convinced that the findings presented have the potential significance that we require for publication in eLife.

Specifically, the theories about possible sources of reported increases in autism need much better justification than provided here, and also need to be reviewed in the context of other putative risk factors. As such, this paper might be more suitable for a specialized journal.

eLife rejects a high proportion of articles without passing them on for in-depth peer review, so that they can be promptly submitted elsewhere. This is not meant as a criticism of the quality of the data or the rigor of the science, but merely reflects our desire to publish only the most influential research. We wish you good luck with your work and we hope you will consider eLife for future submissions.

Best wishes,

Randy Schekman, Editor-in-Chief, eLife

Fiona Watt, Deputy Editor, eLife

Detlef Weigel, Deputy Editor, eLife

In considering that reply from eLife, it should be borne in mind that I had sent them the replies from the previous thirteen journals, including the failure of any of them to find any genuine fault. In that context, eLife put forward two objections.

Firstly the notion that the theories "also need to be reviewed in the context of other putative risk factors". And yet in the paper I had already pointed out that any proper explanation of the autism increase had to account for the now substantial involvement of mercury. And having ruled out mercury from vaccines, that leaves only dental amalgam as the one remaining source of that mercury. In respect of the adult disabilities, one could of course speculate about a great many potential causes which have increased in recent decades, and yet we see here (a) a major increase of mercury, clearly resulting in the autism increase; (b) adult disabilities which are very much characteristic of mercury vapor poisoning; (c) a peculiarly close coincidence of timing of that adult disability increase with the autism increase; and (d) that peculiar system of official falsehoods about the subject. I consider that to be an adequate review of the other putative risk factors. The only alternative would appear to be an endless list of speculations about the many other things that have changed over the decades, and might be supposed to have somehow caused all those disability claims.

The other objection from eLife consists basically of the "skepticism" which I have commented on already. Some of the greatest discoveries in science were dismissed for decades with such "skepticism", so I do not regard it as a meritable objection here.

15. Biometals

Having at this point now given fourteen putatively scientific journals the opportunity to publish this paper, and met only with false objections, I did not see much merit in allowing any further journals to obstruct the publication any further. But before finally turning to other options or none, I noted that the journal Biometals had recently published two papers relating to amalgams, so decided to give them the final chance. After further changing to journal formatting requirements I also added references to Taylor 2013 and Homme 2014 and carefully revised the presentation of the section on mercury causing autism and of the conclusions section. On 26th April I received a reply which contained no other grounds for refusing the publication other than the following:

> Although this is an interesting topic, the manuscript is restricted to statistical data containing no experimental results. Therefore, this manuscript is not suitable material for the journal BioMetals which has an audience of experimentally working scientists. We therefore suggest to submit this manuscript to a journal on environmental health or to a journal with a focus on toxicology which may have the interested readership.

This is of course in the context that they knew I had already sent it to such other journals, and again, no good reason for non-publication was given. Perhaps you can work out for yourself whether they were being honest there.

16. Toxicology Reports

At that time I received notification of the new journal Toxicology Reports which had obvious appropriateness to this paper. So after further formatting adjustment I sent it on 4th May 2014. The editor Dr Lash sent a reply on the 7th May, the essential content of which was as follows:

> "Most of the discussion of published findings provided a conclusion without showing the data that support the conclusion. The final sentence of the Abstract to me illustrates the lack of balance in the presentation. The statement on page 3 that the evidence to support a causative role for mercury in autism is "beyond a reasonable doubt" provides another example of the lack

of balance in the presentation. Accordingly, I am afraid that I must agree with the previous reviews and reject your manuscript for publication in Toxicology Reports."

But yet again, it can be shown that there is nothing there that justifies a refusal to publish this scandalous important precautionary information.

>"Most of the discussion of published findings provided a conclusion without showing the data that support the conclusion."

We see here yet again the familiar objection to many great discoveries, along the lines of "I can't (or prefer not to) see your credible evidential case, therefore it doesn't exist". But numerous other readers have had no difficulty seeing that case. One such stated that "Your paper is important", and "Your work is fine". And when one group of people claim *not* to see something that another group claim they *do* see, the "non-see-ers" have to have some very special grounds to be justified in prevailing in suppressing the evidence which the "see-ers" endorse. And they don't.

>"The final sentence of the Abstract to me illustrates the lack of balance in the presentation. The statement on page 3 that the evidence to support a causative role for mercury in autism is "beyond a reasonable doubt" provides another example of the lack of balance in the presentation."

But both of those statements are firmly grounded in facts presented in the paper. Where is the evidential case that those statements are wrong? There is no such.

Of course certain interest-conflicted readers would prefer those conclusions to not be true but that is not a proper basis for how scientific papers are selected or not.

>"Accordingly, I am afraid that I must agree with the previous reviews and reject your manuscript for publication in Toxicology Reports."

But he was not "agreeing with the previous reviews", because they had came up with entirely different sets of cheap excuses for rationalising the same predetermined decision that they didn't want to put their names to publishing this embarrassing information.

xx. Social Science and Medicine

I decided to next send to Social Science and Medicine in view of there being as much implications about the social context as about the disabilities. The editors replied on 20th June including the following comments:

"At Social Science & Medicine we have to prioritise papers which contribute substantially to one of the major health social sciences and are of particular interest to a wide international readership. I am therefore not forwarding your manuscript for review, as we feel it has limited social science content. [....] This is not a reflection of the quality of your paper, but rather concerns the topic and likely audience."

In view that that is not clearly a false excuse I will not count this journal in the numbering here, hence the "xx" above.

17. Medical Hypotheses

After some reformatting for different journal requirements, and reading of other documents before deciding not to change the text anyway, I sent it to Medical Hypotheses (a journal with controversial recent history of publisher interference).

On 7th October 2014, the editor Dr Manku replied as follows.

Dear Mr Clarke,

Reviewers's comments on your work have now been received. You will see that they are advising against publication of your work. Therefore I must reject it.

I admire the author's efforts, however, I need to mention these points:

The whole text seems like a newspaper article in terms of writing and I doubt whether this is format of your journal or not. For eg. note the statement on page 7 line 38 "cherry-picked selected data" instead of randomly chosen

Page 3 does not include the "introduction/background" title. In fact the whole manuscript does not follow the structure mentioned in "author guides"

Page 4 line 44--> abbreviations such as NHS and DH should be fully introduced at their first appearance

Page 5 line 30--> as the item above for GPs

Page 6 line 21--> I personally don't admire the statement "The famous US dentist Hal Huggins states that ......" which seems more like a TV/Radio report than a scientific citation

Page 6 line 36--> this sentence "Dispersalloy is the most widely used amalgam with over 25 years of proven performance, i.e., since before 1979, but perhaps after their 1974 patent no. 3841860" seems like a commercial copy from the manufacturer which is not scientific

Page 7 lines 2, 13, 23, etc--> using pronouns such as I, My, We, etc is not appropriate

Thank you for your submission, I am sorry to inform you that it has been rejected.

Thank you for giving us the opportunity to consider your work.

Yours sincerely

Dr. M. Manku PhD

Yet again, there is from Dr Mankku zero indication of any actual fault of the science, or even of the content other than some new notion that it "seems like a newspaper article in terms of writing", an observation which curiously was not made by any of the previous readers indicated above. Basically just yet more shallow excuses.

18. Life

After further reformatting for different journal requirements, and delay due to continuing to have to be my own medical consultant and practitioner in absence of a half-decent healthcare system here, I sent it to the relatively new journal *Life*, on 30th November 2014. On the 2nd of December 2014 the Assistant Editor replied with an email indicating that:

"Your manuscript was not given a high priority rating during the initial screening process. ..... Therefore, our decision is not necessarily a reflection of the quality of your research but rather of our stringent resource limitations."

To which I replied:

"Thanks for your prompt reply.

I appreciate that all your other papers relate to origins of life etc rather than medical matters."

The Assistant Editor then forwarded a substantial text of the external editor's comments, as follows (again indicated in bold with my replies non-bold).

"The paper is a review and hypothesis paper (the claim in the abstract that "This is the first-ever study of health consequences of non-gamma-2." is rather misleading) stating the argument that mercury from a specific type of dental filler is the primary cause of autism. The argument is basically that diagnoses of autism have increased, it is alleged that nongamma- 2 mercury amalgam use has increased on a timescale matching the rise in autism diagnoses, and because mercury is neurotoxic the two are therefore linked.

I will chop this up for replies as follows.

(the claim in the abstract that "This is the first-ever study of health consequences of non-gamma-2." is rather misleading)

I had already fully answered that point at the start of my earlier replies to Neurotoxicology. This reviewer makes no advance on my replies here.

"The paper is a review and hypothesis paper (the claim in the abstract that "This is the first-ever study of health consequences of non-gamma-2." is rather misleading) **stating the argument that mercury from a specific type of dental filler is the primary cause of autism.**

The reviewer here misrepresents the essence of the paper, which makes clear even in its title that it is about a lot more disability than just autism.

The argument is basically that diagnoses of autism have increased, it is alleged that nongamma- 2 mercury amalgam use has increased on a timescale matching the rise in autism diagnoses, and because mercury is neurotoxic the two are therefore linked.

The reviewer here grossly misrepresents the case presented. The timing of the autism diagnoses increase is one part of the evidence, but only one part.

The argument is basically flawed in two ways. Firstly, as the author says himself (page 13) that he has no numbers for the use of amalgam in any territory. So the data presented seeks to correlate changes in incidence of autism with the *introduction* of a specific type of mercury amalgam. It is assumed that the amalgam use increased steadily after that. It may do, but there is no evidence of this at all.

Again, this objection had already been fully dismissed in the replies to Neurotoxicology.

but there is no evidence of this [that the amalgam use increased] **at all.**

No "evidence" is needed here. It should go without saying that when a new type of dental restorative is introduced as the new standard then it is going to become more prevalent in mouths over a period of years thereafter. In recent decades it has been the now universal standard "ordinary" amalgam. All this was addressed in the previous replies to Neuropseudotoxicology.

The second flaw is that amalgam use has actually declined substantially in the last decade,

Again I fully answered this point in the Neurotox replies. Again this reviewer merely repeats rather than advancing the discussion here.

especially in Europe as US-style concerns for dental cosmetics mean that patients are no longer willing to have metallic lumps in their teeth. To an extent this has also been driven by consumer concern (whether justified or not) over the health effects of mercury. Thus since the 1990s mercury amalgam use has declined substantially in the UK, even to the point of drilling out old amalgam fillings and replacing them with newer material, largely for cosmetic reasons. This can be readily verified by the obvious lack of metal in the mouths of most young people.

But amalgams are only used in the pre/molar teeth where they are not "obvious".

However autism incidence rates have not come down, even in the under- 10s. In Sweden they have been phased out almost entirely in the time 2000 - 2005 (see http://www.kemi.se/Documents/Publikationer/Trycksake r/PM/PM9_05.pdf) - has the incidence of autism gone down?

Good question. An equally pertinent question is whether (or how much) there has been a decline of the prevalence of non-gamma-2s already in the mouths of the parents of those children (as it is the parents' amalgams that cause the autism). Readily accessible autism incidence data for recent years is a bit patchy (and subject to recency bias) but such as I have seen so far suggests that incidences have generally leveled off at a high level (with prevalence consequently increasing as a lot more autistics are added while only few are dropped out by end of life).

Dentistry today http://www.dentistrytoday.com/ has about 40 articles on materials for fillings, listing hundreds of composites that are preferred over amalgam, again mostly for aesthetic reasons but also functional ones. If this reflects dental practice, autism should also have plummeted.

Firstly, in the UK the NHS provides only amalgams for molars and premolars, and consequently they are still widely used. Similar applies in the US. Of course the fancy pricey new things get a lot more attention, so what?

Secondly, what causes the autism is not installation of the amalgams, but their presence in mouths. Many millions of the things are still in the mouths of the parents, let alone children still having them put in by the NHS and by equivalent organisations in other countries. So it is wrong to predict that "autism should also have plummeted". Though my expectation is that we are going to see such plummeting within the next decade or so, at least in Sweden.

The author makes the equivalent argument very forcefully in the supplementary material with regard to mercury in vaccines as *not* being relevant to autism - autism has continued to rise despite the decline in thimerosal in vaccines. Yes, good argument. So why does the same not apply to autism in Sweden with regard to amalgam fillings?

Because as explained above.

Without some actual measure of amalgam use, therefore, this is a post hoc ergo propter hoc argument that is not convincing, and is just a specific example of the 'amalgam causes autism' argument that has been done to death in the literature and the blogosphere.

Far from it, this is the first ever study of these epidemiological questions, the first ever study of health consequences of non-gamma-2, and the first ever presentation of that evidence. And the comment above also fails to give any recognition to my **confirmed prediction** that the earlier amalgams would have caused an increase of their own, as very starkly confirmed in the Update section and Figure 7. Again this is all entirely new evidence on the subject.

The cheap stereotyping of being "just another" "amalgam causes autism" argument is also noted there.

The paper is also seriously flawed in its presentation of the case, and should be rejected for a complete rewrite even if the basic argument was sound.

Curiously this alleged fault was not remarked upon by numerous previous reviewers. And Dr med. Mutter (author of a notable review) on the contrary commented in emails that it was "important and should be only a little bit corrected" (29 March 2013), and "Your work is fine" (8 November 2013). I am reminded of the comment I made in a letter to Nature (*Nature386;319 (1997)*) that: "The paper involved was described by a reviewer for *Personality and Individual Differences* as well-written, well-argued, and well-documented, whereas a *British Journal of Psychiatry* reviewer reckoned it was of lowest grade in all three respects". In light of this, plus this reviewer's evident difficulty in distinguishing sense from nonsense, I find more credibility in the words of Prof HJ Eysenck (most cited-ever author): "Well-written", and Prof D Horrobin: "You obviously write well".

In the introductory section the author makes a number of highly charged statements, (page 2, lines 21-27) without a single reference or attribution.

Here are the first three of these "highly charged" statements:

"[1] No safety testing was undertaken before or after it was introduced. [2] Patients and the public in general have still not been informed of the change, let alone of the increased levels of mercury involved. [3] No informed consent has been sought, and no warnings have been given of any possible harmfulness."

One has to wonder quite what sorts of references I should be expected to put there. I have now for a decade been challenging so-called experts to provide evidence of safety of amalgams, and am well-aware of what a vacuum of evidence there is for amalgams in totality, let alone in respect of non-gamma-2. Rather obviously I can't cite studies which have never existed. Again, in respect of informing and consent and lack of warnings it is starkly obvious to a UK resident that rather than being informed they are still being disinformed about the change to non-gamma-2. And ditto in the US. Again, quite how do I cite such non-events? The onus has to be on others such as this so-called reviewer to point out evidence that these things did indeed happen. But they never have.

And a better characterisation of those statements is not "highly charged" but rather "stupendously criminally outrageous in their implications".

The author then goes on to list 'untruths', listing a tinyurl address as evidence. Looking through the relevant URL, it seems to be mostly assertions by the author and not responses from the target of his sometimes quite aggressive questions. If I received a list of questions starting with an accusation that I was an unethical, lying weasel who was suppressing data, I would also tend not to try to be helpful.

What a load of shameful rubbish. None of the questions started off with any "accusation of being unethical lying weasels or suppressing data", and anyway they were all addressed to organisations rather than individuals. And even if it were true that any of the questions had been "aggressive", that would still be irrelevant, as many FoI questions are far from what the receivers wish to be reading.   More to the point those were all extremely pertinent and important questions, to which answers rightly demanded to be given.   And easily could have been given if the recipients were indeed honest non-charlatans. The only reason why answers were not forthcoming is the very simple one that those questions exposed extremely criminal charlatanism which could not find any honest answers with which to defend its untruths. (Note I did not call them "lies", though there's a strong bet that's what they should be called.)

Furthermore the reviewer's contention is undermined by the pseudo-responses themselves which do not cite the wording of the questions as reasons for refusing to answer, but instead find other shallow rationales or none.

If this reviewer had the slightest bit of impartiality he or she should at that point be remarking about the outrageousness of those humungous non-answers to massively important questions rather than drivelling about the supposed manner of asking.

The review of mercury an autism is very polemically stated,

Translation: This reviewer is very strongly biased against the conclusions reached and wouldn't recognise a neutral exposition even if it was clearly printed out and highlighted in front of them for ten hours.

but is an OK review of the case for mercury being causal in triggering autism. The statistical argument (page 4, lines 24-26) is not valid, as it assumes independence of data sets, sources of error and bias.

Again, this objection had already been thoroughly discussed and debunked in the reply to Neurotoxicology. This reviewer does nothing to advance from that here.

The statistics of positive *and negative* studies should probably be combined using a Baysian approach if the author wants to do this.

Again, nonsense which was fully discussed in the Neurotox. There were no negative studies.

The statistical nature of this argument also invalidates the logic of the author's next statement that a negative finding cannot invalidate a positive one - epidemiological statistics arguments are not existence proofs, they are evidence proofs, and failure to find evidence *if it is looked for rigorously* is evidence for absence.

Again fully discussed in the Neurotox, with reference to "never having seen the Queen".

The issue is that the author believes that the evidence against mercury is not well done. The case against mercury is not really stated (simply dismissed), and

On the contrary, I debunked all three studies purported to make a case against mercury involvement in autism. And I don't see any coherent grounds for refusing publication there.

there is no discussion of the (many) other ideas about the causality of autism - the author should at least acknowledge that there are other, well argued cases.

On the contrary, I cited my published theory paper which explained that there are many factors in autism causation. And pointed out that because mercury was shown to be a major factor in modern autism, then that ruled out just about everything else as a potential main cause of the increase, so we were left with looking for the source of that mercury. Either vaccines (which I also debunked in an appendix) or amalgams.

The author dismisses reference 38 because they did not prove that the measure of autism in adults was not comparable to that in children. But that was not the point. If incidence goes up in adults and in children in parallel, then some change common to adults and children is most likely to be the cause of the increase. If the numbers are also similar, that suggests (but does not prove) that the measures *are* comparable, but as the author is claiming that the *increase* in autism is evidence for the role of amalgam, then

comparison of rates of increase is valid and relevant.

Again I fail to see any coherent objection to my critique of the Brugha study at this point. In the absence of a means of determining the equivalence of the measuring for the two different age groups, no meaningful data could be derived from the study, and hence it could only be a load of wishwash.

The discussion of UK disability benefits claims is naive in the extreme.

As we will see....?

DB claims are massively changed by changes in policy about what 'disability' means, what specific schemes are available, what the thresholds of duration and severity are, and (critically) what other benefits are available instead of DB.

Any evidence on this point? In the absence of such evidence it is reasonable to guess that no such things have been going on. In fact I'm well aware as a UK resident throughout all that time that there were no such changes of specific schemes or of thresholds, until more recently as indicated by the quote of "caseload growth now controlled". And there were no relevant other benefits available either. More remarkably this reviewer does a great job of ignoring how this curve of the disability claims is a remarkable exponential that remarkably "just happens" to so closely coincide with the autism increase which also "just happens" to begin tellingly just after the change to non-gamma-2. This reviewer would have us believe that some (non-existent anyway) procedural changes "just happened" to produce that increase just such as to "just happen" to have those abovementioned characteristics.

One could equally correlate the number of people on higher band tax with mercury amalgam use, and claim that mercury makes you wealthy.

But I didn't because I was testing a boring rational strongly-suspectable hypothesis rather than an igNobel-prize-winning stupendous discovery silly one.

The political statements that the author quotes (with evident disapproval) illustrate that this is a political posture, not a scientifically testable statistic.

On the contrary, the political statements reflect the strong *opposition* to these increases rather than anything that could be politically causing them.

The arguments about whether British workers are 'workshy' compared to foreign ones is also a) a political posture, not a referencable fact and b) not relevant anyway as by definition foreign workers who come here to work must be fit enough to work.

Many employers have stated that they find UK native workers to be too workshy in contrast to the immigrants. I doubt if this can be adequately explained away in terms of the definitional concept given that the same criteria of "fit enough to work" apply to both sources anyway. And no answer has been made to the point about the ancestors of this nation of workshy somehow having built all those medieval cathedrals in a harsh rainy land and then gone on to create the largest empire in history.

Insomnia, fatigue, memory loss and consequent depression are all plausible results of increased consumption of processed food, increased TV watching disrupting sleep patterns (40+ free channels 24 hours/day) or any one of dozens of other changes over the last 30 years.

Sorry but I don't think this comment warrants any reply. Where are all the studies you have published about these "plausible" explanations of those disability statistics? Where are your answers to the questions on the last page of the text? My own review goes far beyond mere "plausible", it goes to confirming of a massive theoretical prediction (in Figure 7), which is the very essence of hard, competent science rather than "plausible" speculation.

I have no idea on what evidence the author says that fibromyalgia is 'often cured' by amalgam removal, given that a) there are no consistent diagnostic criteria for fibromyalgia and b) amalgam removal is stated to release more mercury into the patient than just leaving it there. There is no reference for this statement.

My own suspicion is that a number of vaguish labels, including "fibromyalgia", "MS", "CFS", and "ME", are all actually just unknowing clinical perceptions of amalgam mercury poisoning which has not been recognised as such (in the context of NHS denialism). Anyway, Andrew Hall Cutler's book mentions fibromyalgia ten times in its index, and here's a ref for some studies which have been done. http://www.fms-sas.co.uk/fmsmercury.html

"The foundation for Toxic-Free Dentistry has compiled statistics from 6 studies on a total of 1,569 patients. The patients reported on their symptoms before and after their mercury amalgams were removed. These included everything from vision problems to depression. Most saw dramatic improvement once the fillings were gone. There are many people who have recovered from chronic illnesses after having their fillings removed; for example, recoveries realized from diseases such as fibromyalgia and CFS. (762 patients used FTFD Patient Adverse Reaction Report to send changes in their health directly to the FDA and FTFD. Dr. Mats Hanson reported on 519 Swedish patients. Henrik Lichtenberg, S.D.S of Denmark reported on 100 patients. Pierre LaRose, D.D.S. of Canada reported on 80 patients; Robert L. Siblerud, D.D., M.S. reported on 86 patients in Colorado.)"

and b) amalgam removal is stated to release more mercury into the patient than just leaving it there.

Yes if done by NHS incompetents. No if done by using competent protocols specifying high suction and separate air supply among other things, in which case a spike of intake is prevented.

Stock was poisoned by *huge* amounts of mercury. The case of acute, massive, severe mercury poisoning is scarcely relevant.

As a person who "just happened" to become chronically severely disabled myself, when I encountered Stock's account it was just like (after so many years) I was reading my own autobiography written by someone else. On what basis was Stock's intake so much more "huge" than that of someone with grams of mercury constantly stored in their mouth for years? Even if you wash your hands in the stuff and drink it it doesn't amount to that much more intake because it enters very inefficiently by those routes compared to breathing and implanting. So Stock's account, collaborated by my own and by Cutler's comments, is eminently relevant there.

The cover letter is an ill-judged and innaccurate rant,

Yes, I can see you'd have some expertise about that.

but I can sympathise with the author's frustration. The list of comments on other rejections shows that the author really does not understand the difference between research and review, and is completely unwilling to take guidance as to how to get his ideas taken seriously.

Which could be why various notable people (Eysenck, Rimland, Horrobin, among others) have so greatly enthused about my ideas.

These documents are not part of the paper and so are not reasons for rejecting the paper, but they do suggest that more detailed comments that I have provided here would be a complete waste of time, and would only result in the author ranting about us to someone else.

Well, that's one prediction this reviewer has got right.

It is a shame that the author has chosen to write what is a polemic instead of a paper.

On the contrary, it is a shame that the reviewer has chosen to write what is a polemic instead of a review.

I think that he may have a good point. Amalgams do emit mercury, mercury is not good for you, dental mercury can be converted to methyl mercury by oral fauna (this has been published), and methyl and dimethyl mercury is *severely* toxic. Phasing them out seems like a good idea. But with no new evidence,

On the contrary, major new evidence is presented in the paper.

highly biased arguments, flawed logic and statistics,

As demonstrated above? Or rather de-debunked above.

and text full of comments accusing opponents of bias, data suppression and radically unethical conduct without any evidence, this is a really poor way to make that point."

On the contrary I do show the evidence, such as it is, for those who have eyes sufficiently unblinkered to see it. My text doesn't make "accusations" so much as state facts which speak for themselves of the bias and suppression and unethicality. And no evidence has been raised in rebuttal.

Preprint servers to the non-rescue

Not being known for my patience or persistence, I thereafter sent the thing to some "preprint servers", which claim to publish scientific papers without first subjecting them to a "peer review" process. Sure, I did have some, ooh, ~slight~ scepticism about how free from "peer review" rejectionism these sites would prove to be.

One option was the F1000 website. But for this article longer than 15,000 words their fee would be at least $2000, and they could well decline it even if I robbed enough banks first.

So I sent it firstly to PeerJ Preprints on 23rd February 2016. I uploaded in both their preferred format (double-spaced single-column with line numbers) and a format with double columns as is typical of most published papers. Three days later, not having had any reply notification, I checked their website which said:

"This manuscript has been rejected as unsuitable for publication. I apologize that we cannot consider your submission. You may find that it is better suited to submission at bioRxiv (http://biorxiv.org/) or F1000 research (http://f1000research.com/)."

Having already ruled out the F1000 option I then sent it to bioRxiv (after adding "?" to the title) and got this reply:

MS ID#: BIORXIV/2016/041517
MS TITLE: Autism, adult disability, and 'workshy':
Major epidemics being caused by non-gamma-2 dental amalgams?

Dear Robin P Clarke;
We regret to inform you that your manuscript is inappropriate for bioRxiv as it is not a research paper being prepared for submission to a journal.
Thank you for your interest in using the bioRxiv service.
The bioRxiv team

And yet this rationale for rejection reads oddly in the context that their website states that:

"authors are able to make their findings immediately available to the scientific community and receive feedback on draft manuscripts before they are submitted to journals." And their Submission Guide states that:

"An article may be deposited in bioRxiv in draft or final form, provided that it concerns a relevant scientific field, the content is unpublished at the time of submission, and all its authors have consented to its deposition."

"All articles uploaded to bioRxiv undergo a basic screening process for offensive and/or non-scientific content. Articles are **not** peer-reviewed before being posted online."

And need I remind you that on sending the same content to numerous "peer-reviewed" journals, they had critiqued it as though it was indeed a *research paper being prepared for submission to a journal*, rather than declared that it was not. So who's telling the truth here?

~~~~~~~

6

Nonsense and yet more nonsense about vaccines

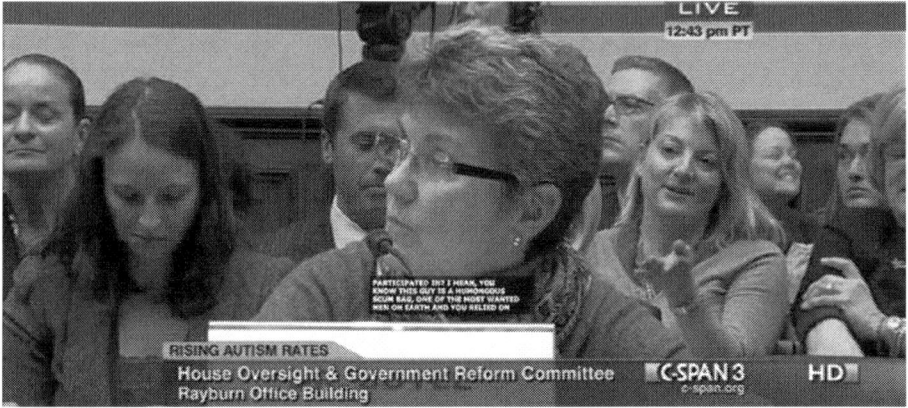

"There's no smoke without fire" – several million undiagnosed fools

For some people there just isn't enough real evil nasty lying going on, so they have to imagine some more into existence to make up the shortfall. This tendency seems to manifest more or less equally in both "sides" of the vaccines-autism controversy.

> *"Boyle suggested manipulating the data by adding 1 and 2 year olds to the data set - kids too young to have an ASD diagnosis - in order to dilute the danger. She belongs in prison."* (Age of Autism, 2012)

But in reality the supposedly incriminating email can be seen to show her suggesting the exact opposite, removing the younger children in order to de-dilute the danger. The supposedly evil email supposedly warranting her imprisonment seems to me to have no unworthy content at all. Rather just doing her job properly (on this point at least).

Meanwhile on the other side of the divide, consider for example an article by "Orac", one of the most rated critics of the vaccine-blamers, titled "The intellectual dishonesty of the "vaccines didn't save us" gambit" (Gorski, 2010). He accuses another author of "it doesn't get more intellectually dishonest than that", for allegedly hiding away and misrepresenting the relevant "Figure 8" (my Figure 6.1 below). And yet that figure in reality rather obviously strongly *supports* the claim of uselessness of measles vaccination, rather than undermining it (which might be why the pro-vax Canadian regime have since stopped showing it to readers of their immunization guide). I think this is an example of a phenomenon which I have repeatedly observed, of self-convinced "skeptical" people who are so blinded by their deluding bias that they can't see the clear evidence even when they are looking directly at it.

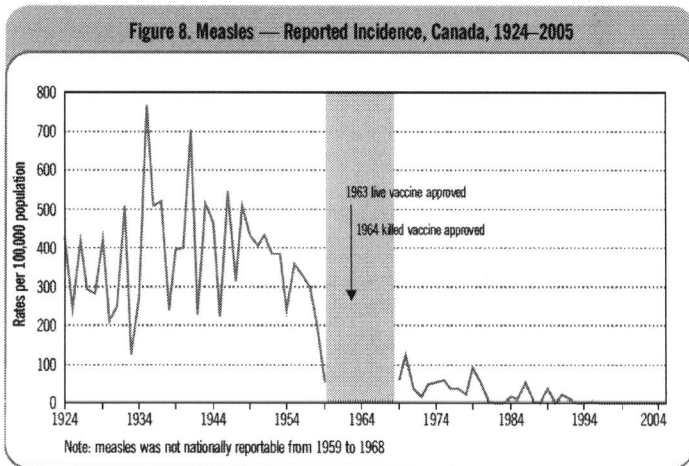

Figure 6.1. Measles data from Health Canada..

And note how the graph shows that Health Canada cancelled the collection of measles data for precisely the nine years just around when the vaccine was introduced, but at no other time. How come they became least interested in the measles data *exactly just then?* Really? Can I be a sucker too please.

Do vaccines cause autism? Few if any other questions in science have generated so much angry dispute and continue to do so. Here two entrenched ideological armies confront each other with no inclination towards ever reaching any compromise. Just about everything one hears or reads on the subject falls categorically into one or other of two camps.

On the one hand the medical authoritocracy insist that it has been clearly proved that vaccines do not cause autism. Many (or even most) even claim that there has not been any increase of autism (re which see my Chapters 2, 3, and 12 here). On the other hand an opposing camp insist in unison not merely that vaccines do sometimes cause autism, but that the increase of autism (aka "vaccine-damaged children") has been proven to be caused by vaccines. Accusations of callous evil profiteering lying fly in both directions.

I disagree with both of these opposing viewpoints. It disappoints me that I consequently find myself in such a solitary position with no congenial group of collaborators to chat with (let alone be chatted up by). But I have to tell it as I see it. The only "personal baggage" I bring to this table is that I originated the antiinnatia theory some years ago. But that theory recognises that a whole variety of factors can be causal in autism, and its coherence and credibility does not have any dependence on whether or not those factors have included some or all vaccines or none. Ultimately my only interest here is to discover the truth and the most credible (and thus hopefully flattering to my reputation) interpretation of the data.

We should first clarify what the question is or questions are. "Do vaccines cause autism?" is not the same as "Did vaccines cause the autism increase?". Furthermore I remind you of what I wrote in Chapter 2 about theories. It is tempting to think that "vaccines cause autism" is one single theory. But in reality it dubiously clumps together a whole group of separate theories of the general form "vaccine x causes autism under conditions z", where x and z can stand for a whole variety of predicates. For instance "MMR can cause autism if given before age 3", or "Thimerosal-containing vaccines can cause autism if the mercury dose exceeds 150mcg."

Paul Offit — the world's leading vaccine expert?

And now, where to begin? Perhaps with one of the most obnoxious books ever written, namely "Autism's False Prophets" by Dr Paul Offit (Offit, 2008). Not least because this highly-promoted volume seems to open a remarkable window on the moral perspective of some of those who defend vaccine "science".

Offit's book is heavily preoccupied with creating unpleasant portrayals of the people whose views he opposes – the "false prophets" of his title. I personally don't incline much towards entering into such "ad hominem" criticism. But in this case there seems to be a huge hypocrisy which cannot be allowed to go unmentioned. Normally in any scientific (or at least medical science) publication, it is considered absolutely mandatory that authors state what real or potential conflicts of interest they may have. Commercial connections for instance. And yet in this book which goes on and on about the supposed unworthiness of Andrew Wakefield, Mark and David Geier, Boyd Haley, and others, this author fails to mention that he himself has personally earned millions of dollars from his rotavirus vaccine patent (which he personally himself voted onto the US vaccine schedule), and apparently stands to earn yet more millions from in due course. Anyway, let's give Dr Offit the benefit of the doubt......

The trouble with authoring a big book is that unless you are painstakingly conscientious (or unreflectingly honourable anyway), you could in any one of the thousands of sentences unwittingly betray an unworthy mentation you would prefer to keep hidden. Let's now take a look at Exhibit A, namely pages 57-59 of "Autism's False Prophets". Note halfway down page 58 where Dr Offit quotes the words of Richard Horton:

"The public is entitled to know as much as possible."

Now note how Paul Offit deals with these words (as shown in Figure 6.2 here). Does he express any agreement with the concept? No, not the slightest. Does he instead express any disagreement with the concept? No, not the slightest agreement or disagreement, or approval or disapproval is expressed by Dr Offit. Or does he present any argument against Horton's claim that "the public is entitled to know as much as possible"? No, not the slightest (and perhaps because there is no defensible argument that could go there). One does have to wonder whether he could be feeling shy of saying what his actual attitude is here. But, in what looks to me like an attack of writer's panic at those Holy Words of Honesty shining embarrassingly out of his page 58, he also fails to hide his true attitude in these pages, as I will now explain.

Offit immediately follows Horton's quoted words with the word "But...". That doesn't exactly come across as a ringing endorsement.

But it gets worse. That "But" is the first word in a sentence which contains two brazen untruths. Firstly it refers to "Wakefield's history of holding press conferences". Here Offit is misrepresenting Wakefield's *one* previous press conference on Crohn's disease into a whole "*history* of holding press conferences" in the plural. Secondly, it refers to "ignoring the warnings of an accompanying editorial". But it was the very same Lancet editor Richard Horton who commissioned and published that editorial which Offit is here blaming that same Horton for "ignoring". The vast majority of scientific papers do not have such an accompanying "warning" editorial. Only if Horton had excluded rather than published that editorial then there might indeed be grounds for complaint against him about it.

contrary.

Richard Horton later published two books discussing his role in the controversy, *MMR Science and Fiction: Exploring the Vaccine Crisis* and *Second Opinion: Doctors, Diseases, and Decisions in Modern Medicine*. Five years after he had published Wakefield's paper, Horton was unrepentant. "There [is] an unpleasant whiff of arrogance in this whole debate," he said. "Can the public not be trusted with a controversial hypothesis? The view that the public cannot interpret uncertainty indicates an old-fashioned paternalism at work. The public is entitled to know as much as possible." But by ignoring the criticisms of several reviewers, the warnings of an accompanying editorial, Wakefield's history of holding press conferences, a British press primed for controversy, and a public distrustful of public health officials, Richard Horton allowed parents to question the safety of a vaccine based on flimsy, irreproducible data. The loss of public trust that followed was entirely predictable. "It was a stunning error of judgment," opined David Salisbury. "It is hard to believe that the paper was properly reviewed. On the link with MMR, it was a complete mess, and had a chance of being correct that was about zero. [Horton] bears a considerable burden of responsibility."

Learning little from his encounter with Andrew Wakefield, Richard Horton has published papers in the *Lancet* claiming that genetically modified foods damaged rat intestines, silicone breast implants induced harmful antibodies, and casualties sustained

Figure 6.2. Part of page 58 of "Autism's False Prophets".

Not satisfied with a double untruth in his first sentence, Offit then goes on to declare that "The loss of public trust that followed was entirely predictable." But wouldn't a more accurate accounting for loss of public trust be that so many people involved have failed to honour Horton's principle that "The public is entitled to know as much as possible"?

Offit provides the coup-de-grace to his own credibility with the way that he not only avoids commenting on Horton's statement but also immediately sets about a vitriolic condemnation of its messenger in the several hundred words that follow it. And also precedes it with a pageful of more dis-enthusiasm against that messenger.

It is impossible for any sane person to study these pages without seeing that Offit has some major personal problem with

Horton's concept that "The public is entitled to know as much as possible". Offit fails to make any direct comment on it, no approval, no agreement, no argument against it, but instead that "But" and two untruths immediately following on as part of an extended raging expression of utter contempt for the messenger who is made out to have behaved outrageously unethically and thereby personally to blame for a (supposed!) major health catastrophe.

So now we can only conclude that Paul Offit does not work to the principle that "The public is entitled to know as much as possible." Which raises the question of what he thinks we should not be told. And of what point there is in reading a book written by someone who prefers that we should only be told a censored account of the scientific evidence.

It appears that there are many who believe that Dr Offit is an evil liar who falls soundly to sleep at night gloating over how rich he has become at the expense of his gullible victims. But I'm not sure that's true, that it's that simple.

Excessive amounts of too-easily-gained wealth tend to delude a person that they are somehow far more superior, intellectually and morally, than they actually are. It seems to me that Dr Offit, along with other such "superior" persons, reckons that human society divides into (a) their minority of superior persons who are properly qualified to handle the full bare information of a subject, and (b) the remaining majority who are inferiors who therefore need to have their knowledge and understanding carefully managed by a process of selective publication. And this can even require telling those simple-minded inferiors some untruths and illogicalities in the service of guiding them thereby to main conclusions which are more beneficial in their outcomes. Thus these superiors tell untruths not with any evil intent but only in order to kindly help their inferiors – or at least that's the self-serving way they see their untruth-telling. So maybe it should *not* be referred to, pejoratively, as *lying*.

I'll here just give this alternative ?ethical? position the name of "info-nannying", and come back to it later in this book.

Offit's book uses a peculiar "shy" system of citation of sources, which gives no citation indications on the text pages, but only in a section at the back (as in Figure 6.3 here). This peculiar system has been used in almost no other scientific/medical books, especially not in any which deal with contentious matters. It is ideal for misleading your readers about what is your mere false assertion rather than what is genuinely evidence-based – as in the following examples?

(The next paragraph contains the word "chelation". This is officially pronounced *key-lay-shun*, but some including myself tend to have difficulty learning this.)

Several of Offit's fallacies are deployed in an attempt to dismiss as pseudoscience the notion that many autism cases have been cured by removal of mercury by chelation. Note that this is a hugely important issue here, the question of whether there is an easy cure for a very serious lifetime disability. And in my experience there has been a great deal of propaganda devoted to pseudo-debunking of perfectly sound safe treatments which just happen to threaten the profits of the medical corporatocracy.

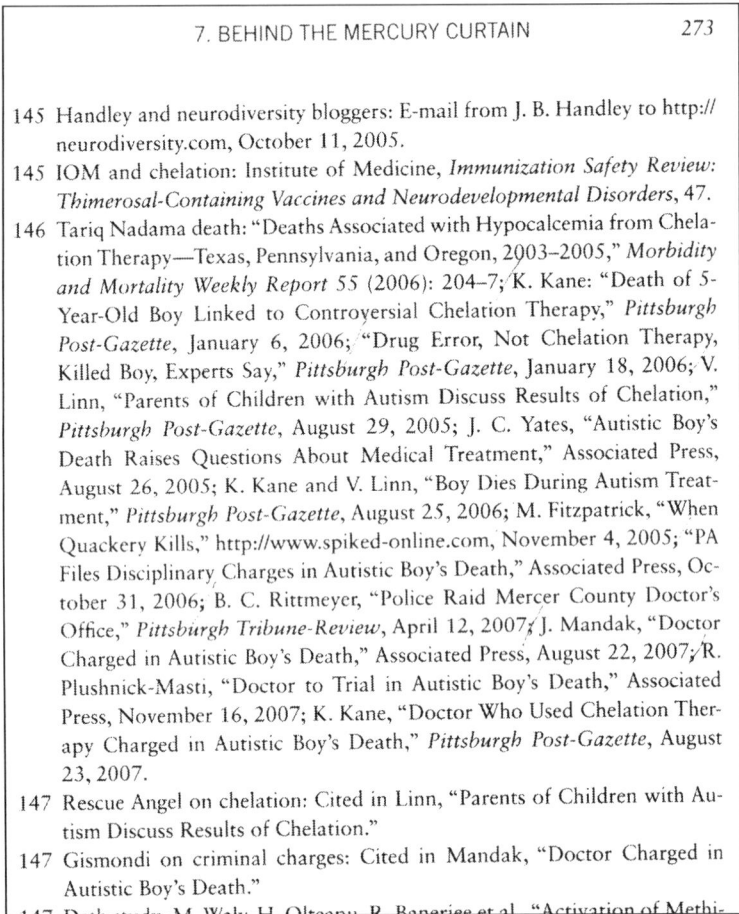

7. BEHIND THE MERCURY CURTAIN   273

145 Handley and neurodiversity bloggers: E-mail from J. B. Handley to http:// neurodiversity.com, October 11, 2005.

145 IOM and chelation: Institute of Medicine, *Immunization Safety Review: Thimerosal-Containing Vaccines and Neurodevelopmental Disorders*, 47.

146 Tariq Nadama death: "Deaths Associated with Hypocalcemia from Chelation Therapy—Texas, Pennsylvania, and Oregon, 2003–2005," *Morbidity and Mortality Weekly Report* 55 (2006): 204–7; K. Kane: "Death of 5-Year-Old Boy Linked to Controversial Chelation Therapy," *Pittsburgh Post-Gazette*, January 6, 2006; "Drug Error, Not Chelation Therapy, Killed Boy, Experts Say," *Pittsburgh Post-Gazette*, January 18, 2006; V. Linn, "Parents of Children with Autism Discuss Results of Chelation," *Pittsburgh Post-Gazette*, August 29, 2005; J. C. Yates, "Autistic Boy's Death Raises Questions About Medical Treatment," Associated Press, August 26, 2005; K. Kane and V. Linn, "Boy Dies During Autism Treatment," *Pittsburgh Post-Gazette*, August 25, 2006; M. Fitzpatrick, "When Quackery Kills," http://www.spiked-online.com, November 4, 2005; "PA Files Disciplinary Charges in Autistic Boy's Death," Associated Press, October 31, 2006; B. C. Rittmeyer, "Police Raid Mercer County Doctor's Office," *Pittsburgh Tribune-Review*, April 12, 2007; J. Mandak, "Doctor Charged in Autistic Boy's Death," Associated Press, August 22, 2007; R. Plushnick-Masti, "Doctor to Trial in Autistic Boy's Death," Associated Press, November 16, 2007; K. Kane, "Doctor Who Used Chelation Therapy Charged in Autistic Boy's Death," *Pittsburgh Post-Gazette*, August 23, 2007.

147 Rescue Angel on chelation: Cited in Linn, "Parents of Children with Autism Discuss Results of Chelation."

147 Gismondi on criminal charges: Cited in Mandak, "Doctor Charged in Autistic Boy's Death."

147 Dark study: M. Weh, H. Olteanu, R. Banerjee et al. "Activation of Methi-

Figure 6.3. Part of a page of Offit's book using the shy citations system.

A first fallacy is Offit's notion that mercury removal could not possibly enable recovery from mercury-induced injury. Offit's rationale is that "Once a brain cell is damaged by a heavy metal like mercury, it is permanently damaged" (page 145). And thus removing the mercury cannot reverse the "damage". And "therefore" chelation for autism cannot work and must be mere quackery.

Firstly, let us for the moment take as accepted Offit's false notion that "damage" of neurons must be involved in autism. Immediately after this critique of the science he presents his scare-anecdote about an utterly irrelevant case of incompetent misuse of *sodium* EDTA (well-known to be a highly inappropriate, deadly, choice of chelator): "And then the unthinkable happened....." (Arrgghh!!!). Curiously he gives *twelve* citations for that ONE utterly irrelevant scare-drivel anecdote (in which he helpfully misleads the reader into assuming that it was the normal *calcium* EDTA), and yet in respect of his key assertion about damaged cells, there is *no* citation of evidence sources whatsoever. But of course that's not really a problem as it is the Infallible True Prophet Offit who is proclaiming it, in whom the reader has been given total faith by this stage. I leave to you to judge whether or not those twelve drivel citations were padded in there to hide the non-existent evidence about "damage". But in my experience that's how propaganda trickery regularly works (see e.g. the UK COT's deliberately deceitful statement against vitamin B6, in respect of which I'm still awaiting that promised claim for libel).

All manner of body cells have extensive systems in place for repairing themselves. They're doing it all the time. So on quite what basis does Offit assert that neurons "damaged" by mercury cannot be "repaired"? And why does he cite no evidence for this key, highly-heretical assertion?

(Offit would perhaps have you believe that he did indeed cite evidence, in his quotation of the IOM saying that "Because chelation therapy is unlikely to remove mercury from the brain, it is useful only immediately after exposure, before damage has occurred." But that sentence is merely theoretical speculation rather than any evidence that "damage" is involved in autism let alone is permanent. And it is common knowledge that considerable brain damage from stroke can indeed be recovered from.)

But anyway, Offit errs more fundamentally, by making that false assumption that mercury neurotoxicity can work *only* by irreparably "damaging" neurons, with no other neurotoxic processes involved. In reality mercury has potential to affect neurons via its pro-oxidant effect, and via its interference with the many enzyme pathways that involve zinc. And last but not least, mercury binds to DNA and thereby reduces gene-expression, which I have long argued is the main way that mercury causes autism.

The mechanism by which mercury causes autism therefore does not have to involve any irreversible "damaging" of neurons. So lowering the mercury levels, such that the DNA has less of it part-time binding and inhibiting the gene-expression required for normal development, would indeed enable recovery, providing it is done before the brain has become too fixed by maturation. Offit's reasoning is therefore doubly incorrect.

You can also see that on page 115 (refs page 269) Offit cites the Nelson and Bauman paper but fails to give the citation of the Bernard et al which it attempted to debunk, nor any mention of the authors' later resounding rejoinder. I leave you to form your own judgement about this selective mentioning of only one side by such a highly-qualified multi-millionaire. Especially given the seriousness of the subject, potentially trying to deprive tragic victims of a uniquely valuable therapy, *and* Dr Offit's heavy financial interest in the question of the safety of vaccines.

Offit further deploys that misinformation there in a second false argument in terms of autism and mercury poisoning being "two disorders". And yet an elementary knowledge of mercury toxicity tells us that there is far from being just "one disorder" that constitutes "mercury poisoning". I can only guess this heroic multi-millionaire was too busy struggling to make ends meet to find the time to properly study what he was publishing about.

A third false argument of Offit is his comparison of autism epidemiology with other epidemiology (on pages 110-111). He states that epidemiology of side-effects of certain vaccines was able to show up even the causation of some very rare hazards (intussusception, thrombocytopenia, and Guillain-Barré syndrome) resulting from them, and so "therefore" the epidemiological studies of autism would have this same power to utterly rule out even very slight involvement of vaccines. But the epidemiology of autism is affected by two starkly obvious major complications which did not affect the epidemiology examples cited by Offit. Firstly, autism is *very* far from being something that can be clearly "yes/no" identified in the way the above-named three conditions can be. Secondly, the autism epidemiology data has huge variance, far from all of it explained, but reasonably suspected to be caused by some changes of awareness and of diagnosis, and or by other environmental factors such as dental mercury (as made clear in other chapters here).

That is, the autism data has a huge level of "noise" in it, preventing hearing of the tiny whisper signal which Offit claims could be clearly not heard. Or in another analogy, the autism data is a very crude unfocussable lens through which to search for the tiny pinpoint he claims ought to be visible if vaccines even rarely caused autism. Or in a third analogy, the autism data is like a choppy sea on which we cannot reasonably expect to notice even a whole cupful of additional water.

So again, we see a third crudely incorrect argument from this highly-qualified, highly-awarded author who has made millions from touting his own highly dubious, highly profitable, liability-evading, forcibly-imposed pseudo-medical products. Sadly it would take up much too much room here to give justice to the full extent of the abysmalness contained in this one book of Offit's, let alone the rest of his output.

But it is important to note that none of that debunking of Dr Offit's hollow rationales can constitute any proof that any autism has indeed been caused by vaccines.

[Update: Offit has now been exposed as falsely accusing a journalist of sending nasty emails and lying, in addition to his including an entirely fabricated interview in his book. (ocregister.com, 2011)]

And on the other hand....

Meanwhile from the opposing camp in this tragic war, we are assured that there is a huge international cover-up of loads of clear proof that vaccines have caused the huge increase of autism, aka "vaccine-damaged children".

You will surely have heard the expression "conspiracy theories", and you will have noticed how it is used in a context of contempt as if such "conspiracy theories" are only believed by silly people with several bits missing from their brains. Conspiracy theory "nutcases", etc.

Most people have little or no experience of politics, campaigning, or what goes on behind the closed doors of corporations. Anyone who *does* have such experience is well aware that conspiracies and cover-ups and misinformation operations are what goes on almost *all* of the time. And the media's cliché expression "conspiracy theories" is just another misinformation tool used to keep the uninformed even more uninformed. Only the ignorant and fools dismiss *all* conspiracy theories.

But you also have to bear in mind that conspiracy and cover-up is the kneejerking norm in politics and corporations to the extent that these people lie and cover up even when there isn't actually any embarrassing truth needing to be lied about or covered up anyway. And so "There's no smoke without fire" is a mantra for the naive rather than the discerners.

So, even if there is evidence or even proof of a conspiracy of deceit on the question, that conspiracy could not constitute any actual evidence on the main question of whether or not any vaccines have caused any autism. We have to look at the specific scientific evidence for that.

Some very notable and relatively competent researchers, most notably Boyd Haley and Bernard Rimland, have taken the view that the evidence points strongly to vaccines being the cause of a huge increase of autism. (And I have already shown you the clinching evidence of the increase in Chapter 3 here.) So I need to also answer the question of why those researchers have ended up at what I consider to be that wrong conclusion. Dr Haley has set out his position quite well in a comment which has been copied to various places on the internet:

"Below [is] my rationale (not exclusive to me) for pointing directly to thimerosal in vaccines as the major cause of the increase (but not the only contributor) .

1. The toxin has to be one that affects boys more than girls.

2. The toxin exposure has to occur before 2-3 years of age, including in utero time (excludes most exposures from eats, drinking and drugs).

3. The toxin had to increase in the time frame of 1988-90.

4. The toxin had to increase in all 50 states at the same time (follow the US Dept. of Education Individuals with Disabilities Act data).

5. The toxin had to be able to cause the pleotypic toxic effects as evidenced by the multiple biochemical abnormalities observed in autism by direct or secondary effect mechanisms. Some examples would be low glutathione levels (Dr. James), aberrant methylation (Dr. Deth), low sulfate levels (Dr. Waring), abnormal urinary porphyrin profiles (Dr. Nataf), low Molybdenum levels, elevated neopterin levels (Dr. Nataf), etc.

I would strongly suggest that elevated mercury exposure via thimerosal is the only causal factor as it can explain explicitly all of the 5 items above."

Haley's rationale there is well-reasoned, but nevertheless flawed. Haley, along with Rimland and others, was aware of the autism increase but completely unaware of the crucial change of dental amalgams to the non-gamma-2 type as discussed in my Chapter 3 here. This was hardly any great offence of incompetence on their part as just about no-one was told about this change anyway. Even most dentists haven't even heard of the change to non-gamma-2 even though they implant the evil stuff in victims' mouths every day.

Haley and Rimland were nevertheless aware of reasons to implicate some new source of mercury in the cause of the autism increase. And because they were unaware of the change of dental amalgams, and being taken in by the ADA's/FDA's simplistic rubbish about amalgam having been "used safely for 150 years", the only change of mercury they could identify was the thimerosal in vaccines.

In Dr Haley's list of five points, "the toxin" can sensibly be identified as mercury. And yet the inference that "therefore" it must be from vaccines is unsound, because it could instead be entirely from the non-gamma-2 amalgams instead. And furthermore, crucially, Haley's point 3 is misinformed. You can see in Chapter 3 that the increase does not just happen in 1988-90, but rather had already started by 1980, and continued long thereafter, and in 1988-90 just continued the ongoing approximately exponential up-curve.

And how *not* to graphically illustrate an epidemic

A picture, or graphical evidence, can often speak much louder than any number of numbers or words (a view you will see reflected in several chapters of this book). And yet many people successfully come to very unsound conclusions on the basis of seriously muddled attempts at making informative graphs.

So I will try to provide a little remedial course here on the correct and incorrect use of graphical data. Please accept my apologies if this section comes over as far too condescending or alternatively far too above your head!

My two graphs on the front cover of this book (basically Figures 5 and 7 from Chapter 3) are charts of time-trends of health statistics, a type of graph which I find particularly interesting. But I've been far from unique in my interest therein. Such charts can be very useful or can be seriously misleading, depending on how competently (and honestly) they are composed.

Important questions which arise in respect of such graphs include the following.
1. How narrowly selective is the extent of the time-axis? (Like, what was happening earlier or later?)
2. Or conversely, has the graph-maker confused the picture by squashing too many decades into too few inches of visual space?
3. Are all the baselines zero or not?
4. Does the graph show the *crude actual numbers* of cases or instead the more useful *ratio* of cases per 10,000 of population?
5. Does the data shown for a particular year mean the number for those born in that year (i.e. the incidence for that "birth-year

cohort") or instead the "actual" number for those alive in that year (i.e. the cumulative prevalence)?

6. Does a particular datapoint reflect hundreds or thousands of cases (in which case it will be very "accurate"), or instead just a handful (in which case it will have a high randomness and margin of error, thus not worth taking too seriously with declarations such as "then it went down again!")?

7. Do any measurement artifacts (such as under-reporting) need to be taken into account?

8. Are the verbal assertions about the graph justified by the actual data-series lines in it?

Generally-speaking, a competent graph should:

1. show all the relevant (or available) range of time-axis;
2. but not much more;
3. have only zero baselines;
4. show ratios per population rather than crude case numbers;
5. show birth-year cohorts rather than cumulative numbers (if the condition is being theorised as due to a peri-natal cause rather than from an immediately-concurrent cause such as fever from infection);
6. be based on reasonably large numbers of cases (at least hundreds) or if not, then at least include some form of error-bars to indicate the lack of confidence of exactness of reflection of the underlying potential reality;
7. have an accompanying indication of any artifacts that might confound the data.

In respect of the first point concerning the time axis, Figure 6.4 here could be useful to look at. This chart was published by Mark Blaxill in about 2001 to illustrate the apparent link between amount of vaccine mercury (thimerosal) and the rate of autism births. It admirably satisfies most of the criteria I've stated above. It gives a very credible impression that the autism was caused by that mercury. Some people are still citing it 14 years later.

But see what happens when I re-plot that same mercury data alongside a fuller (and updated) time-range of autism data, as in Figure 6.5. You can see then that the autism increase was already well under way before the thimerosal increase, and continued upwards even after the thimerosal started going down. The 2001 graph also errs in failing to take into account that the recorded autism rates were declining at the end not due to a real decline but only because the autistics get registered only after some years of delay. You can also see this recency decline artifact in Chapter 3's Figures 3, 4, 5, and 6.

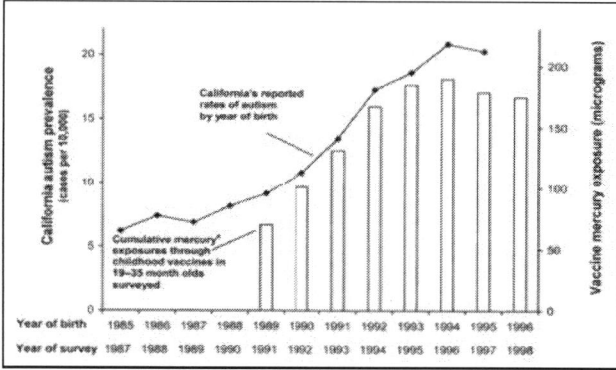

Figure 6.4. Blaxill's ~2001 chart of autism and thimerosal.

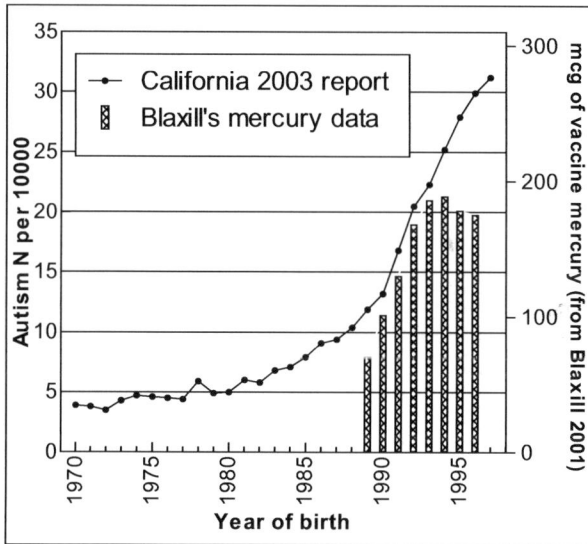

Figure 6.5. My own improved version of Blaxill's chart.

Looking at my improved graph namely Figure 6.5, it is difficult or impossible to discern any impact of the thimerosal on the autism increase which is just a steady approximately exponential (accelerating) curve which just carries on getting steeper and steeper. And can be fully understood in terms of dental mercury anyway (as explained in Chapter 3).

Note that the graphs I have just been talking about use two y-axis scales (the y axis being the vertical axis) so as to give a scale of the mercury on the one side and the amount of autism on the other side. This is a very common arrangement you will need to be aware of in various other graphs in this book and elsewhere.

By the way, it has been pointed out that this California DDS data is not necessarily reliable for making judgements of the causality, as it is merely enrolments rather a scientific survey. However, as I pointed out in Chapter 3, the three prevalence studies in Sweden's Gothenburg collide rather exactly with this curve, from which it can be reasonably suspected to have considerable validity. Besides which, otherwise there must be some remarkable flukes of coincidence in the various graphs I show in Chapter 3.

Turning now to the mistake of counting crude actual numbers of cases rather than ratios of the population, illustrative of this matter is another of the autism graphs which was majorly cited around 15 years ago. Variations of the graph shown in Figure 6.6 here were used for arguing that MMR vaccine (which never contained mercury) had caused a rise of autism in both the UK (lower series) and the US (upper series). There are things majorly wrong with it. Firstly, the use of crude numbers which fails to separate out the impact of a rapid increase of California's population at the time. You would hardly guess it but that California data in that Figure 6.6 is *exactly* the same as the California 1999 data shown in my Chapter 3 Figures 3, 4, and 5. I myself did the conversion of that data from cases to ratios and as far as I'm aware no-one else ever has. And it makes rather obvious that there was not some remarkable consequence of the introduction of MMR in 1978, but only initially a very gradual increase which only years later got a lot steeper.

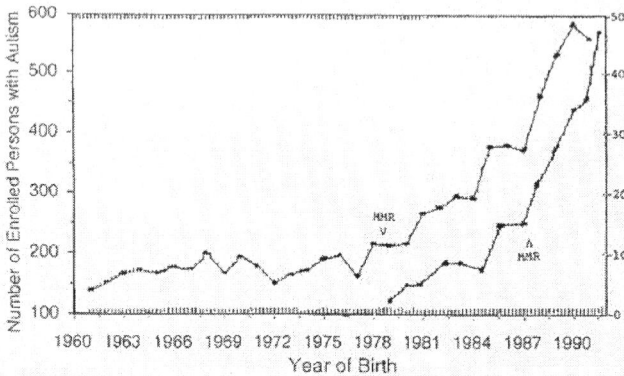

Figure 6.6. A chart of autism data circulating circa 2000.

The same graph commits an even greater offence in that the UK data has a zero baseline (indicated on the right), but the California data is given a baseline far above zero, at 100, thus further misleading the reader of the true relationship between these series. In fact there is manifestly something unsound about that UK data (from GP reports) as it seems to imply that autism was almost non-existent in 1978, contrary to far more credible evidence from other studies.

The mistake of using cumulative data rather than birth-year-cohort data is passably illustrated by a graph recently being shown on some websites, shown here as Figure 6.7. This graph is being claimed to show that the autism increase has been caused by glyphosate herbicide. There is reason to consider the highly-toxic persistent carcinogen glyphosate (aka "Roundup") to be one of the most evil substances ever made and which needs to be criminalised and banned as soon as possible, but I don't see the remotest sound evidence that it has ever caused any autism. It is anyway difficult to seriously consider it as "the" major causal factor because that fails to account for the strong involvement of mercury in most modern autism (as was reviewed in Chapter 3).

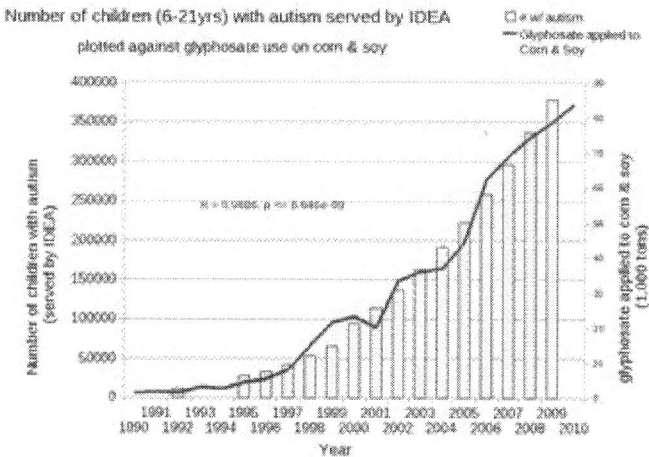

Figure 6.7. A graph of glyphosate and autism, as published on various websites.

To help with understanding the mistake of using cumulative (actual total) numbers instead of birth-year-cohort ratios, the following analogy might be useful. Suppose that you are currently destitute but I kindly decide to pay you a million dollars a year, from now on for the forseeable future. Your cumulative wealth, your "number of dollars", will then rise steeply every year, by about a million dollars a year minus however much you spend of it. But that's even though your income is not increasing at all but instead is entirely flat at one million dollars per year.

Likewise the glyphosate graph of autism goes steeply upwards in recent years and yet the number of infants *newly becoming autistic* increases very much less rapidly. It's just that that number becoming autistic is now at a regularly huge level compared to 20+ years ago.

But maybe the graph is still correct in using the cumulative autism numbers? The graph is stated to be of the number of children aged 6 to 21 years. The problem with that is that it assumes that twenty-year-old children can be caused to become autistic twenty-one-year olds if the glyphosate reaches a certain level. And that is out of line with the normal experience that children aren't becoming autistic at such later ages, but generally in the first two or three years at most, because it's a *developmental* condition. An equally serious problem with the graph is that the increase of glyphosate had hardly got started by 1997 whereas the autism had already been majorly increasing long before then. Again, the graph misleads because it does not include the proper full relevant range of years. The graph gets a wonderful very high correlation between corn/soy glyphosate usage and autism, with very high significance (low p-value) but such a correlation founded on what is in effect a cherry-picking of entirely wrong data anyway is devoid of the supposed implicational capability.

For these reasons, the graph does not even remotely constitute substantial evidence of causation of autism by glyphosate. But does constitute good evidence that glyphosate has *not* been the entire cause of the increase of autism, if any cause at all anyway.

My next example of deficient graph-reading also illustrates the point I made at the start of this book, that there isn't a simple dichotomy between good competent people on the one hand and bad incompetents on the other. Indeed that there's also no neat dichotomy between those who get everything wrong versus those who get everything right. Dr Lucia Tomljenovich resigned from her job rather than follow orders to collude in fraud in a pseudo-study of statins pseudo-medicine. She has since published a paper arguing that aluminium in vaccines has caused a major amount of autism (Tomljenovich & Shaw, 2011). Again an impressively high correlation emerges, from which one could easily conclude this to be strong evidence that aluminium caused all that autism. (Again, I consider injecting of toxic aluminium to be a seriously improper thing to be doing anyway, but the question here is whether it has caused an increase of autism, or for that matter any autism at all.)

Anyway, Figure 6.8 here is their graph as appears in their

paper, and you can see the straight lines which they envisage to be the reality behind their dots. But you might just notice there's just something a little strange about those dots and straight lines.....

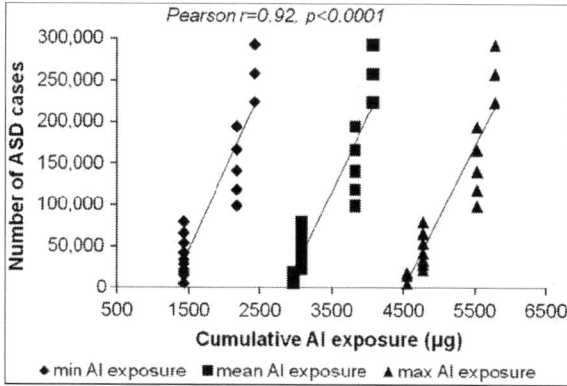

Figure 6.8. Aluminium and autism as per the graph in the paper by Tomljenovich & Shaw (2011).

Actually their original graph is made rather complicated by their conscientiously including three separate datasets, for minimum-, maximum-, and average- possible amounts of aluminium. So I will use some "electronic tippex" from my Office 2000 to convert it to a simplified graph of just the "average" dataset, in Figure 6.9.

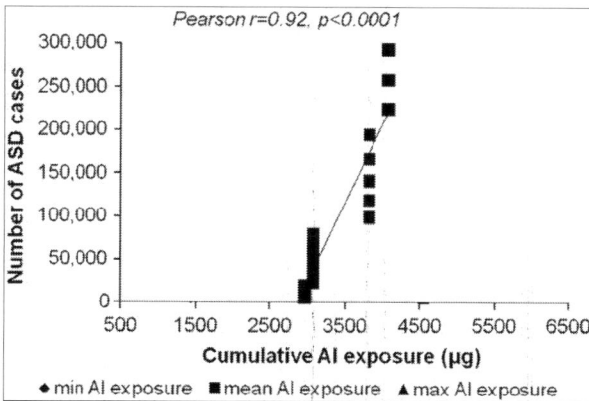

Figure 6.9. My simplification of Figure 6.8.

Note that their graph is not a graph of change of autism over time, but instead of autism plotted against dose of aluminium. There's nothing wrong with that in principle, but...... well, let's see what emerges when I take exactly the same data (kindly forwarded by Dr Tomljenovic) and re-form it into just another of my graphs of how things change over a period of years.

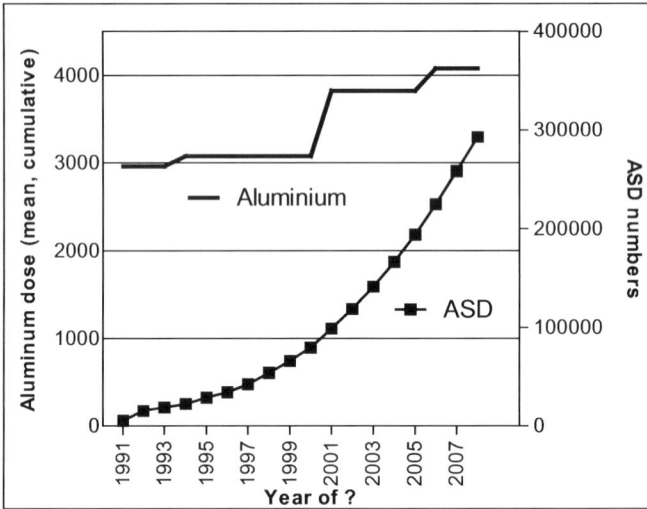

Figure 6.10. My time-series graph of the data of T & S 2011.

My Figure 6.10 shows the result, that is their actual data of changing amounts of aluminium plotted alongside their data of changing numbers of autistics. Can you see what's wrong with it? Well, it should have the autism stepping up in line with the aluminium steps. But it shows nothing of the sort, but instead the autism just curves upwards with not the slightest impact of the aluminium's steps. From this it is difficult to avoid the conclusion that the amount of aluminium is not the slightest bit causal of the level of autism. Again, T&S's data actually proves the exact opposite of what you might have thought, notwithstanding their impressively high correlation and significance level. (Actually science tends not to absolutely "prove" things, but in this and other cases it does get very near to doing so.) (I could correct their raw autism numbers into birth-year-cohort ratios but it would do little to rescue their aluminium theory anyway.) I think the key thing about T&S's own graph is that it needlessly omits the time data, the years for which these observations were made.

I come next to an example of mistake number 2, of squashing too many years too close together to get a proper view of what's going on. You know if you use a telescope rather than a microscope you aren't going to see any bacteria, but that doesn't mean you've found any evidence that they don't exist.

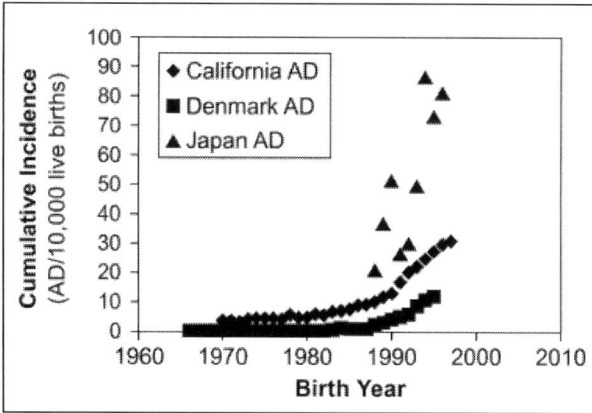

Figure 6.11. Graph from McDonald & Paul (2010).

Much has been made of two papers supposedly constituting really whopping evidence that vaccines caused the autism increase. These are McDonald & Paul (2010) and Ratajczac (2011). The first of these features a very small, squashed graph (Figure 6.11 here), which fits 50 years into barely 2 inches (6 cm). This can be very misleading because it tends to make a gradual upwards curve look like a sudden upward jerking change of direction.

M&P, inspired by earlier claims that autism started rising in 1988, analysed the graph of autism increase to find a changepoint at which a steeper straight line followed after a previous more level line. They concluded that a changepoint had indeed occurred at 1988. The problem with this sort of analysis is that just about any gradual curve can have a couple of straight lines plonked on it, which can then look plausibly correct and indeed calculated to be quite highly correlated. But it doesn't follow that those two straight lines actually enlighten us as to what actually happened. Take a look at my Chapter 3 graphs, Figures 1 to 6. In all those graphs, nothing special about 1988-9 stands out; the exponential increases merely go on getting gradually steeper.

Ratajczak (2011) managed to find not just one but three of these supposed changepoints, each coinciding with one or other supposedly salient change of vaccination protocols. I quote:

> "Autism in the United States spiked dramatically between 1983 and 1990 .... In 1988 .....a spike of incidence of autism accompanied the addition of the second dose of MMR II. .... An additional increased spike in incidence of autism occurred in 1995 when the chicken pox vaccine was grown in human fetal tissue"

Meanwhile, the website of Sound Choice Pharmaceutical Institute gives us basically the same message, accompanied by the Figure 6.12 here which supposedly illustrates its truth:

"In the US, autism has spiked up in 3 distinct years, called changepoints. The first changepoint occurred in 1981, the second in 1988, and the third in 1996. These spikes coincide with the introduction of vaccines that are produced in aborted fetal cells."

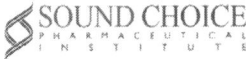

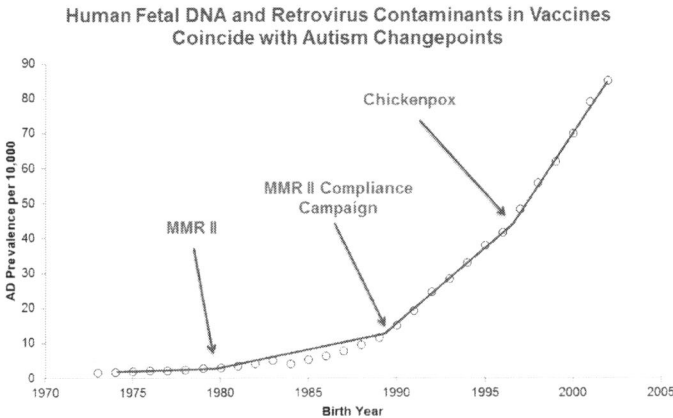

Figure 6.12. Autism graph on soundchoice.org website.
http://soundchoice.org/autism/

In reality, if you had not been already forewarned that those "changepoints" were there, you would never have guessed it from looking at the actual datapoints (e.g. in my increase charts in Chapter 3) without the hypothetical straight lines drawn over them. In the reality before my own eyes there is just a gradually steepening exponential.   But maybe some others' eyes work better than mine.

I have done rather a lot of rubbishing of others' efforts in the last few pages. So perhaps I should correct the balance with a bit of rubbishing of my own efforts for a change. (I should declare a bias at this point, in that I consider cars to be by far the worst invention ever, and that cars should be banned until proven safe, in other words until forever.) Anyway, some of the professional geniuses at California's world-leading MIND Institute have ingeniously thought up the idea that pollution from road traffic could be causing autism or at least increasing the risk a bit. They've published a number of expensively-funded studies of the evidence, in prestigious peer-reviewed journals. Being very clever PhDs and so on, they didn't need to bother doing the simplistic analysis which I will describe in the following sentences.

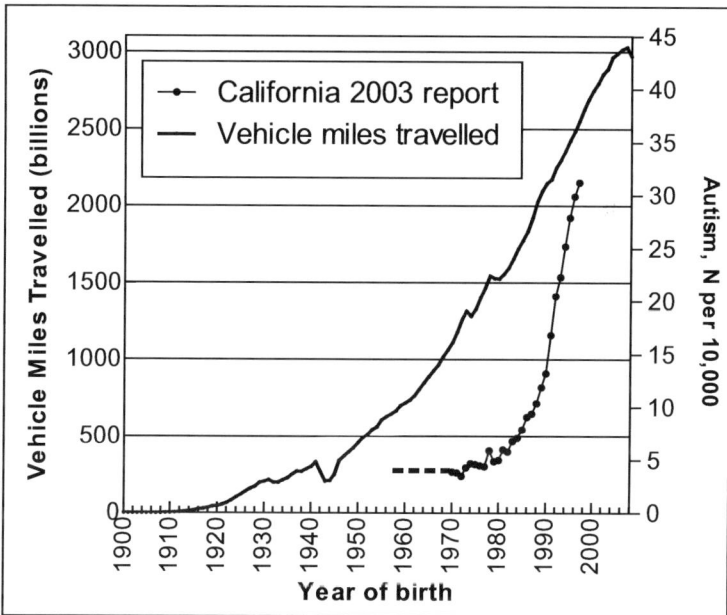

Figure 6.13. My stupid graph of vehicle miles travelled vs. autism.

I took the California DDS autism increase data from my Figure 3 in Chapter 3, and put it alongside the data of vehicle miles travelled (vmt) in the US over the past century or so. I also added in a bit of horizontal line inferred from my Figure 1 in Chapter 3. And thereby produced the Figure 6.13 you can see here. To my simple mind some strange things stood out. The autism increase was concentrated in almost one decade whereas the vmt spread over 80 years. Half the increase of vmt had already happened by the time the autism had started to increase. And the autism increase lagged several decades behind the vmt increase. So it would seem that the traffic pollution would have to be causing autism not in the contemporary generations of infants, but instead in the grandchildren of those exposed to the pollution.

Anyway, to cut a long story short, I compiled a paper reporting these observations. It also included consideration of other possible road pollutants such as MTBE, and more crucially my alternative explanation of the MIND Institute's geniuses' findings of more autism near to busy roads. This explanation was in terms of the fact that people living near to busy roads habitually keep their doors and windows closed to keep out noise and hostile strangers, and consequently get more poisoned by the indoor mercury vaporising from their dental amalgams. (Having myself lived for 20 years six feet from a busy main road junction may have helped to make me aware of this consideration.)

I sent that paper to the Molecular Autism journal edited by Prof Simon Baron-Cohen, but he refused to publish it unless I completely cut out all mention of that alternative explanation. That may or may not have anything to do with the fact that Prof Baron-Cohen himself appears to have never said or written anything about a possible connection of autism and mercury, despite it being one of the noisiest disputes in the whole history of science.

Anyway, the bottom line on this graph of mine is that it was rejected by the peer-review system, whereas the MIND Institute's studies were all accepted in notable journals. So perhaps best not to delude myself that I am a competent researcher.

But sadly I have to add in one more graph of nonsense here. It appears in Polyak et al. (2015) and it supposedly shows clear evidence that autism hasn't really increased but instead there has just been a change of diagnoses from ID (intellectual disability, basically low IQ scores) to autism. (An older name for ID is MR – mental retardation.)

The Figure 6.14 shown here is my direct extraction from the first figure of their paper (which includes a number of other datasets for other diagnoses but in which these autism and ID datasets are the most prominently identifiable and the most talked about). What you see is that while autism goes up, ID goes down quite closely in reverse. And this has resulted in predictably numerous media articles about autism being shown not to have really increased. What these scholars didn't have anything to say about is that they confined their analysis to the years from 2000. And yet the autism increase had been majorly going on for the preceding 20 years, and by starting only at 2000 they pick up only the tail end. Why cherry-pick only those years? Even an unqualified idiot can easily find from a websearch some charts of the preceding years showing that no such contrary trending occurred over all that time, that is through the most intense years of the autism increase. So why didn't Polyak et al. make any mention of that earlier data? Which basically shows their assertion of diagnostic substitution to be untrue. Why no mention of the Croen et al. earlier discussions which debunked exactly the same idea?

This defective paper from Polyak et al. is part of a wider lineage of similarly simplistically-flawed studies supposedly showing that the catastrophic autism increase has not really happened or has not had anything to do with mercury. (Evidence that the increase has indeed happened is presented in Chapters 2 and 3 here.)

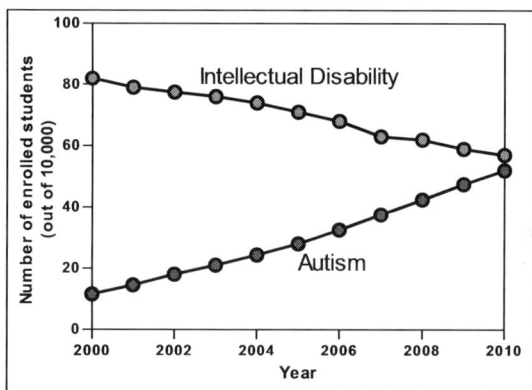

Figure 6.14. Autism and ID data from Polyak et al. (2015).

I'll just add here my own thoughts about this data. The increase denialists of the medical establishment would have us believe that the steep increase of autism numbers in the 1980s and 90s was at the least an overstatement of the reality. And yet medical institutions are famous not for any excessive speed on recognising unwelcome changes, but rather for their slowness in recognising them – as is indeed reflected in the continuing denial exercises such as Polyak et al. here. It therefore seems reasonable to reckon that the increase data was actually underestimating the real increase of autism, such that those various graphs should actually have been even steeper in the 1980s and 1990s, because many of the new autistics were being misdiagnosed as "merely" mentally retarded (intellectually disabled). And that only later in the 2000s and 2010s have these misdiagnoses been getting corrected into autism diagnoses. From this perspective there is reason to suspect that the autism increase may have in reality ended and has now levelled off.

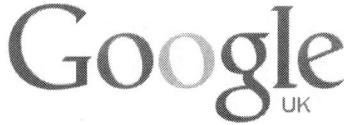

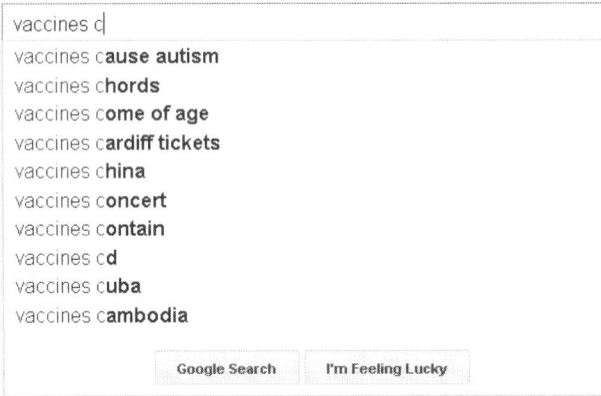

Figures 6.15 and 6.16. The Google search engine's auto-completions of my typing into the search box.

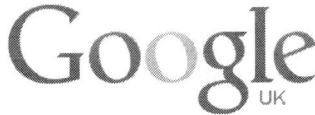

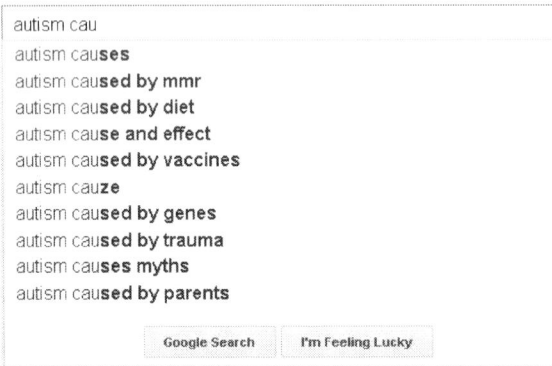

The vaccines-autism evidence

Google's auto-completion prompts as shown here in Figures 6.15 and 6.16 reflect the extent of the notion of an association of these two things.

Part of the problem with the vaccines-autism controversy is that it isn't one controversy but instead as many controversies as you want to make it. It resembles the common experience of gardening in which you finally get rid of all the nettles only to find a week later that a load of prickly thistles have sprung up in their place, followed by couch grass, then horsetail, ...

At this point I remind you of the principle I explained in Chapter 2, that as a professional researcher it is far better if you can blame a gene or virus, as genes and viruses can't get angry or take legal action against you for accusing them. Whereas you should avoid blaming something which some person or company has made or used, because then that company or person may indeed get angry and attack. Well, there is another side to this phenomenon, namely the side from the perspective of the injured person and their family. They conversely would prefer to blame a manufactured product or medical procedure, because they could then (at least supposedly) make a legal claim for injury against those responsible, whereas they could not sue their own genes or a virus.

So, imagine the scene .... Loads of parents are finding their children becoming autistic. Huge mystery of what's causing this. Huge shiftyness becoming all too discernable in the actions of various government officials, corporate officials, corporatised researchers, and authors of books about false prophets. The big questions get asked: "What changed?", and "What did this to my child?".

And one answer which none of them come up with is "non-gamma-2 dental amalgams". Because no-one has even heard of them, not even the dentists. And anyway, babies don't get dental fillings anyway, and the use of amalgam hasn't suddenly started or increased recently anyway. So dental amalgams would seem not to rate even a second look.

Meanwhile there is an industry of outstanding shysters, namely vaccines (as documented by Humphries & Bystrianyk, 2013). And the vaccine schedules hugely increased. And they get given to babies. And the observation of thousands of parents has been that "My child was perfectly healthy until he got a vaccine shot, and then his illness immediately [well, sort-of-immediately] began".

I remind you here again of the parrotting training which professional researchers benefit from. One of the most revered of their parrotting-lines goes as follows.

"The plural of anecdote is not data!!!!!!"

This invocation is rather useful because anecdotes are produced by unqualified non-professionals who need to be regularly shut up as per many previous paragraphs of this book. Competent evidence can only come from proper systematic trials, we are told.   Incorrectly as it happens.   *Very* incorrectly.

There are anecdotes and anecdotes, and like with genes, some are more important than others, and some are more valuable than others.   Consider for instance if I just now saw a nine-legged luminous woman walk into this room.   Well, you wouldn't believe me if I said so.   But perhaps I made a video of it happening, including my expression of amazement.   Could such a report rightly be dismissed as "merely anecdotal"?   You might of course seek to argue that my video was a fake produced to deceive the gullible.   But note that that is not the same argument as saying it is "merely anecdotal".   Hundreds of parents have been reporting that their autistic children majorly recovered after chelating out the mercury with OSR#1 (before the FDA "helpfully" banned them from obtaining it).   Some backed up their assertions with videos.   And their reports have since been supported by actual studies such as Blaukoc-Busch et al. (2012).   Such reports cannot be properly dismissed as "merely anecdotal", any more than the finding of a new species of dinosaur fossil can be reasonably ridiculed as an unscientific "mere anecdote".   (The moon landing was a mere anecdote too.)

But the anecdotal reports of parents blaming vaccines for causing their childrens' autism do not have the same evidential value as those anecdotal reports of the recoveries.   That is because we already know that children become autistic anyway and that almost all children have vaccinations at about that age anyway.   So it would be *expected anyway* that some would become autistic at much the same time as the vaccinations.   It wouldn't constitute any great evidence that the one caused the other.   "My child became autistic in the morning and then later that very same day he got vaccinated – outrageous."   For rather obvious reasons you aren't going to hear such a complaint.

It is sometimes asserted that the parents know "what happened" from direct experience and that that needs to be respected.   But the parents only have direct experience of their own case and a limited number of others they have contact with, and probably biased contact even then.   Ten thousand minimally-informed reports do not necessarily add up to one adequately-informed report.

Another unsound supposed form of evidence is court judgments finding vaccines to blame for causing autism.   Court judgments may or may not be well-founded but they are not evidence.   The evidence is fed into the court via witnesses and documents. The output from a court is merely a hopefully impartial guess from that evidence of whether that particular case was probably caused by the vaccine. Likewise, statements from government officials, or from whistle-blowers alleging fraud, are not scientific evidence.

So what would be scientific evidence? The answer is complicated by that problem, that there is a crude bandwagon-parrotting mantra of "vaccines cause autism", which when challenged splits into any number of separate hydra-heads each with a life of their own. MMR before 3 years old. Thimerosal increasing above 125mcg. Or more thimerosal before 1 year old. Or the interaction of MMR and thimerosal. Or it's actually the Hib vaccines now. Or aluminium. Or a synergy with mercury.

The thing is that it only needs any *one* of those proto-theories to be found to coincide with enough of the facts, and then all those who have been proclaiming that "Vaccines Cause Autism" can rest on their laurels of saying "see, we were right all along", and "children with autism = vaccine-damaged children".

Also you must bear in mind that there are two separate questions in respect of each of these hydra-head subtheories, namely "has vaccine x caused *any* autism cases?", and "has vaccine x caused *a major increase* of autism?" It is my view that we don't have enough evidence to answer any of the first category of questions, that we cannot rule out the possibility that *some* vaccines have caused *some* autism.

So in the following I am going to be only concerned with whether any vaccines have caused *the (or at least a) major increase* of autism.

I'll now try to go through examining as many of these sub-theories as I can manage before going insane myself here. I should point out that the antiinnatia theory (of multiple antiinnatia factors) would be fully compatible with any of these vaccine theories, so I personally have no reason to be biased for or against any here.

Aluminium in vaccines. In the earlier section on graphs, I showed that T&S's data strongly undermines that theory rather than supports it.

Thimerosal (ethylmercury) in vaccines. I've already pointed out the non-existence of the alleged changepoint of 1988 reckoned to coincide with the increasing of mercury in vaccines. My Figure 6.5 fails to see even the slightest impact of the increase and then decrease of thimerosal. The curve is readily fully explainable in terms of just non-gamma-2 amalgams alone (as per Chapter 3). Furthermore, the removal of thimerosal in Sweden and Denmark did not produce any fall of autism (as discussed in Chapter 3's section titled "Increased autism?").

And ditto in the UK and US, even though US levels continuing to be used via influenza vaccines are much lower than the pre-1999 levels.

Bernard (2003) tried to argue that the data from Denmark in reality showed a decrease following discontinuation of thimerosal. But that is predicated on an assumption that the inpatient/ outpatient ratio did not change over some years when autism was apparently rapidly increasing.   Whereas in reality it is highly probable that a rapid increase of autism would cause the inpatient ratio to rapidly fall as well, as inpatient resources would fail to keep up with the unexpected demand. And further objections to Bernard (2003) were explained by Hviid (2004).

Advocates of the thimerosal theory of the autism increase have often cited the VSD (Vaccine Safety Datalink) studies as damning proof, particularly with regard to the non-public Simpsonwood conference which discussed them in 2000.   There may or may not have been some criminal cover-up in this connection, but more to the point is whether there was some real evidence supporting the theory there.   The original version of the data suggested that thimerosal was causing an increase of autism risk between 11-fold and 7-fold. When it eventually got published in 2003 in the AAP's prestigious peer-reviewed trade propaganda rag *Pediatrics*, the risk had been disappeared to nothing.

Rightly or wrongly? The crucial consideration as I see it is that if there really had been that 7- to 11-fold higher level, then it should have been very visible in that time-series graph earlier in this chapter, comparing changing incidence of autism with changing amounts of thimerosal. But there's no sign of its impact whatsoever.

The VSD study author Verstraeten himself claimed that some artifacts had caused the original ratios. That may or may not be true, but I also suggest as a possible key factor the following.

There is liable to be a correlation between accepting/refusing mercury-containing vaccinations and accepting/refusing having great lumps of mercury put in one's teeth (whether due to ignorance, misinformation, laziness, difficulty finding time, bureaucratic inefficiency, concern about healthcare conscientiousness – these would all add to the correlation), and thus vaccine dose is liable to be a strong indirect group measure of amalgam dose, that being the same amalgam which has evidently (per Chapter 3) caused the (mercury-loaded) autism increase. It's notable that the VSD results varied   conspicuously   between   HMOs   (Health   Management Organisations), which is difficult to explain other than in terms of differing compliance levels between them.   Amalgam is a poor-persons' treatment, so would have strong class and race dependence.

Some vaccine-blamers resort to a notion that all these various time-trend statistics of autism prevalence and vaccine usage are fabricated lies anyway – that various governments are all colluding in falsifying their health statistics. In my experience, government health departments are indeed full of deceiving crooks (as per for instance the "claimant count now controlled" distortion of my Figure 5 in Chapter 3). And yet I find it too improbable that all these autism/vaccination statistics have just been concocted in several countries so as to cover up a causation. A problem with such a rationale is that once you start dismissing any conflicting data as just lies, then you can pseudo-justify believing just about anything. You're no longer discussing evidence and reasoning but instead just whatever you prefer to believe. My own independent experience of studying thousands of studies is that the data is almost never outrightly falsified, even though its interpretation is very often unsound. (But pharma corporations' clinical studies of pharmaceuticals are an exception to this rule.)

(This chapter now jumps to the next page so as to keep graphs together with the corresponding text.)

MMR (or MMR AND *other vaccines)*   I have shown in Chapter 3 why the autism increase must be largely something to do with mercury. So the autism increase somehow being caused by any non-mercury-containing vaccines is implausible. Especially as the entire increase data can be more than adequately explained in terms of just non-gamma-2 dental amalgam alone. And the time-series data does little to undermine this conclusion. I've already pointed out the unsoundness of the notion that certain supposed "changepoints" coincided with certain MMR events. I also pointed out how the graph in Figure 6.6 did not justify the conclusion that it showed an effect of MMR. If MMR had indeed caused an autism increase we would expect to see a fairly conspicuous step-up at (or in years around) the time of its introduction. But we don't. Furthermore there is the data from the UK as shown in this Figure 6.17 here, and from California in this Figure 6.18, which in my view leaves the MMR theory all-but written off. In Figure 6.18 you can see that:

(a) the autism in California substantially increased from 1980 to 1987 and from 1989 to 1994 even though the MMR coverage was hardly changing in those years; and

(b) the conspicuous upward jump of MMR from 1987 to 1989 made no discernable impact on the smoothly steepening increase of autism over those decades.

To my eyes this data strongly suggests that the autism increase has had nothing whatsoever to do with MMR. I consider Dr Wakefield an honourable and conscientious person with great competence in gastroenterology, but sadly as confused as too many others when it comes to epidemiology.

In Figure 6.17 you can also see the annotations by the childhealthsafety website, indicating their theory that much increase was caused by a succession of MMR, then DTP, then Hib. I think at this point the debate is getting rather strained. Even with their more elaborated theory the problem remains unanswered of where the mercury has come from.

MMR affecting specifically black boys. This is the conclusion some are drawing from suppressed data recently leaked by the CDC whistleblower William Thompson, which is alleged to show that there was a significant association with autism among black boys even though there was no association in other groups. On that basis some people are advancing a theory that MMR has indeed caused a great increase of autism, but only or mainly among black boys. The problem with that theory is that if true, then the autism increase, and the recent autism prevalence, must have been largely of black boys. And if that were indeed the case then it would have become rather obvious by now. But on the contrary, a study of 1,626,354 children including 7540 autistic found nothing of the sort, and instead white autistic outnumbered black autistic more than three-fold (1897/618) (Becerra et al., 2014).

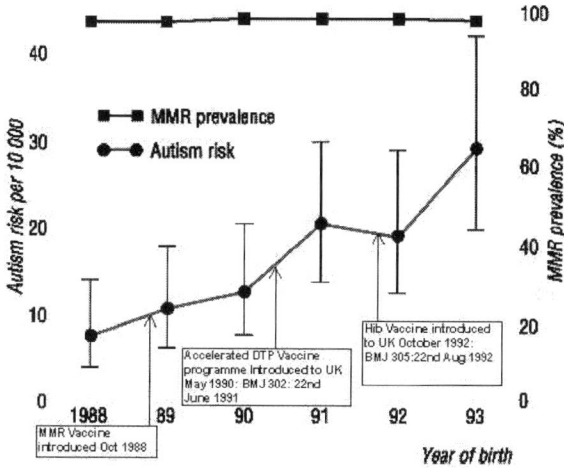

Figure 6.17. Autism diagnoses in UK related to MMR coverage and other changes of UK vaccination schedules. Based on a chart in Kaye et al. (2001) with added annotations by childhealthsafety (2013) website. Vertical bars indicate 95% confidence range.

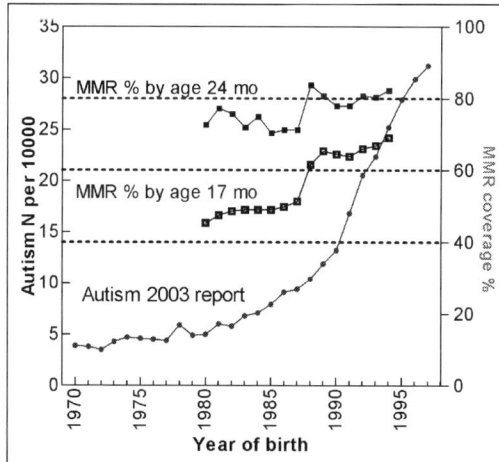

Figure 6.18. MMR coverage and autism enrolment in California. MMR data from Dales et al. (2001) Autism data from California (2003).

Some activists have put together compilations of "16 studies showing vaccines caused autism", or "86 studies supporting the vaccine-autism link", and so on. I've just about managed to stay awake reading through such dossiers but ultimately nothing in them trumps the points I have just made here. For instance, many of the cited studies do indeed show that mercury has been involved in autism, but it doesn't follow that that mercury came from vaccines rather than amalgam. Or animal or in-vitro studies are cited, but such studies can never trump the direct health data facts about humans living in their actual communities and environments. Much fuss has been made in some quarters about some studies of monkeys, but monkeys are substantially different from humans. They grow up and age much faster than humans, don't learn languages let alone pass IQ tests, and no studies have yet shown them having outbreaks of autistic handflapping or echolalia or spinning without dizziness or lining up objects.

The graphs I have cited here make clear to me that vaccines have not been the sole or even main cause of the increase. But they do not have the precision required to rule out the possibility that in perhaps a few percent of cases the main cause has been one or another sort of vaccine. Thus it cannot be ruled out that possibly thousands of parental reports of "vaccine-damaged children" were in fact actually true perceptions of what happened to their child. But neither can it be confirmed. Meanwhile if I were a judge in one of these cases, my inclination would be to side with the parents on the basis of the "Callous Disregard" with which the authorities acted.

I shall also mention here another factor which some researchers have been linking to autism, namely paracetamol also known as acetaminophen or Tylenol®. Some of the evidence suggests a real link, but my own guess is that the causation is primarily due to this ridiculous deadly drug-pusher's profits-generator impairing the glutathione system which is required for lots of important things, not least detoxing of mercury. Thus it makes a person more vulnerable to the amalgam mercury. And the abnormalities of microbiome and immunity are also caused by mercury. The trashy paracetamol is unlikely to account for the autism increase on its own, not least because it is not a mercury source.

This chapter may cause some bruised egos and battered credibilities, of honourable people who have only been doing their well-meaning best in unhelpful circumstances. But the quest for the scientific truth, especially where it relates to such emotionally-salient questions as here, surely has to take precedence over saying that which would be nicer to be able to say about these peoples' proud publications.

I could go on at much greater length here in responding to the yet more complicated confusions built up by those desperately hoping to find a plausible cause (with no hope of identifying the non-gamma-2 of which they are unaware anyway).

I will just add that I consider that the blame for this ongoing tragic complex of disputes lies very much with the deceitfulness of government authorities and of corporatised "researchers" (and more heavily the faceless entities controlling them). The abysmal book by info-nannying millionaire Offit. The gangs of professional liars who have systematically persecuted Dr Andrew Wakefield. The entirely deceitful "retractions" of Wakefield's 1998 case report. The professional "studies" of abysmally low quality published in supposedly leading journals such as Pediatrics and NEJM. It is these who should hang their heads in shame at these abuses of science and such contempt for the abused victims. To say nothing of those faceless anonymous "expert" entities which wrote the cheap filth I replied to in my Chapters 4 and 5 here, in aid of covering up a crime ruining the lives of millions.

And yet this collection of abuses reflects a still larger fact, that behind the epidemics of autism and other disabilities there lies a more fundamental epidemic of sickness, the sickness of a system of medical "expertise" wherein the norm is for deadly deceivers to be showered with honours while the honest are vilified and penalised with false indictments. The Lysenkoism of our time and our place. The *Medical Nemesis* of which Ivan Illich wrote 40 years ago.

But to end this chapter on a more positive point, at least there are those such as Tomljenovic, Humphries, and DeSoto who have been refusing to go along with the corrupt money train. Of which more in a later chapter.

~~~~~~~

7

The peer-reviewed publication
of a still-unfaulted theory

"Robin P Clarke is one of those rare souls with the ability to assimilate and synthesise large amounts of information and generate new and interesting ideas." – Bernard Rimland, founder of Autism Research Institute, founder of Autism Society of America, debunker of Bettleheim's theory, and originator of the modern bio/genetic concept of autism.

"Well worth publishing"
                    – Hans J Eysenck, most-cited-ever scientist.

"Well-written, well-argued, well-documented"
                    – journal's peer-reviewer comment.

"Get your autism puzzle-pieces here!"
                    – Autism research fundraisers.

(You may find this chapter hard to read. I found it hard to write.)

In a preceding chapter I cleared up some serious muddle about *what* autism is in conceptual terms. In this chapter I will set out an understanding of *why* autism is, in terms of causal processes.

A page or two below here I shall paste-in the text of my years-ago-published paper which I re-typed into an Amstrad PCW quite a few years ago, then incorporate some updates and enhancements of presentation. (Puzzle-pieces had no association with autism back then.)

I accidentally came to this theory via some vague impressions I had, that I seemed to have more in common with some historically famous creative people ("geniuses") than with those I met in real life. I did obviously differ from the geniuses in not actually having produced any recognised outstanding works of genius myself. Then my curiosity was increased further on reading that autism was associated with parental high IQ. I wondered what could be the cause of that. I encountered the 1971 theory of Moore and Shiek that autism was caused by "prenatal imprinting". It seemed to resolve the question. But when I showed it to Mike Hunter at Aston University he said he had already read the abstract and dismissed it as no good. I had limited capability of engaging in conversation in those years so I failed to ask him for any further explanation.

But some days or weeks later, when I was as usual still out of bed at a very hushed 3 am. (which I now know is a symptom of mercury poisoning), I wondered to myself what seemed a rhetorical question. The imprinting theory must surely be correct because what other explanation could there be of those links of autism and IQ (and genius)? No sooner had I asked that question than I thought of an answer to it: all three involved reduction of "innate prejudices" (which concept I will clarify shortly). By the next day I had refined that to the idea that they all involved suppression of what I later called "innatons" (meaning innate predispositions, innate preprogramming or tendencies). Let me explain. Autism involved a higher level of this suppression, suppressing valuable innate predispositions relating to communicating and relating (as I knew only three things about autism at that time!). Genius resulted from a more marginal suppression, liberating a person from intellectually-prejudicing innate tendencies such as conformity, self-conformity, pretentiousness, superficialness, wiahful thinking, and presentmindedness (by which I mean the opposite of absentminded-ness). And high IQ was caused by a lesser degree of suppression, only suppressing rubbishy innate junk tendencies ("genetic noise", producing random errors and slowing in the brain – which my first day's terminology would have considered to be random junk "prejudices" (like innately "knowing" that "2 plus 2 equals 5").

The idea was that autism was effectively like a relatively "blank slate" brain lacking some innate human nature tendencies such as recognising other humans as one's own species and interacting with them in conventional ways. I thereafter went off to the libraries to find out more facts about autism, IQ, and genius, to relate to this conception and to test it against. And the more I studied the more I found which fell happily into support of the theory, with nothing undermining it instead.

This eventually resulted in the first version of a paper I sent to journals, which included not only autism and IQ and genius but also various other matters. There followed some further years of self-educated struggling against unknown forces of resistance, during which I concluded it might be easier to get it published if I first separated out the autism part from the rest, and also cut out all mention of the genius part in the hope of avoiding the academic hostility to that concept. Thus resulted a substantial document which was eventually published in the peer-reviewed journal *Personality and Individual Differences*.

This person so contemptuous of theories thus unwittingly became a theorist in defiance of his own intentions.

You need to bear in mind that this paper was originally written for a very different audience some years ago since when a great deal has changed both in autism research and in the wider world. A whole new movement of Neurodiversity pride has arisen, along with some people becoming extremely sensitive to seeming offensiveness of terminology. And I have become much more experienced in writing than back then. And paper-printed journals were very hostile to "excessive" length such that a paragraph about errors and slowing got more squashed than I am happy to see it now.

So for these reasons I am making some very minor changes to the writing, which do not change the actual content or meaning but which make for a better reading experience – it is merely a "translation" to improved language rather than any revision. For the convenience of cynics I will list all those changes near the end of this chapter. In addition I am adding in some update notes in the text, indicated thus: [2014 Update: blah blah...]

Not least I have changed "impairment" to "reduction", and "excessive" to "extreme". This is because some readers would mistakenly assume an implication that the person or their mental functioning is what I mean is impaired or inferior. Also the word "general" is obviously misleading and would be better changed, as explained further on.

I shall also add an introductory outline of the theory here. That is because (strange as it may seem) the original paper never actually gave a summary of the theory itself but only the case for/against it. Instead, after some introductory remarks, it presented a logical argument (guided by some factual pointers), and then followed on with a review of how the evidence stacked up, followed by some concluding remarks. The resulting theory is stated there in the paper but not all in one place or in very explanatory language.

I shall also add an appendix to this chapter relating to the evidence of gene-expression differences in autism.

Finally, just as the paper in Chapter 3 began with an abstract, so does this one here though in this case titled "Summary" instead. Again, you should not let yourself get bogged down by it as you can here just skip to the full article itself. Plus this hopefully enlightening outline which now follows, well, follows after the next bit.

The difficulty of presenting a new concept

Explaining something new to people is often difficult. But it gets much harder when a radically-new concept is involved, and one that is not outrightly simple. The problem is that the terminology does not yet exist for referring to the new concept, and one has to find a way to use the pre-existing set of concept-labels (words) to attempt to describe the new one.

Central to this theory is the concept which I labelled as "antiinnatia" (and antiinnatia factors), and which is the essential thing underlying the autistic syndrome and more. Being a newly invented word, the inclusion of that word in the title and introduction to my paper would have been rather unhelpful, as it would read as meaningless nonsense to all except myself. So I tried to avoid that problem by substituting an expanded wording in the title and introduction, in place of "antiinnatia". Namely "general impairment of gene-expression". I've already told you of my decision to now change "impairment" to "reduction", not due to its being wrong but simply in the context of some people who would start complaining emotionally about my supposedly describing autistics as having "impairments" — such that this theory must be a work of "hate speech" or worse.

But there's a bigger problem, in my use of the word "general" there. It could cause the reader to suppose that I had in mind that all gene-expression is equally affected by antiinnatia, such that autistics would have notable reductions of for instance hemoglobin in blood cells, myosin in muscle cells, collagen in their skin, and so on. Anyone who reads past the first few pages can see that I go on to explain that the reduction is much less general anyway, and instead tends to suppress disadvantageous expressions while leaving advantageous ones unaffected. This theory paper was praised as being well-written, by some very notable readers including HJ Eysenck, Bernard Rimland, David Horrobin, and some anonymous peer reviewers, so clearly this presentational bungle cannot have been too seriously impeding of proper understanding. But never-theless I now consider that that "general" word is less than optimal there, and it appears that the presentation would be improved by replacing it with "evolution-biased". And so in this updated presentation I am also changing the title and introductory sections to remove that problematic "general" word. Meanwhile, the intended meanings are entirely unchanged from the original version.

I should also point out that my meaning of the term "gene-expression" was not confined to the modern narrow sense of generating RNA or proteins from genes (as was already stated in my original). And indeed the picture is now getting even more complicated as it is now clear that the non-"gene" parts of the genome (the "non-coding DNA") are where the main species (and individual?) differences originate anyway. As I see it, the genes are merely the catalog of bricks and tiles supplied by the builders merchants, while the "non-coding DNA" is the construction team and the instructions to them (though somewhat mixed up).

Outline of the antiinnatia theory of autism (and IQ and genius)

(This outline presents only the conclusions without the evidence or reasoning that leads to them. It also does not include any later extensions of the theory.)

There is only one autistic syndrome (including "Aspergers", dyslexia, and so on). There are many individuals each with their own variety of autism causes and outcomes but they all fall within the one syndrome and the one unifying principle explained here.

Autism is not a disorder. Rather it is an aspect of natural individual differences. Exactly the same factors which generally cause high IQ also cause autism at higher levels, and enable potential creative genius in a narrow intermediate range of levels. I have named these factors *antiinnatia factors*, because they suppress or reduce the gene(ome)-expression of innate tendencies or characteristics. Hence anti-innate.

A person with extreme-ish high antiinnatia will be autistic. A person with extreme low antiinnatia will have "ordinary" low IQ. Many autistics also have low IQ scores, but that is caused by a different process than that which causes "ordinary" low IQ, as will be explained.

Humans (and animals in general) have many innate characteristics such as a nose in the middle of their face, eating, breathing, blushing, learning to walk and talk and relate to their own species more than to others. All these innate characteristics depend on gene(ome)-expression of information in the genes(/genome).

Certain factors both genetic and environmental have a tendency to reduce gene-expression not just in respect of individual genes but more generally (though in a biased way as will be explained). The gene-expression processes can be generally reduced by many common factors such as deficiency of energy supply or nutrients, interfering pathogens, gene-expression-controlling regulatory genes, and molecules part-time binding to DNA.

Disadvantageous characteristics are less reliably expressed than advantageous ones. So they are more liable to be suppressed by antiinnatia. These antiinnatia factors consequently have the effect of a quality-controlling filter, preferentially suppressing disadvantageous characteristics while leaving relatively unaffected those characteristics which have a greater evolutionary history of advantageousness. And in consequence of this principle, antiinnatia does not affect the more fundamental aspects of body composition and functioning (which are highly conserved even between different species), but instead particularly affects behaviour and appearance. Thus antiinnatia would not in practice much affect the production of hemoglobin for blood cells, myosin in muscles, collagen for the skin, and so on.

In the normal range the level of antiinnatia has effect mostly in its suppression of disadvantageous "junk" expressions producing errors and slowing of mental functions (and so higher antiinnatia causes higher IQ).

If the level of antiinnatia is much higher than normal it suppresses even advantageous characteristics, thus causing the various features of the autistic syndrome. Most notably, the innate programming for communicating with and relating to other humans tends to be reduced. The autistic brain thus tends to approximate to the notional "blank slate". But there is a twist.

Some human characteristics merely suppress more long-standing characteristics shared by our pre-human ancestors. High antiinnatia suppresses those suppressors with the result that some pre-human characteristics re-emerge in autism (technically known as atavisms). By this means are easily explained such peculiar characteristics as the hand-flapping and toe-walking, and the sometimes occurrence of webbed feet and wide-spaced eyes.

In the original publication of this paper I pre-introduced the concept of antiinnatia with a soundbite-brief description as "general impairment of gene-expression". For reasons explained on a previous page, I have now changed that to "evolution-biased reduction of gene-expression".

Autism is not a condition of the brain but rather of the whole body and beyond. A person can only be autistic in relation to a particular environment (i.e. when their behavior is disadvantageous in relation to that environment such as a highly intolerant community), and cannot be autistic per se. And there can never be any diagnostic test because it is not a disorder anyway.

Finally, it is important to note that this initial paper is considerably strengthened now by major evidential updates such as those in chapters 3 and 16.

Even more finally - the antiinnatia concept is not the slightest bit "controversial". Infinitely more controversial is the utterly crackpot-wacko notion that antiinnatia would not exist or manifest as autism, as is explained at pages 325-26 here.

Author's [nearly-]unrevised reprint of:
Personality and Individual Differences Vol.14, pp. 465-482
(Copyright Pergamon Press)

A theory of evolution-biased reduction of gene-expression manifesting as autism

Robin P Clarke, Birmingham, England,

Summary--This is the first part of a combined theory of autism and general intelligence (IQ).   It is argued that "evolution-biased reduction of gene-expression", produced by a diversity of environmental and genetic causes, is in moderation advantageous in reducing genetic idiosyncracies.   But in extreme it will produce a condition involving atypicalities of appearance and behaviour, with a particular relationship to high parental social class and IQ and with particular sex distributions.   Characteristics and findings relating to schizophrenia, manic-depressive illness, or neuroses indicate that they cannot reasonably be considered manifestations of extreme evolution-biased reduction of gene-expression.   By contrast, characteristics and findings relating to autism accord very well with this conception.   The suggestion is that autism involves primary atypicalities in diverse parts of the brain and in diverse psychological functions.   Random binding to DNA may be a substantial mechanism of evolution-biased reduction of gene-expression.   [2014 Update to the preceding sentence: i.e., would *definitely* cause reduction of gene-expression, and hence cause autism, but only *may* be *substantially* involved (see para. 15)].

~~~~~

[The main concept of this theory is *antiinnatia*, which could be briefly stated to be "evolution-biased reduction of gene-expression". A more precise explanation of what this means will be given further on here.]

It will be argued that the most prominent effect of varying levels of "evolution-biased reduction of gene-expression" is the production of individual differences in innate general intellectual ability, by variable degrees of suppression of certain characteristics that tend to produce slowing and errors in intellectual processing. But that in extreme it causes the autistic syndrome.   The full application of the theory to intelligence and its correlates will be presented in a separate paper.

There have been many theories of autism. But there appear to be no other theories of how evolution-biased reduction of gene-expression would manifest itself.

The present theory differs from other theories of autism in having the following combination of characteristics.

It is founded on an argument from well-established biological principles, providing it with a basis in the context of evolution by natural selection. Indeed, several conceptions that emerged in the course of development of the theory turned out to be already well-established findings, namely the association of reliability of expression with advantageousness, the re-emergence of long-suppressed characteristics, and the conservatism and resistance to change of characteristics other than of appearance and behaviour.

It provides an explanation of why such a severely biologically disadvantageous condition is not eliminated by natural selection, and of why it is a relatively common mode of failure of the brain.

It addresses an exceptionally broad range of findings about autism (and IQ). These include the wide diversity of behavioural atypicalities (listed in table 2), including some particularly odd ones, such as the distinctive hand-flapping and posturing, and also the physical stigmata, attractiveness of appearance, special skills, above-average parental IQ and differentially elevated parental social class, the fourfold preponderance of males among the severely autistic, and the tenfold preponderance among the mildly autistic.

Numerous specialist readers have found not one finding to cast doubt on the theory, nor any flaw in the arguments presented here. This was not for want of hostility.

And yet the theory cannot validly be dismissed as untestable, or as equally compatible with any conceivable findings. Were such a criticism justified, it would be possible to provide some substantiation by substituting, in place of findings about autism, the findings about other conditions such as schizophrenia, manic-depressive illness, or the like, and then rewriting the pages that follow so as to explain all those findings instead. It will become clear that any such explanations would be not merely speculative but absurd and incredible. For example, why should evolution-biased reduction of gene-expression manifest as alternating mania and depression? Why should it first appear in adolescence, as does schizophrenia, and why involve remissions and relapses? Why should relapses be specifically triggered by hostility from others? Why should it be ten times more prevalent among Afro-Caribbeans born in Britain than among those migrating there, as is schizophrenia? Clearly the charge of untestable explain-all is unwarranted.

The above combination of characteristics is very exceptional in a scientific theory. Publication of the theory should not be further suppressed by facile empty innuendos of "speculativeness" or "untestability", but only by substantiated arguments and evidence that prove able to stand up to rejoinder.

Subsequent to the above words, referees and editors of the British Journal of Psychology, recognising the untenability of all other objections, concurred in the view that the theory made no unforseen predictions (and was thus unworthy of publication even as an article). This is simply not true. For example page [220] predicts sequences of changes of SES and IQ distribution in response to certain environmental factors; page [233] predicts certain EEG findings; pages [227 and 233] predict that rigorous investigation will confirm subjective impressions of tendency to intelligent-looking and attractive appearance. But anyway, note that Darwin's theory of natural selection made no unforseen predictions whatsoever. Why is this "criticism" so damning in this case but not at all in Darwin's case?

The scope of the present theory is the whole of the syndrome that includes Kanner's (1943, 1973) syndrome, Asperger's (1944) syndrome, early infantile autism, pervasive developmental disorder, autistic-like individuals, and others who have one or two autistic characteristics. Wing (1988) and Wing and Gould (1979) describe a broad syndrome, the autistic continuum, involving variation in both number and intensity of atypicalities. The present theory is a general theory of that broad phenomenon; it accords with the evidence of diversity of causes and effects, but is not here extended to consideration of details of causal processes in specific cases, because that would be excessively speculative at present.

Evolution-biased reduction of gene-expression

There now follows a presentation of an argument to the effect that evolution-biased reduction of gene-expression would, in extreme, be expected to give the characteristics of autism. Thereafter the theory is related to empirical findings and to other theories and ideas.

[2014 Update: "Phenotype" in the next paragraph is roughly-speaking a posh word meaning the likes of me, you, or some other living thing. In any case don't let this word bother you.]

Gene-expression in its most narrow conception is the transcription of genetic material into proteins. In this paper the term is used more broadly to denote all or most of the processes through which genes affect the characteristics of phenotypes. It hardly needs arguing that these gene-expression processes are affected by environmental factors (otherwise, variation, physical or psychological, would be totally genetically determined). And it is equally well-established that gene-expression is affected by other genes, such as in interactive effects (epistasis) and that some genetic material, such as regulatory genes, and DNA sequences for initiation and termination of transcription, has effect mainly in enabling or disabling the expression of other (structural) genes. There is evidence that regulatory genes are involved in mammalian brain development (He et al, 1989).

It is here proposed that some of these factors, both environmental and genetic, produce an effect of [relatively] substantially general and [sort-of] indiscriminate reduction of gene-expression. It appears that this is an idea which has not previously been postulated let alone investigated, yet it seems very unlikely that such general-acting factors do not exist. Gene-expression depends on processes that have many possibilities for malfunction, with many common factors underlying (for example) all transcription from DNA, all being dependent on, for example, supply of nutrients and oxygen, and freedom from interference by viruses.

As for the idea that evolution-biased reduction of gene-expression can be produced by genes, it will be argued further on that such genes would necessarily be highly advantageous. This makes their prominent existence virtually inevitable when set in the context of a second consideration, namely that the random generation of a mechanism that rather non-specifically reduces gene-expression is very much more probable than the random generation of (say) innate tendencies required for eating or drinking.

One such mechanism of genetically-produced reduction of gene-expression is described by Watson, Hopkins, Roberts, Steitz, and Weiner (1987). This relates to the fact that regulatory proteins (the products of regulatory genes) not only have a strong affinity for their specific binding sites on DNA, but also have a general though much lower affinity for non-specific (random) DNA sequences; thus there is "part-time" binding to "irrelevant" stretches of the genome. The effect of such random binding is to prevent access by activator molecules and RNA polymerases, thus preventing transcription and gene-expression. Obviously, then, a surplus of regulatory proteins (or pseudo regulatory proteins) would give the postulated non-specific, quazi-indiscriminate reduction of gene-expression, but whether this is the principal or even a major process is not clear at present.

For convenience of presentation, processes and factors which produce this relatively general, sort-of indiscriminate reduction/suppression of gene-expression will hereinafter be referred to as *antiinnatia.* Note that it involves both genetic and environmental factors.

The argument that follows proves that antiinnatia must have a quality-controlling effect, eliminating/ suppressing relatively disadvantageous characteristics and tending to leave those that have a history of advantageousness.

(It is contended that the following two statements are self-evidently true.)

In respect of genes producing advantageous effects those producing them reliably will be more consistently selected *in* by natural selection.   By contrast, in respect of genes producing *dis*advantageous effects those producing them reliably will be more consistently selected *out*. Hence in respect of advantageous effects reliability will become relatively preponderant whereas in respect of disadvantageous effects reliability will become relatively rare. That is, there will be a positive correlation between advantageousness and reliability of expression. But this is hardly a radical conclusion; it is well known that dominant characteristics tend to be advantageous and recessives disadvantageous (though biologists have failed to discover the reason just presented (Futuyma, 1986, p 211)).

Thus, characteristics having more evolutionary history of advantageousness will tend to be more reliably expressed, or in other words, less reliably suppressed, that is, will tend to be less affected by antiinnatia.

The implication of this is that antiinnatia has a quality-controlling effect, tending to suppress recently acquired idiosyncracies (which tend to be disadvantageous) and leaving those characteristics which have a relatively substantial evolutionary history of advantageousness.

It should be noted that the idiosyncracies involved can be both (1) idiosyncracies *within* a species, i.e., characteristics uncommon in the species in question; and (2) idiosyncracies *between* species, i.e., characteristics of a species that are uncommon among related species (e.g., language among mammals). Furthermore, antiinnatia has no magic means of discerning advantageousness, present or past, but rather there is the tendency, for the reasons just given, for a history of advantageousness to correlate with reliability of expression, and hence resistance to antiinnatia.

This quality-controlling effect implies that at different levels of intensity antiinnatia affects different characteristics, and consequently it enables not only the explanation of the features of autism but also of general intelligence and its correlates.

Given the tendency of antiinnatia to suppress disadvantageous characteristics and leave advantageous ones, genes for antiinnatia would be highly and persistently advantageous. Furthermore, because of these advantageous effects, the more antiinnatia genes an individual has, the more healthy they will tend to be, and the more effective at getting on in life and in society (i.e., rising in social class, of which more further on).

But beyond a certain level of intensity antiinnatia would be disadvantageous, as considered in the next section.

Extreme antiinnatia

Extreme antiinnatia would eliminate or suppress not only disadvantageous or neutral characteristics but also significantly advantageous, even vital ones. And some of those characteristics could be psychological ones.

Some readers may be sceptical of a notion that humans have innate tendencies or genetically 'hardwired' predispositions. However, such a view does not stand up well to examination. There is general agreement that animals, including primates, have innate predispositions. And it is not very controversial to suppose that heartbeats, breathing, and blushing inter alia are manifestations of central nervous system innate predispositions. Some persons nevertheless would appear to advocate that in respect of just one species, namely humans, certain aspects of the nervous system do not involve innate predispositions, namely those aspects that have to do with 'behaviour' as distinct from heartbeats, breathing, blushing, etc. Arguments and evidence against this peculiar exclusion have been extensively presented elsewhere (e.g., Wilson, 1978).

Let us make this one very modest and reasonable assumption that humans do have innate behavioural tendencies. For convenience of presentation innate behavioural tendencies and the neural mechanisms producing them will be hereinafter referred to as *innatons*. Thus antiinnatia is here conceived of as producing loss/impairment/suppression of a diversity of innatons. Some suggestions of what particular innatons could be lost in autism will be presented later in the consideration of particular symptoms.

It will now be argued that the effects of antiinnatia would be particularly concentrated on psychological characteristics and appearance.

Most significant *physiological* characteristics are of necessity 'specified' within narrow margins; for example blood pressure and temperature. Reasons for this are (a) that the organism's physiology must work together as an integrated whole and this is only possible if the diverse elements are somewhat standardised; (b) fairly small variations, e.g., of blood pressure or temperature, can produce highly significant reductions of functioning with consequent elimination in natural selection.

By contrast, moderate idiosyncracies of innate behavioural tendencies would be advantageous rather than disadvantageous. This is because (a) uniformity of innate tendencies would tend to produce predictability, with consequent vulnerability to competitors and predators; (b) the diversity would tend to make individuals complement one another rather than compete to occupy the same narrow social roles or ecological niches.

Furthermore, moderate idiosyncracies of appearance, particularly of physiognomy, would likewise be advantageous because thereby biologically dominant individuals could mark their identity, and because families of indistinguishable individuals would be beset by problems.

It is well known that the conspicuous diversity (between and within species) of external appearance and behaviour conceals very great standardisation at the levels of physiology, cell types, and biochemistry (Futuyma, 1986). Thus characteristics other than morphology and behaviour tend to be highly longstanding.

It has already been argued that it is idiosyncracies that tend to be relatively affected by antiinnatia. Thus given these concentrations of idiosyncracies in behaviour and appearance we can expect to find extreme antiinnatia manifested as atypicality of behaviour combined with certain peculiarities of physical appearance. And given the highly conservative unidiosyncratic nature of the other aspects, extreme antiinnatia would not manifest as physical illness except perhaps in the severest cases.

Causes and correlates of autism

This section starts with a number of arguments leading to a particular conception of the relationship of autism to certain causes and correlates, then continues with consideration of empirical evidence relating to that conception.

It will not be proposed here that social class and IQ are causal factors in autism; but some explanation of their nature is necessary here for understanding of findings relating to them.

[[2016 Update: There is much scope for the reader getting confused in the next few paragraphs. Partly we are here again up against the problem of novel concepts never presented before, and somewhat outstripping the writing skill I had at the time. The theory posits that autism is characterised by reduction of human-specific characteristics such as language and walking on feet rather than toes, and by emergence of atavisms reverting to pre-human characteristics (such as the hand-flapping and webbed toes). But ironically in the following paragraphs I am also arguing that the antiinnatia causes the person to be more "average" and "typical", with less random atypicalities away from the human average (such as having an extra toe or one eye larger than the other). So antiinnatia tends to make the person closer to the average of the syndrome of "humanness". And yet as the antiinnatia increases further, the person tends to get "averaged" yet more, towards the average mammal, and hence less "human". None of this is intended to have any moral or political significance; I am simply describing the scientific "how it is" (as I see it at least).]]

There is nothing that uniquely and invariably characterises human beings. They usually but not invariably have two eyes, ears, arms, etc., can use language, solve IQ tests, and so forth. But a fair proportion of humans' offspring are born without a brain, or like siamese twins do not have a whole body to themselves. And to define a human as one having human parents poses the equivalent question of what a 'human' parent is. Thus it is evident that humanness is a syndrome. [2014 Update: Meanings of the word "syndrome" are discussed in Chapter 2 here.]

Just as there are variations between persons in the extent to which they have characteristics of schizophrenia or autism, so persons vary in the extent to which they have characteristics of humanness, in the extent to which random mutation and combination and chance events have made them atypical.

Some persons will be relatively distant from the core of the syndrome of humanness by reason of genetic atypicality of appearance or physical or behavioural functioning. They may be lacking in motivations, abilities, or physical capacities. It is obvious that such persons will generally tend to become relatively low in socioeconomic status (SES). This could well be the major reason why SES is correlated with good health and with IQ, even if not the only one.

[2016 Update: Political projects to ameliorate health inequalities have had notoriously limited success since I wrote that. That's not to say we should not keep trying or that I am some sort of Darwinist anti-socialist. This theory has nothing to do with any political biases, it's just neutral science written by a person consigned by society to the lowest of classes as it happens.]

It will be apparent from earlier pages that [so-to-speak-] genes for antiinnatia will tend, by reducing idiosyncrasies, to increase individuals' closeness to the core of the syndrome of humanness, and hence genes for antiinnatia will tend to be genes for high social class, in the sense described above. We would thus expect any cases of autism that are more hereditary than environmental to tend to come from higher social classes. (The co-involvement of heredity and environment will be considered more fully further on.)

There is much evidence that IQ (general intelligence, g) is a factor of individual differences which has major importance both personally and socially, and that in contemporary populations it is in substantial part non-cultural and inherited genetically (see e.g., Eysenck, 1979, 1982; Eysenck & Kamin, 1981; Jensen, 1980). An indication of the great importance of IQ is the fact that a large number of persons differentiated solely by relatively low IQ are so unable to cope with ordinary life that they have to live in institutions for the mentally subnormal. [2014 Update: This appears to be no longer the case, which could be due to the reality of the Flynn Effect increasing of IQs discussed in a later chapter here.]

The processes of genetic mutation and genetic recombination affect us all. They introduce a random aspect into our genes, a sort of "genetic noise", limiting the perfectability of our genomes. At this point I remind you of the concept of innatons explained about earlier. We would expect this "genetic noise" from mutations and recombinations to also cause "noise" in the functioning at the level of innatons. This could be thought of as random junk innatons tending to produce errors or slowing in mental processing, or alternatively as random junk modifications of non-junk innatons.

For convenience of presentation these unhelpful innatons will be referred to as *IQ impairers*. Being disadvantageous, hence un-reliable (as explained earlier), these IQ impairers would be very liable to suppression by antiinnatia. Levels of antiinnatia too low to produce autism would affect the degree of expression of the IQ impairers and hence help to determine general intellectual efficiency, i.e., general IQ. Thus increased antiinnatia would be associated with increased IQ. We would thus expect any cases of autism that are more hereditary than environmental to tend to have parents with above average IQ.

The disadvantageous IQ impairers would not be eliminated by natural selection because of the constraints on its perfecting power such as pleiotropy, recombination, and new mutations.

It has been remarked above that antiinnatia would be caused by both genetic and various environmental factors. Quite properly it is commonly thought that phenotypes are a product of interaction of genes and environment, and cannot be produced by one or other alone; but where a rare condition such as autism occurs it could be mainly due to one or other of two possibilities – a rare combination of genes or a rare environmental occurrence – and findings presented further on suggest that there is in fact something of a dichotomy within autism that corresponds to this.

The suggestion is that similar outcomes should result from the different causes, but this would not be exactly so, for the reason now illustrated with an analogy.

In this analogy machines correspond to people and corrosion corresponds to antiinnatia. If you store a number of machines in a damp room certain parts such as exposed iron and steel will rust, while other parts such as rubber and paintwork will not corrode. In other words there is a consistent syndrome of 'corrosion'. But supposing the machines are placed instead in a dry room, but there happen to be leakages of water through the roof, then while there will be something of the same pattern of corrosion as before, it will be less consistent and less complete, as some parts will be missed by the water while others will be particularly affected. Likewise the antiinnatia syndrome as produced mainly by environmental events could be less consistent than that produced mainly by genes for antiinnatia. Furthermore environmental factors would give a less 'pure' syndrome since they could produce collateral atypicalities peculiar to themselves (such as spots from an infection). [2014 Update: Incoming mercury, even though it is of course an environmental factor, might in its practical effect resemble more the dampness process than the leakage process, if it is pervasively distributed in the trace levels sufficient to cause autism. At higher levels sufficient to kill nerve-cells, it might resemble the leakage process.]

The conception that emerges from all this is of:

1. A relatively consistent syndrome mainly due to genes, and associated with high parental IQ and SES; and
2. Essentially the same syndrome but less consistently manifested and with collateral complications, mainly due to one of a diversity of environmental events, associated with average or below-average parental IQ and SES;

and we shall see that this is exactly what investigations of autism have found, as will now be explained.

A diversity of environmental adversities have been associated with autism and appear to be causal (reviews include Prior, 1987, and Gillberg, 1988). Besides prenatal and perinatal conditions such as rubella and hypoxia, later developments can produce autism; for example Gillberg (1986) reports a case of 'typical autism' produced for 70 days in a 14 year old by herpes simplex encephalitis.

Folstein and Rutter (1988) and LeCouteur (1988) conclude that evidence suggests that genetics has an important role in causation of autism. The first three studies of table 1 add further support to this.

Smalley, Asarnov and Spence (1988) state that the data are not compatible with monogenic, autosomal recessive or X-linked recessive inheritance for all cases; but that there could be multifactorial inheritance, as with IQ. This is further supported by the existence of a continuum ranging from severe autism through the much milder and more common Asperger's syndrome (Gillberg & Gillberg, 1989; Frith, 1991) to normality.

Comparison of autistic persons having neurological signs – suggesting environmental causation – with those not having them finds that they have essentially the same syndrome of behaviours (Garreau, Barthelemy, Sauvage, Leddet, & Lelord, 1984).

But the most noteworthy findings are those relating to social class and parental IQ.

Decades ago it was thought that findings indicated that parents of autistic persons tend to be of above-average social class (SES) and IQ. Subsequently Schopler, Andrews and Strupp (1979) proposed that these results had been entirely due to various factors biasing the sampling of the autistic population. Among other things it was suggested that lower-class parents would have lacked access to the information and expertise required for description and diagnosis of a then obscure condition; and they suggested that later studies avoiding these problems contradicted the earlier results. It will be argued here that sampling bias does not provide a credible explanation of the findings. And anyway, there need not be one absolute yes/no conclusion in respect of all times, places, and subtypes.

Schopler et al did not prove that sampling bias had occurred, but only showed that some conceivable biasing factors were indeed correlated with SES. And their interpretation is challenged by a number of findings, including Lotter's particularly thorough survey, regarding which they could only suggest that Lotter's unspecified criterion of complex rituals may have been biased.

Sanua (1986, 1987) observed that (a) between earlier and later studies there was a broadening of the definition of autism to include individuals with evidence of organic causation or of brain damage; and (b) all the studies that were claimed to show no upper-class bias in fact showed bimodal distributions of SES. He proposed that the bimodal distributions were due to combining of two separate phenomena, 'genuine' autism and similar conditions with organic (environmental) causes. The relationship of this distinction to the theory herewith will be readily apparent.

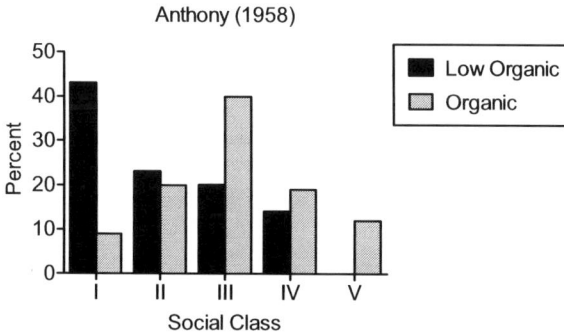

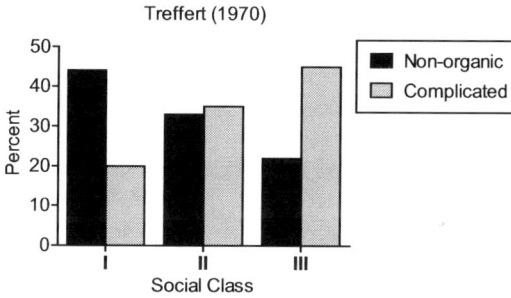

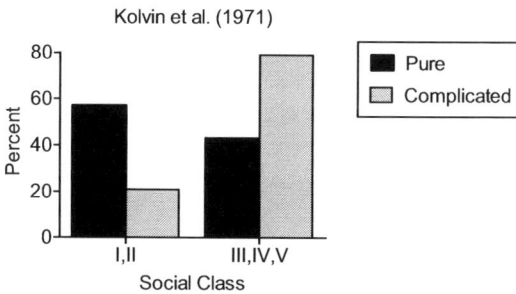

Fig. 7.1. Graphs of social class derived from Table 1 on the next page. (These graphs were not included in the original publication, due to lack of computer graphics at that time.)

Table 1. Social class of parents of autistic persons as found in certain studies [for graphs see previous page]

Author/year/group	N	SES %					p
Anthony (1958)[a]		**I**	**II**	**III**	**IV**	**V**	
Low organic	100	43	23	20	14	0	<0.0005
Organic	100	9	20	40	19	12	
Kolvin et al. (1971)		**I,II**		**III,IV,V**			
Pure	21	57		43			=0.026
Complicated	24	21		79			
Treffert (1970)		**I**	**II**	**III**			
Non-organic	69	44	33	22			<0.007
Complicated	53	20	35	45			
Cox et al. (1975)							
Autistic	19	74	11	16			<0.05
Dysphasic	23	35	9	57			
Fifteen studies[b]							
Autistic (bimodal)	981	42	27	[31][c]			<10^{-20}
Controls	census	17	40	[43][c]			

a   Values of N for this study are estimated/inferred from the percentages; Anthony states only that nearly 100 psychotic children were involved.

b Anthony, 1958; Cox, Rutter, Newman & Bartak, 1975; Creak & Ini, 1960; Gillberg & Schaumann, 1982; Kolvin, Ounstead, Richardson, & Garside, 1971; Lotter, 1967; Lowe, 1966; McDermott, Harrison, Schrager, *et al* 1967; Pitfield & Oppenheim, 1964; Prior, Gajzago, & Knox, 1976; Rutter & Lockyer, 1967; Schopler, Andrews, & Strupp, 1979; Treffert, 1970; Tsai, Stewart, Faust, & Shook, 1982; Wing, 1980; omissions include: Campbell, Hardesty, & Burdock, 1977; Kanner, 1943; Ritvo et al, 1971; Ward & Hoddinott, 1965.

c These numbers in brackets are affected by bimodal distribution and excluded from the calculation of significance.

Three studies of parental SES identify (and compare) groups of organic vs non-organic or pure vs complicated. Their findings are shown in table 1 [and the added graphs]. The probability of all three being due to chance is substantially less than one in 5 million.

Cox, Rutter, Newman and Bartak (1975) did not use organicity as a criterion but did use a comparison group who were dysphasic, a condition they described as comparable in obscurity and severity to autism. Their results are also shown in table 1, and the probability of all four results being due to chance is substantially less than one in 100 million.

The sampling bias explanations were intended to account for the class distributions of autism in general; they were not intended to account for these differential findings. Quite what sampling biases would differentiate between organic/ complicated and non-organic/pure, or autistic and dysphasic? If these differentials really were due to some unknown sampling bias then it follows from the markedness of their results that there must have been a very great preponderance of autistic persons remaining undiscovered.

These results are in line with the general trend which is indicated in table 1 by the aggregated results of 15 studies (including some bimodal distributions); the preponderance of class I over class II has a high level of statistical significance ($p < 10^{-20}$). This suggests that sampling bias has not been a major influence in the generality of studies.

In summary, these findings cannot seriously be squared with a sampling bias explanation, whereas they concur excellently with the theory presented here. And they present the following challenge: what else could be the cause of these differential distributions? Could it be, perhaps, that something in caviar or champagne causes autism and that for some mysterious reason it produces the pure type rather than the complicated? And will this alternative explanation get to grips with many other facts about autism? The objective conclusion is surely that these differentials are powerful support for the theory.

The theory also provides explanation of another characteristic of the SES data, namely the discrepancies between studies at different times and places. Geographical differences may be partly accounted for by the differing distribution of differing persons; for example a rough, noisy area such as Camberwell, London (the location of Wing's study) would attract some sorts of persons and repel others, probably including those with characteristics of Asperger's syndrome.

But there is likely to be a more important process. During the last century there have been considerable unprecedented changes in the environment. These include changes in the chemicals in the air we breathe and in food and drink, and changes in medical technology, not least affecting the prenatal and perinatal environment. And not only is there the aforementioned evidence of involvement of perinatal conditions in autistic etiology, but also the finding of Wiedel and Coleman (1976) of a link with unspecified chemicals.

Now let us consider the effect of such environmental changes on the prevalence of the two categories of autistic persons, namely hereditary and environmental (and note that because autistic persons rarely become parents the autism phenotype is subject to extreme natural deselection).

Suppose, firstly, a longstanding unchanging environment. There would then be a constant ratio of the two categories (genetic and environmental). Suppose that subsequently there is an increase in some ubiquitous environmental antiinnatia factors, perhaps air pollution. Thereupon certain genotypes that had previously been just below the threshold for autism would become autistic, and they would belong to the hereditary, SES-linked category (the environmental factor being ubiquitous). In due course, this new environment would reduce the frequency of high-antiinnatia genotypes in the population, and so the level of hereditary autism would fall again. Conversely, a reduction of the ubiquitous factors would result for a while in the virtual disappearance of hereditary autism, and so on. As regards non-ubiquitous antiinnatia factors, such as obstetric adversities and infections, a different pattern would occur. If a rare perinatal adversity were to become somewhat more common, then obviously, autism of the environmental category would become more prevalent. [2016 Update: This *has* now happened, as shown by Hallmayer et al., (2011).]

Methodologically impressive epidemiological studies are relatively easy to perform in certain countries, notably Japan and Sweden, because of systematic medical data collection covering the whole population. But that very fact attests to the atypicality of those nations in respect of technological sophistication; It follows that studies in contemporary Japan and Sweden could well show only a part of the dynamic pattern presented above.

The only epidemiological survey of the IQ of parents (Lotter, 1967) found substantially above-average scores on the Mill Hill Vocabulary Scale ($p < 0.005$) and the Standard Progressive Matrices ($\chi^2(2, N = 15) = 98.7$, $p < 10^{-20}$). The other studies of parental IQ have given similar, though less marked results (Cantwell, Baker, & Rutter, 1978). Members of Mensa (IQ > 148) have been found to have three to six times the normal frequency of autistic siblings and children (Sofaer & Emery, 1981). though the significance of this is somewhat limited by the small number of cases. Because there is a substantial correlation between IQ and SES, and because this theory proposes similar bimodal distributions for both, these findings must be set in the context of the preceding discussion of evidence concerning SES.

Sex differences in autism and in intelligence variance

Well established findings are that about four times as many males as females are autistic, and that among the less disabled the ratio is even higher, about ten times (Wing, 1976; Lord, Schopler, & Revicki, 1982).

These observations link up with the finding that most intelligence tests have greater variance for males than for females, and that an evoked potential correlate of IQ also has greater variance in males (standard deviation of 59 for males, 50 for females) (Hendrickson, 1982). Hendrickson notes that such a difference corresponds to a male/female ratio of 5.5:1 above IQ 145 and of 47:1 above IQ 175.

There are straightforward evolutionary explanations for greater variance among males. An individual male can have many more offspring than an an individual female, and so exceptionality in a male can make more impact in natural selection. And in a social system where an "alpha male" excludes others from breeding, genes for reduced variance in males would be selected against. [Meanwhile females have only a small number of possible children, so evolution favours them being risk-averse "conservative" and hence more average, hence with that lower variance.]

The relative frequency of different phenotypes depends in substantial part on their probability of arising by random combination of genes and other factors. But the relative frequency of phenotypes also tends by definition to correlate with the relative biological advantageousness of those genotypes that tend to produce them. Hence arises the relative preponderance of exceptionality in males, as indicated by the IQ variances. But the translation from genotypes to phenotypes is, of course, not absolutely directly determinate, but rather involves a spread of probability, through the mediation of environment. Thus there will tend also to be a preponderance of closely related phenotypes (closely related in terms of cause rather than effect). And it will be appreciated that according to the present theory the phenotype most closely related to the highly exceptional individual is the mildly autistic, and somewhat less closely related is the severely autistic. Thus there would be a marked preponderance of mildly autistic males, and a less marked preponderance of severely autistic males, as is found.

What other cause could there be for these observations? [2014 Update: Some have claimed that the preponderance of males is because males are more affected by mercury and or by fetal testosterone. But that merely moves the question on to *why* males are more affected by those factors. They explain only some of the *how*, and not any of the ultimate *why*.]

Emergent characteristics

When this theory was being developed it became clear that some features of the syndrome could not be credibly explained as simple suppressions of innatons, most notably the distinctive rapid hand-flapping alternating with posturing. This led to the idea of "uncovering" (impairment of suppressors) of pre-human innatons, and thence to the following thoughts.

Some differences between a species and its immediate ancestor can be roughly categorised as gaining of a characteristic or losing of a characteristic. A characteristic that has had a long (multi-species) history of advantageousness is likely (as explained above) to be well-established in the sense of being very reliable, i.e., difficult to lose, and in that case losing of the characteristic may most readily result from evolution of a new characteristic that suppresses it. But this suppressing characteristic would tend to be less longstanding, less well-established and hence (as explained above) more vulnerable to antiinnatia. Hence the effect of antiinnatia would be to tend to suppress the suppressor and make the more-established older characteristic manifest again. Thus normal humans could feature suppressed genetic traces of innatons and physical characteristics common among humanity's antecedents, and the autistic syndrome could involve re-emergence of pre-human innatons and physical features.

Lest at this point some readers should be overcome with incredulity, the following should first be noted. Gould (1983) states that "the biological literature is studded with examples of these apparent reversions" (called atavisms) (p. 180). Indeed there is clear experimental demonstration of re-emergence of a characteristic not expressed for more than 80 million years (Kollar & Fischer, 1980; Futuyma, 1986, p 434-6). And a model of DNA organisation (Bodnar, 1988; Bodnar, Jones & Ellis, 1989), with extensive empirical support, shows how information held in DNA "domains" may be suppressed or released by mutations or by environmental factors such as those causing cell differentiation; it also provides a mechanism for atavisms.

There is at least one example of an atavism being produced by both genetic and environmental factors independently, namely the tetraptera mutation in Drosophila. This mutation produces reversion to the four-winged condition that is the norm in higher insects. An identical effect – a phenocopy – can be produced by subjecting normal Drosophila (which have the gene to suppress the extra wings) to either heat shock or ether at a critical stage of development.

However, these reminiscences from evolutionary history could be far from perfect or comprehensive, because of the distortions produced by more recent selection pressures.

Physical appearance in autism

It was argued above that extreme antiinnatia would affect physical appearance, and particularly would reduce idiosyncracies and perhaps also produce emergence of some pre-human physical features. In addition, or alternatively there could be loss of human-specific features (idiosyncracies common to the species), giving tendency towards the average mammalian form.

It was demonstrated by Francis Galton that attractiveness of appearance is largely a matter of averageness, of absence of idiosyncracies. Such results have recently been found to be independent of race and culture (Langlois & Roggman, 1990). Thus because antiinnatia tends to suppress idiosyncracies it should be expected to increase attractiveness of appearance. And in fact, there have been recurrent observations to the effect of autistic persons being of "intelligent-looking", "attractive" appearance. And Walker (1976) found significant occurrences of stigmata as follows: low seating of ears: $P < 0.001$; wide spacing of eyes: $P < .01$; webbing of toes: $P < 0.01$. These stigmata do seem to have a pre-human character but we do not see what might seem more obviously expected, for example fur and a tail. But surely there are other relevant factors involved which account for this discrepancy, namely the complexity and improbability of the genetic coding required for a characteristic, the force of recent selection of the suppression, and the greater importance (in natural selection) and hence reliability of such things as lacks of tails and fur as opposed to slight deviations of form.

Atypicalities of the brain in autism

It was argued earlier that extreme antiinnatia would produce behavioural atyplicalities by preventing or impairing the expression of a diversity of innatons. This could involve primary atypicalities in numerous parts of the brain.

Investigations of brain "pathology" in autism have found a diversity of atypicalities but none of them have been found to be consistently present (reviewed by Prior, 1987, and Gillberg, 1988).

It is not at present possible to discern whether these observed atypicalities are causal of autistic symptoms or are merely collateral occurrences. And it has been argued by Ciaranello, Vandenberg, & Anders (1982) that the causal atypicalities would be in fine details such as elongation of dendrites and axons, synapse formation or establishment of connections with surrounding neural elements. They suggest that "lesions at this stage might be so morphologically subtle as to escape detection with conventional techniques yet have profound clinical consequences".

Goodman (1989) noted that there is a conspicuous lack of agreement about what is the primary neurological "abnormality" (brainstem and reticular formation (Hutt, Hutt, Lee & Ounsted, 1965; Ornitz, 1985; Rimland, 1964), left hemisphere (McCann, 1981; Prior, 1979), mesolimbic system (Damasio & Maurer, 1978; Peters, 1986), cerebellum (Courchesne et al, 1988)), and of what is the primary psychological "abnormality" (social/affective (Fein, Pennington, Markowitz, Braverman & Waterhouse, 1986; Hobson, 1989), recognition/memory (Boucher & Warrington, 1976; Rimland, 1964), handling of complex symbols (Ricks & Wing, 1975), theory of mind (Leslie, 1987), lack of motivation to understand (Frith, 1989)). This led Goodman to favour the idea of a shared vulnerability of several neural systems, involving genetic and environmental factors. Such multiple primary atypicalities had already been proposed by Wing and Wing (1971). These proposals are obviously in agreement with the present theory.

Atypicalities of behaviour in autism

All that remains to be accounted for by the theory is the most significant set of facts about autism: the syndrome of behavioural atypicalities.

Table 2 gives a list of characteristics of autistic persons, based on the list in Wing (1976); I have made additions to Wing's list because it was concerned only with clinical features, and because there have been subsequent developments.

It will be appreciated that with the current limited state of understanding of the mechanisms by which neurons produce behaviour it is not possible to specify the physical form of any of the innaton mechanisms, nor of how they produce their presumed effects. Nor is it practicable to provide conclusive arguments of involvement of innatons in respect of all of the items. But it should be possible to show that there are here a substantial number of atypicalities which can all be plausibly supposed to be caused by loss of innatons, and in many cases strong grounds for suspecting innate involvement.

Turning to Table 2, we come first to atypicalities of communication. A theory of innate predispositions in language has already been proposed by Chomsky (1957) but it is difficult to see any relationship of that theory to these symptoms; hence the present theory and Chomsky's do not seem to offer one another much support at this point. But it seems quite conceivable that Chomsky's universal grammar would not be notably vulnerable to antiinnatia because its mechanism would be relatively simple and hence reliable.

And yet there are a number of facts that strongly point to the conclusion that there is some innate predisposition in language development: (a) language learning is easier for young children than for adults, in striking contrast to the general trend of increase in ability and skills throughout childhood and adolescence – it is surely remarkable that the stupendous task of learning the meanings of words and grammar without the aid of any dictionary or translation can be achieved by children who are in other respects very simple-minded, while intelligent adults take degree courses to achieve a lesser task in non-native languages; (b) humans very consistently develop language competence regardless of environmental impediments and intellectual deficiencies, yet efforts to teach non-humans have consistently failed to reach beyond a very basic level; (c) damage to certain parts of the brain produces impairments highly specific to language; (d) there is a great difference between pidgins and creoles (Bickerton, 1984).

If a person hears utterances in a language unrelated to any he already knows he will not be able to distinguish in what way the various phonemes are grouped into words, since generally speaking words flow into one another without a break, i.e., those spaces between words as on this page do not have a counterpart in the sounds of the language. Would you guess, for example, how to divide up the following utterances in Cornish and Japanese respectively?:

"Unscuberchymblssquythawrukentradhejapelhacusaynuogell."

"Watasiwasukosimoikitakunakattanodesugatootooikaseraretesi maimasita."

Even when forewarned that utterances contain separately meaningful words it must be difficult to discover them, but in the absence of an innate predisposition to search for such words certain characteristics of autistic persons seem inevitable: complete failure of comprehension, and the perfect reproduction of utterances in their

Table 2. Characteristics of autistic persons
(a rearrangement of the table of Wing, 1976, with additions)

A. *Effects of nonfunctioning of innatons*

1. Disorders of communication:
   *Problems in comprehension of speech.
   *Complete absence of speech (mutism) or, in those children who do speak:
   * -Immediate echolalia (parrot-like copying).
   * -Delayed echolalia.
   * -Repetitive, stereotyped, inflexible use of words and phrases.
   * -Confusion over the use of pronouns.
   * -Immaturity of grammatical structures in spontaneous (not echoed) speech.
   *Poor control of pitch, volume and intonation of the voice.
   Problems of pronunciation.
   *Poor comprehension of the information conveyed by gestures, miming, facial expression, bodily posture, vocal intonation, etc.
   *Lack of use of gesture, miming, facial expression, bodily posture and vocal intonation to convey information.
   'Pragmatic' deficiencies of verbal communication (see text).
2. Problems of motor imitation: difficulty in copying movements; muddling right-left, up-down, and back-front.
3. Erratic patterns of eating and drinking, including consumption of large quantities of fluid *[also category C]*.
4. Lack of dizziness after spinning round.
5. *Apparent aloofness and indifference to other people, especially other children.
6. *Lack of imaginative play or creative activities.
7. *Attending to minor or trivial aspects of people or objects instead of attending to the whole.
8. Socially immature and difficult behaviour.
9. Failure to use gaze, facial expression, posture and gesture to regulate social interaction. (a)
10. Rarely seeking others for comfort or affection. (a)
11. Rarely offering comfort or responding to others' distress or happiness. (a)
12. Rarely initiating interactive play with others. (a)
13. Rarely greeting others. (a)
14. No peer friendships in terms of mutual sharing of interests, activities and emotions – despite ample opportunities. (a)
15. Lack of reciprocal eye-contact and social smile in first months.(a)
16. Normal attachments not present when expected. (b)
17. Rarely imitating, even when motivated. (c)

18. Deficit of joint attention behaviours (i.e., showing an object or pointing). (c)

B. Less direct effects of nonfunctioning of innatons

19. Abnormal responses to sensory experiences (indifference, fascination).
20. Spontaneous large movements, or fine skilled movements, or both may be clumsy in some children though others appear to be graceful and nimble.
21. *An unusual form of memory: the ability to store items for prolonged periods in the exact form they were first experienced.
22. *Intense resistance to change, attachment to objects and routines or a repetitive, uncreative interest in certain subjects.
23. *Absorption in repetitive activities, stereotyped movements, self-injury, etc.

C. Emergences of long-established innatons

24. Abnormal responses to sensory experiences (distress).
25. Abnormal responses to pain and cold.
26. The use of peripheral rather than central visual fields *[and or category A]*.
27. Looking at people and things with brief flashing glances rather than a steady gaze *[and or category A]*.
28. Jumping, flapping limbs (i.e. alternate handflapping and posturing (d)), rocking, and grimacing.
29. A springy tip-toe walk without appropriate swinging of the arms.
30. An odd posture when standing, with head bowed, arms flexed at the elbow and hands drooping at the wrist.
31. Erratic patterns of sleeping and resistance to the effects of sedatives and hypnotics *[and or category A]*.
32. *Inappropriate emotional reactions *[and or category A]*.

D. Other suppressions of relatively idiosyncratic characteristics

33. Immaturity of general appearance and unusual symmetry of face. (Attractive appearance, and intelligent appearance, and or stigmata such as low seating of ears, wide spacing of eyes, and partial webbing of toes. (e))
34. *Skills that do not involve language, including music, arithmetic, dismantling and assembling mechanical or electrical objects, fitting together jigsaw or constructional toys. (Some very retarded can read words out loud. (f))

* Items essential for diagnosis of autism as described by Kanner (1943).

(a) Rutter & Schopler (1987). (b) Volkmar (1987). (c) Sigman, Ungerer, Mundy & Sherman (1987). (d) Walker & Coleman (1976). (e) Walker (1976). (f) Silberberg & Silberberg, (1967); Snowling & Frith, (1986); Welsh, Pennington, & Rogers, (1987).

---

entirety as semantic units. And it is remarkable that some autistic persons can read in the sense of translating from printed letters to speech (which 14% of the population of the USA cannot currently do), yet completely lack comprehension (Silberberg & Silberberg, 1967; Snowling & Frith, 1986).

Probably there is also a predisposition towards forming of a conception of and monitoring of the mental state of others, of their intentions, information, assumptions and points of view (this has been conveniently labelled a "theory of mind") [2014 Update: though only some years after I had started mentioning that concept myself in earlier versions of this paper sent to journals and others.]

Its absence could manifest not only in the mixing up of 'you' and 'I', but also in certain 'pragmatic' failures of communication (pragmatics being defined by Bates (1976) as use of speech and gesture in a communicative way, appropriate to the social context).

Pragmatic deficiencies identified by Paul (1987) and Volkmar (1987) are:

1. Lack of use of non-linguistic knowledge in interpreting sentences (e.g., "Colour this circle blue" is only understood if preceded by "I'm going to tell you to do some things").
2. Difficulty in judging how much and what pieces of information are relevant in response to enquiries. (e.g., "Did you do anything at the weekend besides raking leaves?" "No".)
3. Difficulty in identifying the topic initiated by the other.
4. Failure to establish joint frame of reference, e.g., beginning discussion without providing adequate background information.
5. Failure to take social norms or listeners' feelings into account (e,g., "You're very fat").
6. Reliance on limited conventional stratagems of conversation or stereotyped expressions (e.g., "Do you know about Cambodia").

The notion of "theory of mind" is also supported by experiment-al evidence of inability to attribute false beliefs to others (Baron-Cohen, Leslie, & Frith, 1985; deGelder, 1987; Leslie & Frith, 1987); and quite how does the "theory of mind" come about anyway except innately?

Leslie (1987) has proposed innate mechanisms (an expression raiser, a manipulator, and an interpreter) to account for pretend play and the manifestations of "theory of mind". This scheme seems unnecessarily complex – all that is required is innate concepts (or preparedness for concepts) of others having beliefs and attitudes, coupled with the awareness, possibly innate, that such beliefs do not have to be true or logical.

Baron-Cohen (1988) observes that Leslie's innateness theory accounts well for some findings about autism, while others are better explained by Hobson's (1989) theory of innate mechanisms for expression of emotions and their recognition in others. But the theory presented here accounts not only for all these findings but also for the many others indicated in this paper.

It seems likely that the development of language and non-verbal communication depends on not only the abilities of comprehension and expression but also on motivation. Probably a motivation to influence others (to get them to help, etc.) would be an inadequate basis for the learning of communication skills if not accompanied by a motivation towards informing and expressing for its own sake. Only a small proportion of human communication consists of appeals, requests, or inducements to perform desired actions; informing and expressing predominate. Deficiency of such a motivation is suggested by the lack of joint attention behaviours (item 18), the tendency to communicate only to request some favour, and the complete absence of expressive gestures even though instrumental gestures are used (Attwood, Frith, & Hermelin, 1988). Deficits of joint attention gestural behaviours (pointing, showing) are found to predict subsequent language development in autism (Mundy, Sigman & Kasari, 1990). Such motivation and behaviour would presumably either be innate or a consequence of innate reward contingencies.

It also seems parsimonious to assume that nonverbal communication involves in humans as in animals, innatons for its generation and reception.

Certain other characteristics of autism appear to relate to processes that must have an innate element, as will now be considered.

As with the other sensory organs, there must be some innate neural mechanism for detecting and interpreting movement of the fluid in the balance-sensing labyrinths of the inner ear, and deficiency of that mechanism would prevent dizziness caused by the inertial flow of the fluid after spinning (item 4).

A number of the features listed in table 2 could be explained in terms of deficiency of imitating, namely poor control of pitch, volume, intonation and pronunciation, deficiency of non-verbal communication, problems of motor imitation, erratic eating and drinking, lack of pretend play, and the various atypicalities of social functioning (items 2, 3, 6, 8-16, 18, and parts of 1), though it seems more likely that most of these involve loss of specific innatons. But surely, the normal tendency to imitate must itself be innate, and hence all the abovementioned must be dependent one way or another on innatons. It might be objected that imitation could be learned by operant conditioning, but this would still depend on something (namely innatons) providing specifications of what constitutes 'reward', 'punishment', and 'imitation'.

Indifference to some sensory experiences could occur if innatons for interpreting or reacting were impaired. And how else could the orienting response arise other than innately?

The clumsiness of some autistic persons could be due to dysfunction of innatons either directly involved in controlling or coordinating movements, or involved in providing the feedback required for appropriateness of the movements. The alternative gracefulness and nimbleness will be considered further on.

The unusually accurate memory (item 21) can be understood in terms of a lack of innatons that normally produce categorisation, coding, grouping, compartmentalising, or other processing of data. For example, normals remember sentences not as strings of letters or sounds but as strings of words. Hermelin and O'Connor (1970) found that unlike normals, autistic persons do not find meaningful sentences easier to remember than meaningless ones. And the intense resistance to small changes in the environment (as opposed to a complete change of environment) could well be a result of the difficulty the unprocessed memory has in adapting to such partial change – the need to start the memorising all over again. Perhaps there are innatons in normal memory processes for the avoidance of such problems.

It seems reasonable to suppose that a person having many or all of the characteristics of items 1 to 18 and 24 to 32 would find life confusing and unpredictable in many ways. This would result in stress and distress that could be alleviated by reassuring, predictable data, and items 19, 22, and 23 are probably in part a manifestation of this seeking of predictable, reassuring data (perhaps in item 19 "fascination" may be a slight misinterpretation). This accords with the finding that these behaviours are more frequent in unfamiliar circumstances (Runco, Charlop, & Schreibman, 1986).

It has been proposed (Lovaas, Newsom, & Hickman, 1987) that a number of autistic behaviours including these latter involve self-stimulation, and result from the resulting "perceptual reinforcement". This is consonant with the above but fails to explain why certain peculiar behaviours have this self-reinforcing quality exclusively in autism (e.g., the distinctive handflapping, of which more below), or why the behaviours are characteristically repetitive and predictable. Surely, the repetitiveness/ predictability is because the reassurance is rewarding hence reinforcing; and surely the particular repertoire of behaviours available for reinforcement depends on what innatons the individual has – which ties in with the idea that autistic persons have emergences of pre-human innatons.

A number of autistic characteristics seem strongly suggestive of emergences of pre-human innatons; indeed that is how the idea originated. There now follows a presentation of specific instances, then a consideration of the general merits of these explanations.

Autistic persons' short periods of rapid hand-flapping and posturing are suggestive of the bursts of running alternating with rigidity that are seen in birds, squirrels and rats in certain wild contexts.

We do not see foot-flapping such as would produce running, presumably because it has been substantially suppressed by natural selection. However, the mean periodicity of the hand-flapping rate (0.26 seconds) and its mean duration (1.76 seconds) and the mean duration of posturing (1.85 seconds) (Walker & Coleman, 1976) all correspond well to the characteristics of the squirrel and rat behaviours (though these same measurements are re-reported as 0.25, 3.51, and 3.67 seconds by Coleman, 1978).

[2014 Update: Online video of *Purgatorius*, a rat-like ancestor of humans for 160 million years. Online video of 8-yr-old Anthony mentioning that hand-flapping ("stimming") is often accompanied by equally-uncontrolled moving forward. Both observations are remarkably in line with the explanation given above.]

Item 29 suggests the walking manner of a nonhuman primate, in addition to which walking on toes rather than heels is the norm in mammals.

A species idiosyncracy of humans is their upright posture. Most animals stand on four legs, and when such animals stand on rear legs alone they characteristically position their front legs ready to meet the ground when they fall down to it, and they position their heads drooping downwards since otherwise their eyes, ears, mouth, and nose would be pointing upwards. It seems that these same predispositions can be seen in autistic persons (item 30).

Innatons are probably also involved in ensuring that eating and drinking are regulated to the requirements of the digestive system. Innatons more appropriate to animals of different size and with different digestive systems could cause the abnormalities of eating and drinking.

Regarding item 24, a case has been reported of extreme distress induced by the presence of a silver teapot (Wing, 1976), and a similar case involved a silvery spoon with an ornate end. It is well-known that phobias are usually evoked by evolutionarily long-standing stimuli rather than by guns, electric wires, etc. It is notable that in both the present cases a silvery object with one plane of symmetry and of complicated shape was involved. In the pre-human world there would have been no teapots or spoons, and such a shape would usually be indicative of an animal, and if a silvery one, perhaps a reptilian predator just emerged from water.

The jumping, rocking and grimacing of some autistic persons may be a reappearance of non-verbal communications/expressions of pre-human primates.

These notions of emergent innatons are not very testable at present but at least they provide explanation of a number of very peculiar phenomena in terms of a few well-established biological principles, as indicated earlier. The alternative to these explanations is to suppose that by some freak of improbability "it just so happens" that abnormal brain functioning produces this particular pattern of hand-flapping and posturing resembling a common animal behaviour, and "it just so happens" that it also produces this particular standing posture resembling that of four-legged animals, and "it just so happens" that it also produces the manner of walking of most mammals, and "it just so happens" that it also makes infants scared of teapots and spoons that resemble animals in their plane of symmetry, . . . (not to mention all the other facts about autism here integrated together by antiinnatia). In the past fifty years no other alternatives to these "just so" non-explanations have emerged. [2014 Update: Nor in the subsequent 20 years either!]

It might be casually supposed that emergence of innatons could just as credibly account for any conceivable atypicality; but, then, supposing that autistic persons walk on their heels, adopt the postures of ballet dancers, and flap their tongues rather than their hands, what are the equally credible explanations?

It is not necessary to suppose that all the behavioural atypicalities are primary manifestations of lacks of innatons or emergences of pre-human ones. The suggestion of Carr and Durand (1987) that autistic persons' aggression and tantrums occur because of lack of any more appropriate means of expression is fully compatible with this theory.

Two remaining characteristics in table 1, namely gracefulness and nimbleness, and special skills, seem rather unlikely concomitants of a severe pervasive disabling "disorder", but they are quite in harmony with the theory presented above. They may be simply accounted for as further manifestations of the "quality-controlling" effect of antiinnatia, as already exemplified by the attractive appearance of autistic persons and the link with high parental IQ and SES. This may also be the cause of the finding that many (though not all) autistic children show relatively great imagination and productivity in drawing (Boldyreva, 1974).

An important fact about autism is that while a significant minority of autistic persons are of average to high IQ, the majority are markedly subnormal with IQ below 70. According to the present theory all these autistic persons have the characteristic that normally produces high IQ, namely high suppression of IQ impairers, as explained earlier. But if the extreme antiinnatia also suppresses certain other innatons necessary for effective mental functioning, such as innatons for language skill, then low IQ will nevertheless result. Unequal impairment of different IQ-aiding innatons would account for the notoriously uneven scores on intelligence sub-tests (Lockyer & Rutter, 1970), which is exaggerated in some individuals (idiots savants), probably by constant selective practice and social reinforcement of their single competence.

Certain EEG waveforms have been found to show marked correlations with IQ (e.g., Ertl, 1968; Ertl & Schafer, 1969; Shucard & Horn, 1972; Hendrickson, 1982). The theory of IQ associated with this theory of autism includes a mechanism which in computer simulation reproduces the shape of these waveforms; in this mechanism interindividual differences in the waveforms are determined by the degree of suppression of the IQ impairers. Thus it is to be expected that idiots savants and autistics would have waveforms such as are usually associated with high IQ despite being of low or unmeasureable test-measured IQ. This could be a useful aid to diagnosis.

Concluding discussion

Numerous other theories of autism have been proposed, but none of them address more than a fraction of the findings presented here, and few attempt any explanation of why such a severe disorder exists and is not extremely rare. So with good reason there has continued to be a widespread view that the syndrome constitutes an unresolved mystery. The present paper has argued that extreme evolution-biased reduction of gene expression can be expected to manifest as atypicality of behaviour and appearance, with certain relationships to high parental SES and IQ and environmental factors, and a peculiar sex distribution. The autistic syndrome is shown to accord fully with the requirements, whereas other psychiatric syndromes cannot be credibly conceived as doing so. A remarkable diversity of facts about autism challenge the theory, but they all prove consonant with it. Thus, though no scientific theory can be absolutely proved correct, the reasonable conclusion is surely that the autistic syndrome no longer presents a mystery, except in respect of many important details yet to be fully elucidated.

An obvious shortcoming of the theory as presented here is that it provides little or no description, physical or chemical, of the mechanisms of the innatons and antiinnatia. This is unavoidable at present because so much remains unknown about, on the one hand, the precise brain mechanisms that produce behaviour, and on the other hand, the processes controlling gene-expression. If such detailed information becomes available then according to this theory it may be possible to develop drugs to adjust gene-expression such as to prevent or cure autism. Research to date in neuroscience and gene-expression does not seem to indicate any obvious starting points for investigation, other than the possibility of drugs to reduce the prevalence of proteins that tend to bind randomly to DNA. Perhaps other fruitful starting points could be provided by the etiological factors associated with autism. For example, information emerging about the molecular-biological effects of rubella and herpes virus, or of atypicality of the genome associated with autism, could be interpreted in the light of the theory.

The theory does not imply that there is no value in psychological forms of therapy, such as holding therapy, special learning programs, or specially modified environments or routines.

It has been suggested by one of the this journal's reviewers that the present paper has to a substantial extent unwittingly retrodden the same ground as Rimland's 1964 book, and arrived at mostly the same conclusions.

At a time when autism was widely thought to be caused by inappropriate behaviour of parents, Rimland argued against that theory in favour of the conception, which accords with the present theory, of autism resulting from genetic and non-psychological environmental factors.

He also argued that the findings of above-average parental IQ and SES were not attributable to sampling bias. However, his conclusion was subsequently seemingly discredited by the accumulation of subsequent studies that showed no relationship anyway (Schopler et al, 1979, and subsequent). Rimland further proposed that an excess of genes for high IQ tended to produce a vulnerability to autism. The theory presented here concurs with this, but goes further by presenting an explanation of why this would be so, in terms of antiinnatia and IQ-impairing innatons.

The present theory also differs from Rimland (1964) in his positing a single primary disability (inability to relate new stimuli to remembered experience). The fable of the blind men and the elephant comes to mind (they described it in turn as like a tree trunk, a snake, a leaf). Over the years a number of suggestions have been made of what might be a primary psychological or neurological 'abnormality' in autism (listed earlier). Quite possibly most of these are correct as partial accounts of aspects of autism. And their authors were not unreasonable in doubting the validity of other aspects of the then uncertain syndrome. But the suggestion of the present paper is that more or less the whole of the "elephant" has been genuine all along.

Finally, a few words about criteria for evaluation of theories.

There has recently become widespread a view that to be worthy of publication a theory must present precise and readily testable predictions. I agree that these are worthy qualities in a theory, and regret that that presented here is still at some points deficient in this respect. But it seems to me that there is a more important quality that a theory can have, against which precision and ease of refutation are only secondary. This is what we might call its degree of harmony with the totality of facts, its explaining power, the degree to which it encompasses a whole spread of observations within a scheme of a few basic postulates, and integrates them with the canon of existing understanding. Should any reader think this to be an easy quality to obtain, I commend to their consideration the numerous previous theories of autism, of which only a few have been cited here.

There is no reason to presume that reality has been specially designed for the convenience of investigators conducting empirical tests, and those who effectively make that presumption censor themselves from any understanding that does not conform to their preconception.

References

The references cited in this paper were in the original publication listed at the end here as usual in a scientific paper, but as this is incorporated in a book chapter they have here been merged with the list at the end of the book instead.

List of changes made from the originally-published version.

{In addition to a number of notes indicated thus: [2014 Update:....]}

general > evolution-biased [in numerous instances]
impairment > reduction [in numerous instances]
excess > extreme [in numerous instances]
abnormalities > atypicalities [in numerous instances]
hypotheses > conceptions
hypothesis > interpretation
impairments > suppressions
excessive > extreme [in numerous instances]
that > which [in numerous instances]
exposition > presentation [in numerous instances]

Given the existence of innatons and genetic diversity (from mutations and recombination), we would expect to find various odd innatons which interfere with effective mental functioning by producing idiosyncratic errors or slowings. >
The processes of genetic mutation and genetic recombination affect us all. They introduce a random aspect into our genes, a sort of "genetic noise", limiting the perfectability of our genomes. At this point I remind you of the concept of innatons explained about earlier. We would expect this "genetic noise" from mutations and recombinations to also introduce "noise" in the functioning at the level of innatons. This could be thought of as random junk innatons tending to produce errors or slowing in mental processing. (Or alternatively characterised as random junk modifications of other innatons.)

these > these unhelpful innatons
highly sensitive to > very liable to suppression by
Thus ... high > Thus increased ... increased
that is > [none]
[none] > as will now be explained
hypotheses > explanations
hypothesis of sampling bias > sampling bias explanation
Now > Now let us
(note > (and note
environment: there > environment. There
[none] > (genetic and environmental)
; there are additions to Wing's (1976) table > based on the list of Wing (1976); I have made additions to Wing's list
hypotheses > notions
hypothesising > suspecting
is > being
hypothesised > [none]

come about > come about anyway
some readers > one of this journal's reviewers
hypothesis > theory
discredited (so it seemed) > seemingly discredited
hypotheses and > [none]
hypotheses > postulates

Appendix: Modern hi-tech studies of autism causation

Since the original publication of the theory, technology has developed to the extent that changes of expression of specific genes in autism can now be studied. A meta-analysis of such studies was given in a 2013 dissertation by Carolyn Lin Wei Ch'ng. At first thought you might suppose that this should conspicuously confirm the reductions of gene-expression which this theory has as its main premises. And yet an unclear picture emerges instead.

What you need to bear in mind is that the overall amount of reduction by antiinnatia would be very small even in autism. A 50% overall reduction of gene-expression would just about certainly result in gross non-viability rather than ("mere") autism. A more likely level of reduction in autism could be something like 0.1% or even much less, as per the first graph of the last chapter here. And the autism atypicalities would not be caused by body-wide reductions of major protein outputs such as hemoglobin, collagen, and so on. Instead they would be caused by very specific tweaks of special factors in a small minority of neurons or associated glial cells, such as to no longer pre-program those neurons to connect in specific ways to manifest as innate predispositions (innatons).

Researchers would only find these atypicalities if they were analysing the correct very few neurons and targetting the correct small minority of RNA transcripts involved therein.

But there is already considerable difficulty in the relatively rough and off-targetted analyses they are doing. The brain is an extraordinarily complicated and little-understood thing very inconveniently enclosed within a solid skull and not at all suitable for prodding around inside until after death anyway. And so these more challenging studies could be analogous to searching for plastic needles in live haystacks encased in blood-filled "skulls" of concrete. I would like to think that my ideas could someday be triumphantly confirmed with such observations, but it looks like it may be forever impractical. And indeed likely that the entire quest to identify the precise cellular-molecular details of what has "gone wrong" (or more properly "gone different") in autistic brains may never succeed.

And meanwhile there could be better directions for autism research to concentrate on, as can be inferred from Chapter 3 here.

But before I "sign off" this chapter, another line of molecular analysis needs to be discussed. A reader might think as follows. Surely if the theory were correct, then it should be possible to identify the "antiinnatia genes" which it claims to be causing higher risk of autism and high IQ. And yet this doesn't seem to be happening. Instead, there has been at best limited success in identifying any genes clearly and majorly causal of either autism or high IQ, let alone being "antiinnatia genes".

I suspect a first part of the problem is that (as indicated in my original publication) there would be not merely a handful of "antiinnatia genes", but many, something like thousands or more (including variations in the non-coding DNA, hence not strictly "genes"). A minority of those variants might have effect mainly in increasing or decreasing the antiinnatia. But many might be primarily contributing to some other xyz, such as basic cell structure, while meanwhile also affecting the antiinnatia to some extent.

A second complication is what we might call "pseudo autism genes" (and again also including the non-coding DNA). As follows. Let us suppose there is a genetic variation which specifically causes increased shyness (or muteness, or mental incapacity), even though it is not an antiinnatia gene and does not tend towards causing the autism syndrome more generally. Nevertheless, the only thing that autism researchers will be able to see is that that genetic variation is associated with the "diagnosis" of autism. And they would not know that that association is only because a person being more shy (or mute or mentally incapacitated) is more likely to be "diagnosed" as autistic as a result of their shyness (/etc.) and hence "diagnosed" as a result of that gene, even though it is not at all associated with increased antiinnatia or causing actual autism (*per se* rather than "diagnosis" as autistic).

And a third and most important part of the problem relates to a point I made in the opening pages of this chapter. Namely that the main differences are likely to not be mainly in the *genes* (i.e. those lengths of DNA which are code from which proteins are produced), but in other parts of the genome, namely the "non-coding DNA".

This relates to another major mistake in the history of DNA science (alongside the misunderstanding of mutation discussed in Chapter 2). The mistaken wisdom supposed that the information for production of a human or other living entity was contained mainly in its genes, that is the parts of the genome which consist of code which gets "translated" into proteins. The newer understanding, not least since the major ENCODE study, is substantially otherwise (as discussed by for instance Mattick 2013; Parrington 2015; Carey

2015; Maimon 2013). And in fact in retrospect (or in my own case "meanwhile-spect", as I didn't think much about the subject until writing this book!), it is rather obvious that the genes are more like equivalent to just the catalog of components available from the builders merchant, sizes of bricks and tiles available, rather than any instructions from the architect (blind or otherwise). Or more accurately, more like equivalent to a collection of moulds for producing those bricks and so on. And the pattern of "expression" of the genes would also not determine the design, just as merely "expressing" 900,000 bricks, 80,000 tiles, and 40 glass panes would leave much uncertainty about the building that could result from such "expression". Rather, in this newest understanding, it is the "non-coding DNA" which contains most of the information on the "design" or instructions for construction of the organism. It is notable that the differences between species are far more in that non-coding DNA than in the coding "genes". This also answers the mystery of why autism has such a strong "genetic" component (about 1/3 even in Hallmayer et al. 2011) and yet the genomics studies struggle to find the relevant "genes".

(The whole terminology here has got in an even worse muddle than the autism "disorder" nonsense.)

The problem for researchers is that they have even less understanding of the functional significance of most bits of the "non-coding-ome", than they do of the genes. In respect of the actual genes they can at least relate them to the corresponding proteins and then delude themselves that they thereby understand what that gene "does" for the organism.

Meanwhile I should mention that Rett syndrome, which has often been mistaken for autism (or maybe is a sort of autism?) was in 1999 shown to be due to defect of the MeCP2 gene, and *"In fact, the majority of genes that are regulated by MeCP2 appear to be activated rather than repressed."* (Chahrour et al. 2008). Hence the disability involves de-activating of lots of gene expressions. Which was and is of course the central concept of the antiinnatia theory.

Oh well, I'm writing this as the very last bit of this book (gasp!), and I can now latest-update that Casanova et al. (2016) have just now reported that:

"we find that the majority of genes that confer high risk for autism are located within the nucleus and function as nuclear epigenetic regulators."

and

"it is clear that the majority.... are tightly linked with general dysregulation of gene expression, "

Well, what a surprise. (~~~~~~~)

8

Years and years of careerlessness caused by official expertise

"The NHS is our priceless national treasure"
                                    – Everyone who's anyone in the UK

"....we both agree that he would be unsuitable for a university course. There must be many other students that merit the privilege of a scarce place and who would benefit from and respond to the opportunities provided by the University".
        – Confidential letter from doctors to university department

Previous chapters have presented a generalised picture of millions of victims. In this chapter and following ones I present the same matter from the perspective of one particular real person, namely "David".

"David" prefers to remain anonymous for the following reason. Even though the following will just state the facts of David's case, many people will nevertheless react by imposing attitudes onto these facts, such as supposed anger, resentment, negative "complaining", "look at what a tragic victim I am", or the like. But I repeat it will just state the facts. If anyone can really reckon those facts to be justifying any such attitudes then the problem is with the facts and that reader's mental aberrations about them, and not with the person reporting them.

The following will be presented in David's own words. So in the next few chapters "I" will mean David, starting from the paragraph after next here. If you have passably memorised the preceding chapters here, some facts about mercury may ring out loudly at certain points, but you hear them with the benefit of my educating you, and these "bells" did not ring for David until many years later than they should have.

There won't be room for anything like a full biography here. The following is limited to aspects of David's life that are most pertinent to the subject of this book and so you won't find a balanced account of his life here.

My case, by "David"

As a child, I, David, was very conscientious about my health-care. At age 12 I decided I was not going to eat sweets in future, though in fact I'd rarely eaten them before then anyway as I'd always preferred healthy things such as vegetables and proteiny foods such as milk, black pudding, and nuts. At age 15 I had one last aspirin (painkiller) which as usual made no difference to my headache and I decided never to take any drugs again (as indeed I didn't). (Indeed I had already lost faith in pharma by age 10 when I discreetly dumped some medicine I was prescribed.)   And even though I didn't get much toothache I made sure I regularly attended the dentist for treatment anyway, in order to ensure a good future for my teeth and general health. There are so many people who are unwise and casual and sloppy about their health, and self-abusing, but I was about as far as you can get from that.

People are individuals and have differing notions of what they value or want or expect from life. For instance, some want to get married and eventually teach their grandchildren a few things. Some others have no interest in children, or even prefer to have only homosexual relationships. Some resolutely do not want to have any children, whereas some others value them above just about everything else. Some say that it is better for the planet and society to choose not to have children, but I say that such a choice effectively leaves the future monopolised by those who do not care or cannot be bothered (for genetic or cultural reasons or both), which hardly sounds like a better sort of future to me.

Although I was an "intellectual" person and with high aspira-tions I was not a "swotty" person (the sort that works slavishly hard like a dog to please his teachers). Rather at the grammar school there were constant complaints that I was not making enough effort. And yet I easily got high results in exams. In the exams at age 14, in a class of 32, I came first in maths, first in physics, first in chemistry, first in geography, third in French, fifth in Latin, and "He achieves this standard with little effort" (first in physics) and "Not enough effort" (Latin).

The overall life-plan aspiration of myself, David, is a very "normal" one. I am a very "intellectual" person, and highly talented, with rare creative capabilities, and with high aspirations, and it is as inevitable that I should pursue a career as a researcher or discoverer of ideas as it was inevitable that Bach or Beethoven would become composers. So I will naturally go to university by the usual age of 18, get my first degree at 21 or sooner, then go on to excel in masters and doctoral degrees before proceeding on to professorships and so on. I will become very famous and respected for my great ideas. Meanwhile, being friendly and social and good-looking I shall develop the respect of a wide circle of friends, as I consider the company and respect of good friends to be one's greatest treasure. I shall get married at about age 25, and look forward to seeing my grandchildren someday.

Or so it would have been. What happened in the event was entirely different.

Not long after those routinely-excellent exam results, mysterious things started happening. I don't recall the full timing or order of events and no records were made by myself or others. But one of the first things was that I could no longer wake up in the morning. I had originally been going out at 7 am to do my "paper round" – local deliveries of newspapers – but I ended up doing the deliveries at more like 10 am, and after months of failing to get back to the earlier hours, I gave up doing the paper round.

And I developed a crippling problem with writing. I later named this a "writing phobia", though looking back now I'm not sure it was properly a phobia. At school we had to write essays but I could not decide what words to write. In desperation I mentioned this problem to my mother but none of us had any idea what to do so I just struggled on much as I was also struggling on with trying to wake up in the morning. In due course I twice failed the English Language exam which pupils took at age 16. And without a pass in that exam it was impossible to get into *any* university course.

My exams at age 16 were fairly disastrous and all I could do was hope to resolve that I would somehow make up for them in my A-level exams at age 18.

But it soon became clear that that was not heading towards happening. I found I could no longer remember things. And my sleeping problem aggravated to the extent that I rarely got to school before the afternoon, if even then. I felt nervous, embarrassed by my serious difficulties, and "strange" (stressed?). My life had transformed into a constant nightmare with no end in sight. My school reports expressed mystification: "*A rather enigmatic personality* who does not seem to be putting his heart into the work in which he could do so well...". "We all know he has some good qualities. *Why does he fail to show them here?*". "*His attitude and behaviour perplexes me.*" "*His enigmatic personality....*" "A tragic waste of outstanding ability."

I also developed severe reactions to hair-washing and bath-ing (this in the era before people had showers instead). These reactions were not anything visible or measureable but were very harsh sensations as if something was going horrendously wrong in both body and mind. And therefrom I was soon also phobic of hair-washing and bath-ing.

My memory and attention deteriorated to the point that I could not get to the end of a sentence before I had forgotten its beginning. This not only made communication virtually impossible but also thinking. For this reason I resorted to using pencil and paper in an attempt to assist my thinking. Over the next eight years I used a series of about eight secret "thinking books" with which to assist my thinking. Note that these were not diaries or personal "notebooks" but rather crutches for a crippled mind(?)(brain?).

I developed a whole load of mysterious symptoms as per the following list. But note: NO psychotic/schizophrenic symptoms at any time throughout these years of severe mental disability - so it is clear that I have very low propensity to becoming psychotic.

(a) <u>Extreme deficits of memory and concentration</u>. By age 20 this was so severe that I could not get to the end of a sentence without forgetting its beginning, and so reading, writing and listening became nearly-impossible (and I rarely did much speaking anyway).

(b) <u>Much fatigue, lack of energy</u> (mental/physical) for no evident reason.

(c) <u>Extreme indecision</u> ("<u>procrastination</u>"). What most people can decide in moments could take weeks for me to decide.

(d) <u>Severe reaction to hair-washing and bath-ing</u>. Consequent phobia of washing and obvious consequent severe social problems. In 2003 I (incorrectly) thought I had established that this was sensitivity specifically to hot water storage systems and so I adopted use of shower and kettles in substitute.

(e) <u>Extreme instability of circadian cycle</u>, such that I was no longer able to get to school on time, and ultimately at best only able to arrive in the afternoon, and in twenties regularly unable to get up before 4pm (in the days when banks and offices closed by 4pm). Eventually I read a science report in The Times which enabled me to invent and construct an effective light-entrainment system which eased this problem substantially thereafter, but still a significant problem. (That Times report enlightened me that my previous attempts had failed because the light had to be very bright to have an effect.)

(f) <u>Extreme shyness</u>, <u>extreme tendency to blushing</u>, <u>various phobias</u>, including severe agoraphobia/social phobia and phobia of writing (and consequently failed English Language O-level twice) and of communicating in general (obviously now much reduced from earlier). I would stay in my bedroom till no-one was around before hurrying out; would crouch down to avoid being seen through the window.

(g) <u>Inability to adapt to abrupt changes of temperature</u>, such that on entering any public building in winter I always became extremely overheated and sweaty however many clothes I took off.

(h) <u>Blank mind</u>, like writers' block applied to life in general.

(i) <u>Prolonged crash *after* exertion</u>.

(j) Several years of <u>IBS</u>, later managed by regular consumption of glutamine and avoidance of gluten products (wheat etc).

(k) Constant <u>adrenal deficiency</u> such that I had to take bottles of salty water with me everywhere for many years.

(l) <u>Muscular weakness</u> to the extent that I could never do press-ups, pull-ups or squats (until improved in recent years following heavily enhanced nutrition).

(m) <u>Exciteable, restless, irritable</u> (zinc/copper ratio keeps this down).

(n) For many years used to get <u>delirious</u> (non-psychotic), used to get <u>hyperactive</u>; both ceased after I started colloidals containing trace lithium.

(o) <u>Watery sore eyes</u> and painful <u>hypersensitivity to daylight</u>.

(p) <u>Dry skin</u> (subsequently reduced by coconut oil and humidifying).

(q) Slight <u>jerkiness of fine movements</u> (which I noticed was increased by wind-less days; reduced by installing large nose-level ventilation slots).

(r) Eyebrows red with <u>eczema</u>, constant for 20 years.

(s) Disappearance of outer ends of eyebrows.

(t) Female-pattern hair-loss.

(u) Low temperatures down below 35C *(s,t,u = three hypothyroid features)*.

(v) Easily getting confused, silly mistakes.

(w) Persistently unpleasant effect from drinking alcohol (so lifelong non-drinker).

(x) Periodontal disease.

(y) Food allergies.

(z) Depression (till age 25).

(aa) Excessive salivation, waking up choking several nights a year.
(bb) Migraines (till age 25).
(cc) Hot flushes, extreme sweating.
(dd) Neuritic pain (like gnat bites).
(ee) Joint pains.
(ff) Clumsiness (sometimes hopeless at sports).
(gg) Excessive breathlessness on exertion.

My secret thinking books record the many attempts I made to understand what had happened to me and to find out how to overcome at least some of the many problems.

No one else ever did anything to help me or suggest what may have caused this transformation, other than many suggestions that I was "not trying hard enough" in various respects. Basically my own fault. And it's important to factor in that I had grown up in a context of the standard Christian philosophy of mind-body dualism, and for that reason I could have no notion that my difficulties of thinking could be caused by anything to do with one's physical bodily health or the environs thereof.

I could only suppose I had made some error in my thinking which had taken me down a wrong path psychologically. The best I could speculate was that some sort of "stress" was causing the continuation of my problems and I just had to work to get over it. Just "try harder".

I was regularly given the benefit of other peoples' ignorance. For instance I was recommended to "just" wake up earlier with an alarm clock, or "just" go to sleep earlier. If only. I did try arranging a six-day week of 27-hour "days" with a view to getting up and going to college on the sixth day. Which I indeed did but the next day I woke up three hours later and so it had been a complete waste of time. And it had been such a horrible experience that there was no question of repeating it.

Or it was suggested that I could overcome my memory problems by (oh!) "just" keeping a diary and "just" keeping notes. This would-be expertise from clueless superiors overlooks the fact that as a memory-less person you don't remember where you left your diary, don't remember to make the note anyway, don't remember to check you diary, and wouldn't remember where the diary had got left in the meantime anyway.... And so often I had slaved away for hours at making careful notes of something, only to then spend further hours striving unsuccessfully to find those notes again, and then yet further hours making the notes all over again.....

Another problem with lack of memory is that you can't remember people. Which apart from massively impeding social functioning is excruciatingly embarrassing. I resorted to never asking people any questions about themselves and just vaguely smiling hellos at everyone I met. And this in the context that any competent book about socialising will explain that asking questions is exactly what you *do have to* do.

Thanks to a very concentrated effort on the one stupid subject I eventually managed to just about pass the crucial 16-year-old childrens' English Language exam at third attempt at age 22.

Meanwhile I formed a view that the world's most important problems were social-political rather than technological. So I was most interested in social causality but could not see any scientifically-sound useful courses or education in that direction. It appeared that a proper social science would have to be founded on psychology (a premise outrightly rejected by sociology schools). So I sought to get admitted to psychology courses, not in connection with my own (psychological?) problems but in connection with my intellectual interest in developing a scientific study of social causality.

After a few years I managed to get marginally better (or rather give an impression thereof) and at last persuaded a quite notable university to let me into a psychology BSc course five years late so-to-speak. But within a couple of months I was becoming overwhelmed by the same problems again, and ended up just sitting in my room trying to decide what to think, but getting nowhere. I was not in a position to make the connection at the time that that student room had almost no ventilation – just a door at one end and a minimal metal window usually firmly sealed closed at the other. I failed all the exams and my attempts at persuading them to let me continue the course got nowhere.

Some months after being dumped from the university, a crucial "turning-point" event occurred in my life. How crucial? Well, I would have been dead several times over by now if it were not for that fateful night. So you wouldn't have this book to read, among other things.

At the time I was renting a room in a house with some more successful people (had jobs and qualifications etc.). I was in a seriously bad way at the time, with numerous peculiar symptoms such as soaking sweats and phobias and insomnia, which were mysteries to me. I was suspecting that nutrition might have some power to ameliorate these symptoms but that presumably it would just be too complicated for anyone to find out whether that would be the case.

Anyway I was yet again awake till late into the night. And so I was sitting in the kitchen at 3 am. when I noticed a book on a high shelf with its cover wrapped in paper (so the title was not visible). I took it down and opened it.

It turned out to be called Let's Eat Right to Keep Fit, by Adelle Davis. It was full of detailed factual information about the effects of vitamins on health. For instance it didn't just say "vitamin x cures problem y". Instead it said there was an experiment with prisoners testing a B6-deficient diet and they developed symptoms x, y, and z. My memory was nearly non-existent at the time but I read the pages over and over again many times till I remembered at least the key points.

In the next month or so I encountered another book, Manual of Nutrition, published by the regime here in the UK. It was a slim volume, the spaced-out contents of which can be fully summed up as "Just about everyone gets enough vitamin A; just about everyone gets enough vitamin B1; .....". And maybe just about everyone also recognises enough uninformative bee ess if they try hard enough.

I ignored the official advice and followed instead the carefully-argued heresies of Adelle Davis. My health rapidly and hugely improved, though as I knew nothing about mercury toxicity at the time and the book mentioned neither mercury nor the crucial anti-mercury nutrient selenium, it should not be surprising that the improvement was far from 100%. Experts will tell you that Adelle Davis was a dangerous charlatan. And who am I to disagree, notwithstanding that I know of various people who used to be 10 years younger than myself, but subsequently became 10 years older than myself instead.

The following paragraphs I could expand rather a lot if I have time and energy to get back to them.

Over the years and decades I struggled again and again and again and again to make progress in formal education, but again and again I was too exhausted and too encumbered by the various problems to ever succeed to any significant extent, nowhere near getting back into a university course. False hopes were raised again and again and again only to be again and again shattered by the grim realities of exhaustion and other continuing pathology.

I eventually managed after a year of the greatest of efforts to get a B grade in physics, but so what, what piddling use would that be for anything "career"-wise?

Likewise my many attempts at enterprises to somehow earn money invariably fell upon the same obstacles. Meanwhile for years I pretended to be an unemployed person "available for work", because from my most thorough reading of the leaflets there appeared to be no other way I could get social security payments. Eventually unemployment claimants became required to keep applying for jobs and attending interrogations to prove they were. I don't recall quite what happened but I can only suppose that employers started complaining about the jobcentre sending them a person who was clearly completely incapable of doing any job. Anyway, I somehow ended up being transferred to disability benefits instead.

At which you may think that it is so cushy to have a life of leisure along with a guaranteed income. Free time to enjoy all day long. For some persons with only the most minimal of aspirations that may be the case. In my own experience, surviving on minimal income can be a full-time "job" in itself anyway, especially if for most of the time you are too exhausted or dazed or nervous to be able to do anything anyway. The person with money just solves their problem by simply spending money whereas the poor person has to spend many hours travelling in hope of finding something affordable and trying to decide where best to invest what little they have in terms of clothes, household essentials and so on. I've never owned a tv or bought any furniture, let alone owned a car or house. And how does just about everyone define themselves except in their answer to "what do you do?"? And what's my answer to that question? How about: "Oh, I'm a chronically mentally spasticated disabled person." "My, how wonderful, I've always wanted to meet a mentally disabled person and hopefully even to marry one!".

Even though I was a mental wreck and a discard from the education system I did not cease to be an "intellectual" person and highly creative and highly curious. One thing that intrigued me was a reported link between high IQ and autism, and my impression that creative genius might have some similarity to the latter. In the course of wondering about that, I chanced by accident to suddenly think of a new theory of autism and IQ and genius. Subsequently a number of further theories came to me. Indeed I have always been plagued by so many good ideas of which I could hardly find the energy to chase up more than a few. And I meanwhile see so much half-baked rubbish being written by more-energetic "highly-qualified" and supposedly ultra-brilliant others.

Unable to make progress by any other means, I tried at least to make progress by writing up my theories and getting them published. This was made difficult by the fact that I had had barely a few weeks of university education and had a writing disability. But over a period of years I persisted in working at the writing and re-writing and sending to journals, and eventually even famous professors started saying of this person who was unable to pass that most basic of English exams, that "You write well". And three of my medical theories got published in "peer-reviewed" journals - namely those of autism, bipolar, and dementia.

But if you don't have even a first-level "degree" or even a remote prospect of getting anywhere near one, then no matter how many people say "you write well", so what?

Over the years there have been a number of relatively positive moments, but the shadow has always been there constantly that I am still alone, still a complete failure, the most despised of persons, and with false hopes being shattered again and again and again. Where can there be the joy of attending any event, going on a trip or whatever, if one does not have one's (non-existent) partner to share it with? Let alone one's non-existent family.

Decades after this situation began, I happened upon yet another false hope. I decided that my problems had been and were being caused by contaminated hot water systems (due to lack of lids on tanks - now a legal requirement). Confident that I had found the problem at last, I did some plumbing and wiring and installed a shower. But before long I was again finding my false hopes shattered, again found myself still plagued by the same familiar symptoms, even after so many years. I could barely cycle two miles without becoming clapped out for a whole day afterwards. And the thought occurred to me that....

.... it was as if I was being poisoned.

And yet, obviously I was not being poisoned. I wasn't taking any drugs, I wasn't using any household chemicals (not even soap), I wasn't consuming any junk foods or drinks. And there weren't any dubious chemical industries in my residential locale. So of course I couldn't be being poisoned.

But meanwhile one of the greatest revolutions in history was taking place, namely the development of the internet or more exactly the world-wide-web. By this time a huge and hugely-increasing number of websites were becoming accessible on the web. The problem with the web is that any rubbish can be written there. Anything, including the truth. At last. Somehow I picked up from some forgotten website(s?) a vague notion that mercury from my twenty dental amalgams could have been the cause of my decades of disabilities. So it seemed I could indeed be being poisoned – by the amalgam in my mouth.

You may of course wonder why such a possibility had never occurred to me at any time in all the preceding years. What a fool!

But firstly note that no one else ever suggested it either. Not even any health, ahem, experts. For instance after I was dumped from my university psychology course the department staff recommended I consult the university's medical centre, and there was no suggestion of any poisoning then. And five years later, when I went back to that medical centre in hope of getting their support for my readmission, again there was no suggestion. Many years later in 2012 I decided to obtain my medical notes as part of conducting the requests detailed in the next chapter. It was only thereby that I came to learn of a letter that had been sent to the psychology department from the university GP many years earlier at that time of seeking readmission. I quote: *"....we both agree that he would be unsuitable for a university course. There must be many other students that merit the privilege of a scarce place and who would benefit from and respond to the opportunities provided by the University"*. But again no suggestion of any possible toxicity.

When I was a teenager a psychiatrist had ruled out a diagnosis of schizophrenia. And again in 2010 consultant psychiatrist Dr Pradhan ruled out a diagnosis of schizophrenia. And for decades I regularly saw the dentists and students who were replacing the amalgams in my mouth. But at no time did anyone even suggest a possibility of any sort of poisoning.

And furthermore I was familiar with the content of psychiatry textbooks and journals. I knew about depression, phobias, other neuroses, schizophrenia, bipolar, delirium, dementia, autism.....(I'd even had theories published about these). And yet it seemed that I had my own peculiar "David" disease which was not in any textbooks but instead somehow unique to myself.

I did once or twice hear of some controversy as to whether amalgams might cause problems (never specified). But the only thing I ever heard of it was that there was no evidence whatsoever and that it was just silly scare-stories from people who were evidently a bit daft. From those notions I made the reasonable inference that *even if* there were any harmful effects of amalgams they must be something very subtle (and I never heard what sort of symptoms they might be anyway). And so amalgam could hardly be the cause of my life being so utterly de-railed for decades. (And note that even now in 2014 all the official "experts" and their pseudo-qualified GPs are still absolutely insisting that it is impossible for any symptoms ever to be caused by dental amalgams anyway.)

And so I had to wait through decades of illness until the internet and web were developed and those websites finally gave me the hint that perhaps I was indeed "being poisoned".

It would be nice to be able to say that that was anywhere like even nearly the end of this story, but.........

Ten years of further abuse (and still ongoing)

To discover, or more exactly to start to suspect, that you have some severe poisoning, might seem an unhappy discovery. But after decades of having one's life oppressed by an unrelenting mystery, there is a great relief in at last having - even just possibly - solved that mystery and now seeing everything become comprehensible at long last.

You may think that from there onwards it is a simple matter of "just" researching the evidence about mercury poisoning and getting the required help or self-help. But I knew nothing about toxicology beyond the usual vague knowledge about cyanide and arsenic and so on. And knew nothing about mercury other than it being that boring silver liquid in barometers. To usefully research such a field of which one has no prior knowledge would necessarily be a daunting task to a mercury-fatigued person. Worse, even though I had previously been granted a library borrowership by Birmingham University, subsequently just about all the journals and associated indexes had become electronic and accessible only to university members and no longer accessible anywhere by subhumans such as myself.

Of course I could by this time now do instant websearches of for instance "amalgam harm" and so on. But from these, while I did encounter various assertions about how bad amalgam was, I could not find anything by way of solid detailed information or evidence base on which it was founded. It seemed that amalgam was being reckoned to vaguely cause just about everything, just as allegedly also did candida or Lyme disease or electric fields EMF radiation or chronic fatigue syndrome. (The situation now ten years later is very different, with huge amounts of information about amalgam poisoning, not least my own documentations.)

I was very ill at the time and I'm not sure whether I did that websearching before or after my turning point with the dental school hospital. They proposed yet another amalgam replacement. At which I wrote to the head of the dental school querying what evidence there was that it was not harmful. The reply from Professor Trevor Burke cited as supposed evidence eight documents including the childrens' amalgam trials which would be published a couple of years later. I replied back pointing out that the documents were full of absurd self-contradictions and irrelevances and in no way constituted any scientific evidence of harmlessness. I didn't get any further reply. From then on the clinicians shooed me away from the students and other victims over to a private section and agreed to just sort out a glass ionomer for that remaining hole, finalise my treatment, and then discharge me from their register (after being a patient there for many years).

Thereafter I continued to try to research the subject of mercury poisoning and of how to persuade anyone to remove the twenty amalgams, including several crown-sized ones. It would surely cost thousands, which a benefits-dependant simply doesn't have for even the most important of purposes.

In the course of this research I soon learnt two further key facts. Firstly that mercury randomly binds dose-dependently to DNA and thereby impedes gene-expression. This was notable because I had said in my autism theory 20 years earlier that such binding would cause autism. And the second fact was that there had been a change in the 1970s to a newer type of amalgams, non-gamma-2, which emitted 20-50 times more of the mercury vapour. Which would perhaps explain why autism had apparently increased in recent years. So I became occupied with trying to progress that research.

But after only a few months my life was thrown into further turmoil by the harassment operation organised by Nic Bliss and our 20-20 Housing "Co-operative" (www.2020housing.co.uk). Which I coped with for two years until I was then suddenly evicted into homelessness by redacted cheap lies redacted in this edition.

In that context it took me some time to get together my first attempts at persuading anyone to help me with my "crackpot" notion that I myself had been poisoned by the UK government's harmless amalgams. But please be assured that the delays due to these factors were minor by comparison with those produced by others.....

How the NHS "treats" its patients

As I said, after having lost decades my life to this scam, I was shooed aside by the Dental Hospital staff, and finally discharged from being registered there.

Later that year I got over to speak to the receptionists of an NHS dentist, Dr Morse, who was listed as someone who did mercury-free dentistry. I was told they couldn't help me unless I either paid many thousands of pounds or got a letter from a doctor saying I had a (local) allergy to mercury. Which was of course not what was the case in respect of myself. Expeditions to two other dentists were equally unproductive.

In 2006, I got together some evidence which I showed to my GP Dr Daniell. On following up she responded that she was unconvinced but would "as a precaution" refer me for removals to the Queen Elizabeth Hospital (now replaced by the grand Queen Malala hospital). Thus began the wild-goose-chase.

2004

- Requested Dental Hospital to show evidence of safety; defective response from Prof Burke; then they failed to answer my rebuttal; they abruptly shooed me away from their other victims of disinformed consent.
- **Dental Hospital said I should see a doctor instead**.

2006

- **GP Dr Daniell made referral to the QE Hospital** for amalgam removal "as a precaution".
- **QE Hospital said they could not do the removals**.
- **Referral switched to Dental Hospital**.
- **Dental Hospital Consultant Stephen Chambers said a student would do the removals**.
- Six months later, on attending the student appointment, was told that **Dental Hospital could not do the removals after all**.

    Stephen Chambers sent to my GP a **secret letter containing three nastily-calculated libel lies** (that I had concealed my previous registration; had concealed that there had been a "lengthy" correspondence; had been discharged several times with insinuation of unworthy reasons).

2008

- 20ᵗʰ March: (after two relocations due to homelessness), new **GP Peter Wright of Karis asserted that there was no basis for amalgam referral, supposedly on grounds of secret letter from Dental Hospital**. In reality that libellous letter from Chambers contained not the slightest evidence about mercury except for accidentally confirming my severe memory difficulty which is actually a most pathognomic symptom of amalgam poisoning.
- 3ʳᵈ Sept: Harley Street dentist el-Essawy found I had world record 460mcg/m³ oral mercury vapour (unprovoked, open mouth) and recommended melisa test of immune cells reactivity.

2009

- Harley St Melisa test positive 3/3 mercury.
- New GP Dr Peter Gini of Broadway Health Centre said **I should see a dentist instead**.
- NHS Dentist Deborah Morse said **I should see a doctor instead**.
- Dr Gini said **I should instead get the dentist to send a request**.
- **After a lot of chasing, eventually the dentist's request was received by GP's fax**.

- **Dr Gini wrote back saying he didn't have anything to say about it.**
- **I raised again with Dentist D Morse in a first letter, detailing three violations of directions for use of amalgam (including gold in occlusal and proximal contact).**
- **Dentist replied that not her responsibility to do anything about.**
- **I sent letter 2 in reply.**
- **Dentist again not her responsibility.**
- **I sent letter 3 in reply.**
- **Dentist again dismissed the matter,** citing defunct Healthcare Commission.
- **Dentist's phone never answered.**
- 19<u>th</u> October: Eventually I travelled there myself and **the Practice Manager told me they were not contracted to do or refer for Advanced Mandatory and so approval from Contracts Manager Steve Connelly was required.**
- **Steve Connelly said the dentist must do the referral instead.**
- **Dentist practice manager again said Steve Connelly must do it (as not normally NHS funded).**
- **Steve Connelly said I should get a letter from a doctor**
- 10<u>th</u> December: I asked (GP) Dr Verma for a referral to a toxicologist; she said she would have to confer with Dr Gini.

2010
- 29<u>th</u> January: I was told that Dr Gini was referring to a toxicologist.
- 22<u>nd</u> April: Dr Verma said an (unrequested) referral to Dental Hospital had been declined.   And that **referring to a toxicologist would not be useful**, and it would be better to refer to a psychiatrist.
- 11<u>th</u> June: First appt with psychiatrist Dr Pradhan.
- 1<u>st</u> October: **Dr Pradhan declared that there was no capability for diagnosing mercury poisoning** anywhere within the Birmingham/Solihull MHFT.
- So I immediately went back to the GP clinic. GP Dr Zaman phoned toxicologist **Mrs Khan who (under direction of "distinguished" "Professor" Allister Vale) proposed a urine mercury level test**, which even GP Dr Daniell had ruled out as useless 4 years before (and Dr Verma had too on 22nd April).

- So I myself phoned Mrs Kahn. She explained that a urine test was the standard test for occupational recent mercury intake, and that it would (supposedly) indicate whether there was currently significant mercury input from the amalgams. Re which so what, given that I had huge vapour measurement and fully positive Melisa results and a whole army of ruinous chronic symptoms unexplained any other way. She refused to discuss this baseless pseudoscience any further (re which see Freedom of Information request in Chapter 3), proposing instead that I could discuss it with my GP (though they consistently refused to do so too).

- 9th November: I took a letter to Dr Gini questioning the pseudoscience of Mrs Khan's proposed test.

- 10th November: **Dr Gini wrote back that "....this is a dental problem....please arrange to see any dentist of your choice.** Unfortunately we cannot take this any further."

- 11th November: I delivered a reply to Dr Gini, indicating the absurdly conflicting words and deeds of the various people abovementioned, all in conflict with Dr Gini's own last letter. Later the same day I attended an appointment at which **Dr Gini then said that there was a directive from the PCT which prohibited him from dealing with "dental matters".** He said **I would have to enquire of the PALS of the HOBtPCT** about this.

- 15th November: An email from the PALS stated:
"I can trace no directive from this PCT regarding the issue that you raise."

- The same day I enquired by letter of Dr Gini to clarify quite what was the directive to which he had referred.

- 22nd December: A letter (16 Dec; PM'd 21 Dec) arrived from Dr Gini's receptionist which **requested me to make an appointment for a blood test.** (Re which further pseudoscience see Freedom of Information request in Chapter 3.)

- 23rd December: I sent a reply questioning the need or value of a blood test which would also be baseless pseudoscience (as per the quotations above). And also pointing out that I still had not been told what was the directive from the PCT that Dr Gini reckoned was constraining him.

- 29th December: A reply dated 29th Dec from Dr Gini at last included the supposed directive which turned out to be from BENPCT, a letter of 30th Sept 2009 headed "Re: Patients with dental problems that access GP services.", and which turned out to be manifestly irrelevant to my own case, being concerned only with typical dental problems properly investigated primarily by dentists such as painful teeth.

- And yet Dr Gini's letter again repeated the fallacy that I should instead see a dentist about my "dental and allied problems". His letter concluded with **"We .... do not intend to respond to any other communications from you about your dental amalgams."**

2011

- 12ᵗʰ February 2011: I sent a carefully documented report to the PALS of the HOBtPCT, requesting proper diagnosis and treatment action.

- 23ʳᵈ March: I received a reply from the PALS indicating that **my (*non*-dental) problems had been referred exclusively to their dental advisory panel** (with no expertise in psychiatry, neurology, toxicology, etc); which is logically equivalent to them referring the autopsy of a suspected murder only to the local union of murder suspects (whose official view is that no murders have ever been committed and the whole concept of "murder" is just a big scare story).

(Note the following incoherences in the above. Dr Daniell (2006) and Dr Verma (22ⁿᵈ April) had rightly said that the toxicologists' tests would be no use. And yet Dr Zaman and Mrs Kahn under the "expert" advice of "Professor" Allister Vale all asserted that they would be useful, even though they could not provide the slightest rebuttal of my demonstration of their quackery. (I learned that "Professor" Vale later proposed the same quack tests for another victim near here, David Jary.)

After they had failed to fob me off with BSMHFT's "birds are highly unlikely to have wings" quackery and then with SWBHNHST's testing quackery, Dr Gini then immediately changed the subject on to BENPCT's "dental problems" nonsense. But if the latter had any validity then why had they first got those other pseuds involved?)

- Following that reply from HOBtPCT's PALS, I filed an extensively-documented complaint to the HOBtPCT about the various above nonsenses.

- 18ᵗʰ October 2011 I eventually received a reply of this date from Denise McLellan, the Chief Executive of the Birmingham and Solihull NHS Cluster. I first should make clear that that letter is extremely misleading. And it completely failed to address any of my challenges to the pseudo-expertise. No rebuttal of my debunking of SWBHNHST's proposed quack tests. No rebuttal of BSMHFT's "birds are highly unlikely to have wings" pseudoscience. No acknowledgement of the gross inappropriateness of referring a decision about mercury poisoning *only* to their *dental* panel (with no toxicologists or psychiatrists). Instead just going along with all these nonsenses and endorsing BENPCT/Dr Gini's deceit about "this is a dental matter" and now adding in two further deceits of her own: her slimy falsehood that he "tried to" "refer" me to a dentist when a <u>referral</u> was exactly what they consistently failed to provide in all these years (when everyone in the UK (except this NHS Chief Exec of course) knows exactly what "referral" means). And the second slimy falsehood of just stating that "Dr Morse suggested that you approach the PCT to ask to consider funding your treatment" without adding the continuation that my request for that funding failed precisely because Dr Gini still refused to provide A REFERRAL.

I then tried to make a "complaint" via the NHS complaints system. But it became clear that that would be a complete and utter waste of time, not least because the NHS works with excellent coordination for purposes of denying honest treatment to its victims but as soon as you try to make a complaint it instantly falls apart like horsetail weed into innumerable separate "trusts" to which separate complaints have to be made with no consideration of how they logically have to be related together. Bear also in mind how mercury poisoning disability makes it difficult to initiate an effective complaint. Just surviving has been as much as I can do let alone also conducting a fruitless unending campaign to get truth from this horde of liars.

... and now just yet another episode along this road ...

While it is important to remove the source of the mercury (if possible), it is also important to take other measures to remove the mercury that is already in the body, at least if the patient has accumulated a large amount over time as I have – huge 460mcg/m3 for several decades. Furthermore, a few months after the mercury source is removed, the body transitions from "lockdown" mode into "let it leak out" mode, at which symptoms can start all over again due to the re-mobilised mercury, as explained on page 52 of Cutler (1999). Whether the amalgams are removed or not, it anyway makes sense to take such measures of "detoxification" as are effective.

This toxin removal phase can take decades if left to natural processes, so some form of chelation may be required. But the options for chelation have been problematic. There are some questionable natural options such as chlorella (of which sadly more later). Otherwise there have been poor-quality chelators such as (at best) DMSA and ALA, neither of which bind the mercury properly so they are very complicated to use and present a risk of severe side effects from re-release of the mercury (and removal also of needed nutritional elements).

I am now at liberty to take some of these dangerous products. Or I could just carry on being horribly disabled and costing the taxpayer thousands per year for more decades to come. Or alternatively I could, or rather COULD, take the infinitely more sensible option of obtaining a prescription for a relatively new product which has been specially engineered to bind mercury strongly with a 180 degree bonding pair, and which has been extensively found to be entirely harmless and to be extremely effective.

But I then encountered yet more of this charlatanism in the form of Dr Zaman's insistence that "we" "cannot" allow me a prescription of this ideal product.

- 29ᵗʰ July 2013 I gave to Dr Gini's receptionist a documented proposal for a "Specials Prescription" of the harmless relatively new product, NBMI (previously known as OSR#1 before pharma-propagandising organisations such as "Quackwatch" campaigned to get its sale criminalised). Ten days later I had had no response so I arranged an appointment to see Dr Zaman.
- 13ᵗʰ August 2013 I attended the appointment with Dr Zaman. Dr Zaman first stated that "**We can't** prescribe that". Note that he did not say "**I am not willing** to…" Instead he presented it *as though some NHS rule prohibits all of* "We" *from doing so*. Which is untrue (unless there is indeed a conspiracy of secret rules of course).

When I queried his assertion, his first excuse was that he had no experience of prescribing it. But that is certainly a bogus objection because on that basis no-one could ever make a specials prescription because by definition they would first have to prescribe it with no prior experience of doing so.

Dr Zaman then started going on about what terrible side-effects it supposedly might have, even though there was ample evidence basis for believing it would have none whatsoever, and in any case should be tried out (however cautiously) as a treatment of the severe injuries these crooks had imposed on me. In any case it's not as if I would be forced to keep taking it, or had been brainwashed by TV adverts propaganda.

On further pressing, Dr Zaman came closer to his real problem, namely that supposedly I could not be mercury poisoned anyway (as all his pseudo-expert colleagues had supposedly proved), and that there was supposedly no clinical evidence of mercury poisoning because I had refused the pseudoscience blood and urine tests (which none of these pseuds had ever even tried to rebut my debunking of nor even answered those FoI questions). In reality I had the substantial evidence of the exceptionally high vapour input levels (and that for *decades*) and the 3/3 positive Melisa immune cell test results but these charlatans preferred to deny any sound evidence anyway, along with the evidence of the huge catalogue of mercury-typical disabilities which supposedly "just happened" for no particular reason.

There is here thus yet more serious deviation from appropriate clinical conduct:

(a) Dr Zaman first deployed the falsehood that "We can't prescribe that".

(b) Dr Zaman next deployed the patently illogical bogus excuse of no prior experience with NBMI.

(c) Dr Zaman thereafter failed to have regard to the fact that the treatment was not being requested for a trivial or temporary condition but instead for chronic severe disabilities such that the option should not be lightly dismissed on very far-fetched grounds of supposedly insufficient evidence of harmlessness.

(d) Dr Zaman was indifferent to the fact that I was left with several far from safe alternatives to resort to in consequence of his violating my right to obtain this ideal harmless option. If unable to obtain this product I could also manufacture it myself even though that requires a dangerous process (involving chloroform fumes and highly exothermic reaction).

(e) Dr Zaman falsely dismissed the diagnostic words of dentist Dr Harvie-Austin, when it was clear that the latter's reference to "definite tolerance issues with the mercury" was explicitly about my "*system*" and was based on that same list of systemic symptoms detailed here.

(f) Dr Zaman then insisted on ignoring my substantial genuine evidence of high mercury load, and instead imposing the dogma of the pseudoscience tests even though he was well-aware there has been no attempt at justifying them against my demonstration of their incompatibility with the actual evidence. He refused to discuss my proof of their complete and utter incompatibility with evidence, just as the pseudo-toxicologists Mrs Khan and "Professor" Allister Vale had consistently refused to.

Dr Zaman then stated that my remaining option would be to complain to the PHSO. And indeed clearly there would be no point in trying to first take it any further with the local NHS or NHS complaints system at this point.

So at this point the story moves on logically and chronologically to the next chapter here, about the PHSO complaints system.

And yet there's even more needs to be included here first, notwithstanding that it has come after my turning to the PHSO.

[NBMI/OSR#1 is now officially registered with names Irminix and Emeramide, and has passed FDA safety testing.]

Following my complaints about the preceding nonsenses, the Broadway Health Centre wrote to say that Drs Zaman and Gini had de-registered me due to "a breakdown of confidence".

I was at this point in much doubt whether it is worth being registered with the NHS anyway, but in the event just to be "safe" I re-registered, with Dr Surdhar at the Five Ways Health Centre. I immediately got prescribed some daily statin due to apparently being about to drop dead from a heart attack. No mention of any possible side-effect downsides or whether there really was a problem other than a "dangerous" cholesterol level (as discussed by Gøtzsche (2013), Kendrick (2014), and others).

Subsequently, on top of the mercury "non"-problem I developed some additional "non"-problems which again no-one helped me with, as discussed in a later chapter here.

But Dr Surdhar did give me yet another free statins prescription without me even having to ask for it. So at least someone is looking after my healthcare. [David's story has now continued quite a bit further downhill, but we have to stop and print this book at some point .....]

NHS Choices!

P.S.: I strongly suspect that the cytotoxic mercury from amalgam also damages a person's facial bone structure such that it becomes disfigured and the person thereafter looks less "classy" than they really are. This seems likely anyway considering that the amalgam is implanted in their face so it would cause most damage thereabouts. I have noticed that some people's faces rapidly become less attractive in their early 20s and I suspect that may be the cause for them too (though only at a later age and much more subtle extent in my own case, due to "strong" genes (as per Chapter 7)).

~~~~~~~

9

The NHS complaints-denial system and the PHSO

"Not only are investigations fixed. But whistleblowers are being threatened by overpaid useless management."
— Richard Farrell-Adams (2015)

"The Ombudsman's conduct in investigating complaints is not too clever either. They refuse to investigate many well founded complaints and have a curious attitude to evidence."
— Rory Graham (2015)

"When you make a complaint using the PALS service inevitably the "professional" clinicians support each other in their statements. Nobody has to admit to a mistake because they don't need to – they justify each other's reasoning in the decisions they take regarding a patient's care. All complaints are reported to Monitor. A very low figure of upheld complaints reflects very well on a Trust. Truth and integrity are sacrificed. NHS culture is rotten to the core."
— Bilbobanks (2015)

The UK charity *The Patients Association* has got here first. They have recently published damning reports describing both the PHSO and the NHS complaints system as "not fit for purpose", and documenting that others have encountered exactly the same utter pseudism as I was going to document here myself.

The PHSO is the Parliamentary and Health Services Ombudsman, the final resort for those who have been left still aggrieved by the NHS's own pretence of a complaints system.

The English words "complain" and "complaint" have very negative connotations, implying selfish negative unconstructive people who fail to appreciate their good fortune or give due gratitude for the efforts others are making on their behalf. In any case, I am not a person inclined towards complaining. Instead I am a person inclined towards challenging of charlatanism and appealing against outrageously unsound decisions, and yet in the language of the NHS and PHSO the only procedure for this is called making a "complaint".

In a preceding chapter I mentioned that Dr Zaman concluded his fiction-filled rantings with the notion that my only remaining option was to complain to the PHSO. Dr Zaman deserves an award for 100% consistency, because he was incorrect even with that notion. I duly sent a carefully-prepared detailed complaint to the PHSO, at which the PHSO replied that I had first to go back to Dr Zaman's practice and the other NHS "trusts" to "complain" to them again. That was despite that it was already crystal clear to me that there was not the slightest danger that any of those organisations would have any inclination to start responding to me with any honesty or rationality any time ever.

In respect of that point, I should explain that concurrently with the ongoing nonsenses of my own case as described in the preceding chapter, I was also pursuing the wider truths and falsehoods via a series of FoI (Freedom of Information) requests. Any public body in the UK is required (at least in hopeful Wonderland theory) to answer such requests and to do so within a month, subject to reasonable criteria. Meanwhile a few years ago some clever people set up a website called "WhatDoTheyKnow", which enables users to make their FoI requests publicly online for all to see, and with the entire exchange on public record thereby. I chose to use that website for all my requests.

My first FoI request was inspired by Dr Pradhan's declaration that there was no capability for diagnosing mercury poisoning anywhere in the entire BSMHFT (Birmingham and Solihull Mental Health Foundation Trust). A few weeks after that I had chanced to encounter Dr Pradhan again in the local Tesco store, and raised with her my mystification about that notion. Her response was merely that she was as baffled as myself. So I made a FoI request to BSMHFT asking what capabilities they had for diagnosing mercury poisoning. The essence of their reply was that they had no such capabilities because "Chronic mercury poisoning is highly unlikely to present in a psychiatric setting".

That reply made me even more intrigued because it was so obviously the very reverse of a major truth. It is on a par with the notion that "Birds are highly unlikely to have wings". So I put in a further FoI request, as to why they had made that statement and on what scientific basis and from whom and how it had originated. You can see that FoI request copied into the Appendix to Chapter 3. You can see how my counter-evidence takes up several pages. And you can see that they failed to answer it (other than with some drivel which did not really answer it, as my reply explained). And its source was some unspecified "professor of psychiatry", not quoting any scientific literature.

As was indicated in a previous chapter here, the very essence of being a professor is excellence in efficiently parrotting the established wisdom of their expertise subject. Any genuine non-charlatan professor would be delighted to immediately rattle off a list of references justifying such a basic statement as "Chronic mercury poisoning is highly unlikely to present in a psychiatric setting". That's what they excel in doing. It follows that the persistent failure over a period of years to supply such a response in the face of overwhelming counter-evidence constitutes fully adequate proof of a charlatan lie. And four years later I am still awaiting that expert evidential justification of "Chronic mercury poisoning is highly unlikely to present in a psychiatric setting".

It should be obvious from the preceding that (a) there was/is something *very* seriously wrong with BSMHFT, and (b) they were/are not minded to face up to that serious wrongness but instead prefer to pretend it isn't there. So what could be the point of wasting yet more of my shrinking lifetime on going back to them with a "complaint"?

My "success" with that FoI request to BSMHFT led me to follow up with others.....

I was intending to continue this chapter with a summary of the way my complaints were treated by the various NHS "trusts" and the PHSO. I wanted it to show you the huge extent of the abusive lies-excuses dumped upon just one of the victims of these scam organisations. But my personal case correspondence alone would fill a larger book than this one, and I'm not sure how soon if ever I could complete the task of transforming it into a sensible number of pages here. And that voluminousness is not due to any verbosity on my own part but instead due to these bureau-rats' endless capacity for finding new ways of wasting their victims' limited time and energy.

In any case, the opening quotations here of the words of others adequately tell the essence of the story. The NHS complaints system and the PHSO ombudsman system are both outrightly criminal scams, heaping further callous abuse on those who have already been abused by the pretended healthcare system and its pseudo-experts. I'll just mention that the NHS functions with excellent coordination for deceiving and abusing patients (and it even leaked out that my case was "well-known" to NHS confidentialitycrats in the area), but as soon as the victim tries to raise any objections it instantly splits into its innumerable supposedly independent "trusts", which he has never even known the existence of before (BSMHFT, SWBHNHST, HOBtPCT, BENPCT, SBTPCT,....), all of which must be formally "complained" to separately and then complained about separately (shattering any coherent big picture), not that it's worth trying to get any honesty out of any of these taxpayer-sponging crooks anyway.

Just one detail of this abuse I will state here. The PHSO demanded that I must indeed first complain to BSMHFT (and all the others) before returning my desperately urgent complaint back to themselves. So I duly sent a carefully compiled complaint to BSMHFT, clearly titled in large bold at the top that it was *a complaint*. After further unenlightening communications to and from them, it was only after eleven weeks that they wrote to confirm that they had now worked out that my complaint, clearly titled "Complaint [etc.]......" was indeed *a complaint* (rather than a lottery ticket or curriculum vitae or annual report or whatever). But even after those eleven weeks they still did not confirm it as a complaint about what I was actually complaining about (namely the false expertise), and they still took seven more weeks to finally issue a baseless blank declaration that my complaint was unfounded. And still they have never done anything to answer my challenge to their "Birds are highly unlikely to have wings" claptrap assertion.

If I find time to do so, I may compile all my correspondence with the PHSO and other complaints pseudo-systems into a dossier to be downloadable from one of my websites such as www.pseudoexpertise.com or www.robinpclarke.com.

~~~~~~~

10

The hideously ugly *un*-truth about bloodletting and leeches

Nun weiter denn, nur weiter, mein treuer Wanderstab!

In my experience, some of the most important things one learns are learnt not by intention but by accident.

Everyone knows how in the past, medicine was dominated by outright pseuds whose favourite "therapy" was extracting the blood of the patients in their care, not least by means of leeches sucking the blood out. Whereas we now understand that to be a primitive load of rubbish now thankfully consigned to the history books.

Until recently, I "knew" that too. But then I had a misadventure as follows.

I had been making great progress in overcoming the problem of too much mercury making me ill, as per earlier chapters here. The NHS had been proving completely useless in any respect of helping me with this. My request for the prescription of the ideal antidote, NBMI, had been blocked by the quack excuses from Dr Zaman and "Professor" Allister Vale.

Meanwhile over a period of 18 months of constant experimenting I had been finding that the only thing that was stopping my terrible sore eyes and extreme photosensitivity (and other symptoms) was doses of the anti-mercury nutrient seleno-methionine of at least 1600 mcg. With lower doses the mercury symptoms were back within a day or two. I was thinking that a person with high mercury levels would likely need and tolerate that high dose or even more anyway, but this was uncertain frontier science so there was (and is) always the question of possible selenium toxicity. (By contrast the NBMI refused me by the NHS "doctors" has no such toxicity problem.)

In that context I was on the lookout for anything else that might be credibly safe and useful for countering the mercury. Now I need to make clear at this point that Dr Mercola is *not* a villain of this piece. Few people in the medical world have impressed me so much with their honesty and thoroughness of research, even though

I do have one or two points of contention even with Dr Mercky. Again it's not Dr Mercola's fault that......

.... I had the great misfortune to read an article by the aforesaid expert. Like many others, he recommended chlorella as a measure against mercury. Chlorella is a sort of food, an algae. Dr Mercola wisely included a cautionary note which no-one else did, as follows.

"So for men using chlorella, you want to have your blood iron levels checked regularly to ensure the iron in your blood is staying within healthy levels. The simple best screen is ferritin. Ideally it should be between 20 and 80 ng/ml. Levels over 150 or higher become problematic and should be treated by blood donations or therapeutic phlebotomies." [Meaning in essence exactly the same as the bloodletting of old.]

So, thought I, that's no problem, I'll just ask the NHS to do that ferritin test and if necessary have those therapeutic phlebotomies.

If only.

Concurrently with taking the chlorella, I was also continuing experimenting with the amount of selenomethionine (SeMet) I was taking. Selenium is known to have a special binding affinity with mercury, producing an inactive compound. But it is also reckoned to be toxic in relatively low levels. The usual doses are 50 to 200mcg a day. But I theorised that as I had such exceptionally high levels of mercury, therefore I might need exceptionally high levels of Se to counter it.

I had for some years been taking 600-800mcg, but by mid 2014 had concluded that high Se was a most crucial factor in countering my horrible mercury symptoms, the most "obvious" of which was light sensitivity. You can "wonder" whether you really are tired at moment x, but you don't need to stop to "wonder" more than a second whether your eyes really are killing you just because you have moved towards a window.

So I switched to Healthspan brand, ten of their tablets a day (= 2000mcg). This just happened to more or less coincide with also starting the chlorella. I soon started getting odd bumpings, twitches, in my chest. I wondered if this might be caused by excessive maltodextrin from those Healthspan tablets (which say only take one a day, not ten).

I then learned about Revici Patent Selenium. This was designed by the great Prof Revici to be specifically taken up by cancer cells, which are then killed by that selenium. So I stopped the selenium tablets and tried the drops of Revici instead. After ten days it had become all too clear that the Revici selenium was completely ineffective for countering mercury, and indeed did only go to cancer cells (of which I hadn't got any anyway). I was getting really bad recurrence of mercury symptoms, not least getting emotionally labile, and in danger of getting angry. But I didn't want to go back to the Healthspan tablets which might have been causing those chest twitches (in reality heart errors known to be caused by iron overload, but I didn't know that at that time).

So, with expenditure of much time and money and a bit of my mechanical wizardry, I set up my own system for filling capsules with selenium yeast. I started out at about 3000 mcg (300 mcg ten times a day). And yet that chest twitching continued.

Meanwhile, after about a month of the chlorella, something really weird happened. The chlorella was a dark powder. Suddenly I found that my urine contained a dark cloud of particles, followed by my kidneys being painful for 24 hours along with being unable to pass any urine for that 24 hours. It seemed that somehow the chlorella was getting out via the urine, and clogging up the kidneys in the process.

I (correctly) guessed that it would be best to drink a lot of water till the system hopefully started again – which it did after the 24 hours.

None the wiser of what was really going on, I restarted the chlorella at a more cautious level. Then I had another of these episodes, the dark cloudy in urine and the 24 hours painful system blockage.

After two months of the chlorella I hadn't yet got round to seeking a ferritin test, and I decided I should stop in case the iron was indeed starting to build up as Mercola had suggested.

A month after stopping the chlorella, I had yet another of these episodes of the dark cloudy in urine and 24 hours of painful blockage. This time it was difficult to believe it could be the chlorella coming out a month after I had stopped it. So I did some research and it emerged that what was really going on was myoglobin getting into my urine. That manifests as that dark cloudy and it causes acute kidney failure which was what I had experienced those three times. And myoglobin is one of the main iron-containing molecules in the body.

So at this point, I realised I already had an iron overload problem. And a bit more study explained to me that the bumping twitching in my chest was actually the heartbeat error characteristic of iron over-loading in the heart. Anyway, at this point the NHS experts would obviously help me to get that iron out again (not least as it was their fault that I had got the mercury problem in the first place and their further fault that I had had to resort to the chlorella to counter it).

If only.

I successfully persuaded my GP Dr Surdhar to order a ferritin test. The result was 140, in contrast to the 20-50 level recommended by Dr Mercola and by the various iron overload organisations. But as far as the NHS is concerned, if you have ferritin below 150, then you cannot possibly have any iron overload problems and cannot be referred for blood removal or even to a haematologist. I could get blood removed via donations, but that was only allowed once every twelve weeks and far too slow for reducing an iron overload problem.

A huge amount of further time was then wasted on trying to find anyone else who would help me get the iron out. Failing on that front, I then I spent another week or two working out how to do it myself instead. And resorted to getting the needles ("blood collection sets") and other bits to do it myself.

But I have a great aversion to sticking things in my arms let alone my veins. And a first attempt got only 220ml out before it clogged, and a second attempt (with an extension I made from an extra blood collection set) only 110ml. Far too little.

Meanwhile I was very exhausted by the iron poisoning. And slowly cycling or walking only a mile was again now my exercise limit. And hair started falling out rapidly.

The combination of mercury and iron poisoning is an "interesting" one. A very important factor against mercury is regular vitamin C in relatively high doses. But the same vitamin C does a great job of picking up the ruinous iron from your diet and depositing it in your heart and liver and so on. So it becomes like learning to hop on neither foot.

And then it got worse. Those who eat and cook liver will be familiar with the very distinctive (and repulsive) smell of liver going off. Fresh liver never has that smell, only liver that has been over-cooked or is going off. And I started to smell that exact smell in my urine. And then I developed a pain in my right abdomen where the liver is. And I found I could only eat a little before getting pain.

Finally, some days later, I noticed that my urine had become slightly green. I hadn't thought that was possible. Surely only plants have anything green in them?

Again I researched and found that green urine indicates that there is bile in the urine, and bile comes from the liver. Well, I'd always assumed that bile would be yellow or brown rather than green, so it was not as if I had had any reason to expect that green urine.

And yet as far as the NHS experts were/are concerned, I still really can't have any problem of iron overload because my ferritin is only 140.

At this point I tried to explain to these dolts with an analogy.

Suppose your house has been flooded by an overflowed river and your furniture and carpets have been damaged by the water. Next day the insurance inspector comes and tells you that any flood damage must be confirmed by a "river level test" (aka a serum ferritin test). And the inspector can see that the river level is fifty centimetres below your floor level, so "therefore" you cannot possibly have any flood damage needing correction. Of course, in the real world, to put your house in order it is not sufficient for the river level to be below your house level, but there must also be further drying out. Which in respect of iron overload damage is the lowering further down to the level of 20-50 ferritin recommended by numerous iron overload organisation people. All the more so in the context that that ferritin test was only taken *after* those three episodes of myoglobinuria had expelled some of the iron.

On my further nagging of Dr Surdhar he agreed to make a referral to a haematologist at the City Hospital. In due course I phoned them and they (Christine Wright and Richard Murrin) told me that I hadn't got an iron problem anyway. Eventually I made progress under my own advice by a combination of 12-weekly donations and taking IP6 powder.

Anyway all that above here is the "how" of how I came to accidentally unearth yet another branch of NHS nasty pseudo-science. And this one is a real whopper too.

I had never had any of those problems, of heart, liver or kidneys, in all those many years before starting the chlorella. Any idiot other than an NHS-trained pseudo-genius can see that I had a serious life-threatening problem of iron overload needing urgent treatment by blood removal. And yet, yet again we see utter nonsense from the NHS pseudo-experts. And yet again a peculiar indifference to the serious problems of the patient. None of these jokers are asking or suggesting why I have these problems which I see as serious and unprecedented in my history. Just as with the mercury, I just get fobbed off.

Why this indifference?

A common theme established by many critics of modern medicine is that it has become dominated by making corporate profits rather than making patients healthier. And there's something really weird about that therapy I was seeking there. Bloodletting was one of the world's most major medical practices for at least 3000 years. It was considered important by the ancient Chinese, ancient Egyptians, ancient Greeks and Romans, and the medievals right up to and into the scientific revolution. But then that long-honoured practice became rapidly transformed into the most derided of ridiculous quackeries. Why that?

A first serious problem with bloodletting is that just about anyone with a knife and bandage can do it. It's not like a drug which they can make money from a controlled supply of.

A second serious problem is that no corporations are needed for its supply.

And so a third serious problem is that it has almost zero potential for generating corporate profits.

And a fourth, even more serious problem, is that it is a very effective and harmless optimal preventer of some very serious illnesses indeed. And that seriously cuts into the profits of the corporate cancer industry, and the corporate profiteering industry of liver transplants, heart surgery, kidney dialysis, and so on ad healthy nauseam.

And so with the rise of corporate capitalist "healthcare", the 3000-year-old expertise of bloodletting found a very hostile enemy. That enemy could not easily prevent people from bloodletting one another, or prevent possessing the tiny needles or blades required. So instead they deployed the credibility of their "expertise" to make it out to be a ridiculous pre-scientific stupidity instead. But here let's look at the real science of therapeutic bloodletting.

Most people know that iron is needed in the hemoglobin of the blood to carry oxygen and prevent anaemia. It is also contained in myoglobin in the muscles to provide a ready-to-go store of oxygen for a sudden burst of movement – a bit like the cache memory in a computer. In a healthy body all the iron is entirely contained in such proteiny containers because unbound iron is a seriously horrible substance to have in your body. Have you ever tried sucking or licking a piece of iron or mild steel? Or a rusty nail? It has to be one of the most revolting of tastes, to which perhaps only copper compares (unless you are anaemic perhaps).

The problem with unbound iron is that it is an extremely strong catalyst of oxidation (like the rusting of iron that produces rust), and unwanted oxidation is a ruinous process in the body. So it is important not to have more iron than can be kept bound in those protein complexes to keep it under control and away from biomolecules which would otherwise be damaged by it.

A further crucial fact about iron is that a man's body has no normal means of getting rid of an excess of it. Well, that is apart from the unpleasant means of myoglobin getting in your urine and causing acute kidney failure as I experienced myself three times.

So as people get older they build up more and more iron. Older people have higher iron and older women have increasing iron too, though older men have the most. And it is well-established that excessive iron causes various problems. These include the heartbeat errors which I developed, liver damage, pancreas damage, and primary liver cancer. In my own case of course I also had much fun with kidney failure. Iron overload also weakens the immune system, causing liability to serious infections. And bloodletting has for centuries been reckoned to counteract that problem. You can now understand why primary liver cancer is much more common in men than women, and yet rare in men under 45 years old. And why women live longer than men.

As Levy (2013) comments: "What happens when the vast majority of the population is abnormal? The answer is that a grossly abnormal laboratory result, like a ferritin level of 390 to 400 ng/cc, is simply declared to be normal."

So now you can understand why my becoming seriously ill from iron overload was not really a problem other than in my head. That river level test proved me wrong.

P.S.: One of my chronic disabilities is that I keep thinking of practical inventions which are beyond my personal means to set up to manufacture to marketable standards. In August 2014 I filed a patent application for a novel container for one or more USB flash pen drives, basically a DVD case with built-in USB socket or cable, so that it is much harder to lose your important data, and more convenient to store it. (And yes I am well aware that some people fail to see that such a product could be found valuable by others.) Unfortunately immediately after I filed that patent application I became very ill as described in this chapter, and being thus plunged into a new unfamiliar field of mystery and misinformation, and becoming very exhausted by the dual toxicities, I just had to abandon trying to find support for developing the invention, not least the £9,000 to get some samples made (without which I would have negligible chance of interesting anyone). But meanwhile my UK patent application GB2529457 is still alive and now published, and if anyone in China or wherever feels like giving it a go as a change from their drives helpfully shaped like frogs or snails, then please don't let me stop you.

PP.S.: An excellent new book about iron overload has been published in 2016: "Dumping Iron" by P.D. Mangan.

~~~~~~~

11

"Did the UK Committee on Toxicity lie to the government about vitamin B6?" (co-authored with Bernard Rimland)

"The COT report on vitamin B6 is the worst piece of pseudoscience it has been my misfortune to come across"
– Dr Guy Matthews MRCS LRCP FRCPath (Commons, 1998)

"this travesty of science, one of the worst applications of pseudoscience that I have ever encountered."
– Prof. Arnold Beckett (1998)

"The COT report on vitamin B6 is an appalling document"
– Dr John Marks MA MD FRCP FRCPath FRCPsych
(Commons, 1998)

The quotations above here are condemnations of exactly the same criminally crooked document as this chapter is about. And that's a document written by the head of a UK medical "school" no less. (Namely "Professor" H Frank Woods BSc BM BCh DPhil FRCP(Lon) FFPM FRCP(Edin) Hon FFOM CBE) In which case, quite how could this system of pseudo-education get any worse than it already is, notwithstanding its insistence on the supplying of references of good character by anyone seeking admission thereto?

This chapter contains an unpublished paper which was mainly written by myself (in 1997-8) though with some input and collaboration from Bernard Rimland (founder of the Autism Research Institute) communicating by fax (as he didn't yet use email).

I had been aware that Rimland had got a number of studies done of the use of vitamin B6 in treatment of autism. I'd also corresponded with him in respect of the autism theory and also of the book "Let's Stay Healthy" which I had identified as falsely attributed as Adelle Davis's "last book" by pharma's anti-nutrition propaganda deceivers after her death (and Rimland replied that he actually happened to be on the board of the Adelle Davis Foundation, such is the small world of competent science).

This vitamin B6 matter began with the Consumers' Association, which was the publisher of the famous consumer advice magazine *Which?* in the UK. The head of the Consumers' Association was "Dame" Sheila McKechnie, who has since then died. I was surprised to read in an obituary of her a statement that she had been given an award "for services to the pharmaceutical industry", as if it had been some sort of charity work. If you've been awake through previous chapters of this book you'll be aware that the multi-billion pharma corporations are not exactly desperate for donations and are full of lying greedy crooks peddling deadly poisonous crrap while pretending to help their victims. And they are very hostile to nutritional supplements because they undermine their profitable patented junk drugs.

Vitamin B6 is an especially strong instance of this because it provides a non-patentable very cheap and harmless cure for many cases of depression, anxiety, insomnia, obsessions, epilepsy, migraine, headaches, pre-menstrual tension, and more. Well, it would provide that treatment if the patients were informed of it, but in practice much effort and millions of dollars is put into selling profitable poisonous junk and approximately none into informing people of better but less profitable alternatives.

Anyway, round about 1995, no one was complaining about vitamin B6, until Saint Sheila McKechnie's Consumers' Association spontaneously started raising a fuss about possible danger of toxicity (Woods, 1998). In the words of Professor Beckett: "In 1995, the Consumer's Association, a non-scientific organisation that had recently been castigated by the Advertising Standards Authority for ill-informed reporting, expressed concern to MAFF about dosages of vitamin B6 currently in use. The reasons for this concern are not clear: no member of their organisation had complained to them about B6. MAFF referred the matter to COT...." (Commons, 1998).

The UK government has (or at least had) an advisory committee, the Committee on Toxicity (COT), which was constantly declared to be independent though in reality it consisted entirely of people paid by the big pharma corporations. "Professor" Woods was its chairman and very much in charge.

In response to the Consumers' Association's "concerns", the COT published a first statement on vitamin B6. There were considerable complaints about that first statement, so the COT went on to "review" the matter then published a second statement on vitamin B6 in June 1997. That statement, like the first one, recommended banning of doses higher than 10mg, due to supposed evidence of harm from higher doses. This in the context that many people with stressful lives can need more like 100 mg to sort out their stress. Being well aware of how the "dangerous" doses of vitamin B6 had hugely positively transformed my own life, I perceived the COT's statement as a deliberate attack on my own healthcare, a criminal assault against myself (and millions of others), indeed attempted murder by this regime of luxuriating "distinguished" liars.

Note the resolute confidence of tone with which Woods asserted the supposedly clear soundness of his conclusions (the same as referred to very differently by those quotes at the top here):

> "We are clear that we have not seen any evidence that would convince us that there is a need to alter our advice, and we have every confidence that our conclusions are justified given the evidence available to us." (Woods, 1998).

Given that this was their second statement following challenges to their first, and on a matter of major public interest, one would reasonably expect that they would take extra care in preparing that second statement. You will see from my unpublished paper that they indeed did take extra care, namely extra care in contriving the presentation of their second statement with a view to deliberately deceiving its readers. (And you'll also see something more at the end of this introduction to our paper.)

The COT statement against B6 provoked the largest public protest in UK history, with about a million letters of objection. Campaign groups were founded such as the Alliance for Natural Health (ANH). Some pseudo-campaigning (controlled opposition) groups were also set up to wastefully divert objectors' time and energy. The fact that the leading retailer Holland & Barrett had become owned by a pharma corp helped in those pseudo-campaigning operations. (It's in the nature of pseudo-campaigning groups that they also attract non-pseudo- people as they don't of course present themselves as being pseudic.)

I was well aware of the history of anti-nutritional propaganda and the charlatanism of the COT and decided to study their alleged evidence. Thereafter I decided to write a paper to send to the Lancet journal. I got Dr Rimland to co-author so as to give the paper more "credibility" to the editor. I gave it the title you see in this chapter's heading. Dr Rimland was reluctant about the L-word in there but I coaxed him into going along with it cushioned by the question mark ending.

Then I mailed in the required four/five paper copies. The editor thereafter contacted me on *four* occasions proposing that I reduce it to the 500 words limit for a letter, even though that would obviously be useless for presenting a meaningful evidential case on such a serious subject.

After some months, the editor informed me that all four/five* copies of our paper had been "lost". (*I could have sworn it was five copies but a document I wrote in 2000 says it was four; it could take xyz minutes to verify the actualité from my archives, but xyz might turn out to be hours.)

Meanwhile I phoned "Professor" Woods to see if he was capable of giving any honest response on the matter. Which turned out to not be the case. His rambling evasive reply included the notion that the vitamins industry was nearly two million pounds-worth but no mention of the multi-billions of the drugs industry. So I compiled a 4 x A5 leaflet of more-or-less the same content as this paper here, and titled it "**The head of Sheffield Medical School lied to the government about vitamin safety**" (Clarke, 1998), and included all my contact details. I printed out 150 copies and got the train to Sheffield, where I handed out the copies in the medical school, dental school and general campus, plus a copy (and letter) to the Vice-Chancellor's fancy office as I wouldn't want anyone so important to feel excluded. The latter duly sent me a reply rambling on about being "*sub judice*", a legal principle of no relevance to civil litigation anyway. Unfortunately I am still waiting for the *judice* to get out from that *sub* and it appears that the litigation limitation time has now run out more than a decade ago.

I also put up a website (of which there were vastly fewer in 1998), containing not only the content of that leaflet and paper, but also uploads of the COT's other statements for comparison (as discussed in my leaflet and this paper). A few months later a new law was introduced enabling libel claimants to sue the internet provider hosting the website they were complaining of. So "Professor" Woods sent a letter to demon internet demanding that my content be removed, whereupon demon sided with cowardice. I decided I didn't want to support an internet provider which caved in to liars so I dumped my demon account at that point. Numerous *free* internet connection services had started up by then anyway.

On 23rd May 1998 the Lancet at last published something about that matter, an editorial fudgily titled "Still time for rational debate about vitamin B6". That editorial referred to my website and myself in the following terms:

"The [chairman] is Prof Frank Woods, and a telephone conversation with him is detailed on a website put up by one of the pro-B_6 groups. There, Prof Woods, interviewed by a research scientist who felt obliged to say he was calling as a journalist (such is the cloak-and-dagger world of food supplements), said that he had investigated the committee members' conflicts of interest and that any suggestion of the committee "being deliberately misleading and untruthful" was nonsense."

I have to question the imputation there that I was acting under false pretence of not being a research scientist, given that I have never earned so much as a penny for researching or sciencing anything whatsoever and I've not exactly been stalked by any researcher recruitment headhunters in any of the years before or since.

The Lancet also published several letters from others, not least one from Prof. Arnold Beckett (1998), which included those damning words I quoted at the top of this chapter. Woods published no reply. Woods's claptrap was also torn to shreds in a parliamentary committee, and the crooked conspiracy to ban vitamin B6 ended up abandoned in the face of the huge opposition.

I later compiled all my information and sent it to the police at Bournville Road station in Birmingham. On later phoning them about it, they replied that it was not a "police matter" but a "medical matter" instead. On that same principle they presumably were also dismissing all fraud cases as not being police matters because they were merely "accounting matters" or "financial matters" instead.

In the unpublished paper that follows here, I referred to four other statements issued by COT which I compared to their B6 statement. On web-searching now for [COT statements 1997] I see that there are now listed a total of eight other statements published that year, and another two the previous year (and the one for chlorine listed but not downloadable). The peculiar anomalousness of the B6 statement is even clearer now, in that none of those other ten statements have the peculiarly hi-tech irrelevant introductionary section (giving the impression to the reader that the matter is beyond their expertise), and nor do any of them use the peculiar confusing fully-in-text citation system (which I have anyway never seen used in *any* other document).

Meanwhile, in the process of writing this chapter here, I just thought I'd do a websearch check up on what "Professor" Woods is up to nowadays, if anything.

I see that in 2001 he was made a CBE "for services to the Committee on Toxicity of Chemicals in Food, Consumer Products and the Environment". (A CBE is higher level than MBE and OBE.)

And in 2007, Sheffield (cough....) "University" awarded him an honorary degree of M.D.

And, well, have a guess. I mean you wouldn't predict that this professor awarded a CBE and that honorary doctorate would do anything less than exemplary, notwithstanding my strident assertions of him being a callous lying deceiver collaborating in a nasty conspiracy.

It turns out that in 2013 he was appointed Chairman of the Governors of the *430-years-old* St. Bee's School. And within a year its closure had been organised in the face of (yet another? Surely not?) huge protest and accusations of deceitfulness and secrecy and lack of transparency and bad faith. But please don't take my word for it as I am obviously biased here. Rather take a look at their statement here with over a thousand signatures in support.

The Charities Commission is right now conducting an inquiry into the affair. Why do people keep ganging up so unfairly on poor Professor Woods? Well, that's what happens when you reward a callous criminal with a CBE and honorary doctorate rather than a prison sentence. One does have to wonder how much further grief he has been causing people in the intervening 16 years since I exposed his gigantic crime.

~~~~~~~

"An Open Letter to the Governors of St Bees School

On March 13th 2015 you announced your intention to close St Bees School with the loss of around 150 jobs, with 300 children having to seek their education elsewhere at unacceptably short notice and with no impact assessment on the local and wider community.

You also took this action under a **cloak of secrecy** – without consulting with staff, a legal requirement under the Employment Act, without consulting with the charity's stakeholders, contrary to Charities Commission Guidance 2010, without attempting any effective fundraising and without proper consideration of credible attempts to keep the school open, again contrary to the Charities Commission Guidance 2010 where closure is noted as being the last resort.

The School's objectives include "other associated activities for the benefit of the community". As of today you still have not formally notified representatives of the Community such as the Parish Council Committee, Local or County councils or the former MP of your decision to close nor have you consulted with them.

Instead what you did was **mislead** stakeholders and the Rescue Team in terms of the timing of the EGM, in respect of your comments about the finances and the markets and in **not giving access to vital information** to the Rescue Team **as you indicated you would do**. Instead it seems that your efforts were to ignore or delay the rescue attempts, not only by the Rescue Team but also several other options including a free school, Keswick merger and international schools.

Whilst the Rescue Team and others were finding a way to keep the school open, you were hastily terminating contracts of employment and supply and rushing to sign over the pupils to other schools, making rescue harder.

You did not undertake any impact assessment of the consequences of your actions on others. As a direct result you have motivated parents, alumni and members of the community to demand your resignation and to complain to the regulator, the Charities Commission. The Charities Commission have consequently launched an investigation into your actions, actions which have severely damaged the school's reputation and damaged the wider reputation of charities as consultative bodies.

We now demand the board of Governors resign with immediate effect.

This letter is accompanied by a petition, which supports our demand for your resignations, signed by over 1,000 people representing parents, alumni, pupils and the wider community.

Quite simply, as Governors you have lost the trust and confidence placed in you by the school's stakeholders and your position has become untenable.

In addition, in the interest of **openness and transparency**, we would request you answer the following questions:

Firstly, why there was no serious consideration given by the board to the options for keeping the school open, especially given the Rescue Team and the Society of Old St Beghians managing to secure a £2m funding package?

Secondly, even though it was apparent from the 2013 accounts that the school was making losses, why did you continue to increase the level of bursaries and invest in facilities and infrastructure instead of reducing overheads and undertaking effective fund-raising?

Thirdly, how much is the closure of the school costing? Considering the cost of the termination of employment contracts, enhanced severances for employees to waive their rights, the costs of advisors including a consultant brought in specifically to close the school, the employment of a PR company and lawyers fees to sue a parent for using a publicly available photograph on his Facebook site in support of the school. The significant financial loss you have created will damage the charity severely.

We are now demanding a new set of Governors are installed in order to give full and fair consideration of the future of St Bees School. This new board will engage with all stakeholders to find a way of keeping the school open and retaining its future as a centre for education excellence -whatever form that may take.

Your behaviour has been **shameful; reminiscent of some sort of 'secret society'**. We suggest that in order to retain some semblance of dignity, as a Board, you resign with immediate effect and let others who are more engaged with stakeholders take your place.

Save St Bees School Campaign and over 1000 others. **"**

~~~~~~~

Before presenting our unpublished paper I will just mention a letter written by Stephen Terrass of Solgar Vitamins UK, which makes various compelling points, not least the following.

"....Cigarettes kill over 100,000 UK citizens every year. Vitamin B6 has never killed anyone, and in the doses that you seek to ban for free sale, it has never been proven to harm anyone either. Never mind the scientifically proven health benefits of B6 (which pertain primarily to the levels that are to be banned). So in a few months time I, and every person living in Britain, will be able to kill ourselves with lung cancer from smoking, but we will no longer be able to exercise our health freedom by purchasing a beneficial nutrient in harmless dosages.

Paracetamol kills hundreds every year, and this, too, will be available for free sale in every corner shop, every petrol station, and every supermarket - but not B6. The list of examples of this nature is considerable, but I suppose the tobacco and especially the pharmaceutical giants can make a lot more threatening noises against restrictions than health food stores or vitamin companies. Yet, how many peer-reviewed studies can you cite that show that smoking does not cause lung cancer, or that paracetamol is not the cause of hundreds of deaths from liver failure each year? Not one....."

Please note that the following unpublished paper uses a different type of citation method than elsewhere in this book, namely a numbered list referred to by the numbers in brackets (=

"parentheses" for language experts).

Did the UK Committee on Toxicity lie to the government about vitamin B6? (of which all four copies "lost" by the *Lancet*)

Robin P Clarke and Bernard Rimland [written in 1997-8]

Abstract: The statement on vitamin B6 from the UK Committee on Toxicity contains a high proportion of incorrect and misleading material. Its flaws are not merely in details but in its most essential contents. The committee not only produced this outstandingly defective work but also steadfastly stood by it against heavy and informed criticism. It is very difficult to see how this could have been due to straightforward errors or misjudgements. Furthermore there are some most remarkable peculiarities in the presentation as compared to other statements from the committee. It is here hypothesised that the committee carefully contrived its statement to mislead policymakers. The hypothesis can be tested by seeking a credible rebuttal from the committee.

~~~~~~~~~~~~

The British government is currently preparing legislation to restrict the sale of vitamin B6. In this it is acting on the advice of the Commitee on Toxicity (COT) whose chairman is Professor H.F. Woods. It will here be argued that the statement on vitamin B6 produced by COT contains a high proportion of untrue and misleading material, and that these flaws are not merely in details but in its most essential contents. We cannot easily dismiss these incorrectnesses as simple inadvertent errors. The statement was written for the purpose of enabling a government policy restricting the rights of the public, and was defended by Professor Woods in the face of heavy and informed criticisms.

We will here firstly consider the scientific merits of the COT's statement (*1*), then consider its peculiar presentation and other matters.

Several sentences proclaim that the authors are approaching the data in a discerning manner. The committee dismiss numerous studies on grounds of abnormal genotype, insufficient subjects or durations, or for dating from 1940. Curiously the discernment greatly relaxes in respect of studies that appear unfavourable to B6.

It is normal in a literature review to cite the strongest, soundest studies at least. The COT statement cited six papers in their support (*2-7*), and dismissed a seventh citation (*8*) as too old and lacking in detail.

The statement's conclusion that 10 mg is the safe limit is built on two pillars as it were, the one being the human data and the other the animal data. Under careful examination both these pillars prove to be vapor.

Fundamental to the human data pillar is the study by Dalton and Dalton (2). COT concentrated four of their six supporting citations into a key sentence asserting the relevance of this study: "The observations of Dalton and Dalton are also consistent with the reported symptoms of patients in other studies undertaken at higher doses which contained objective measures as well as subjective observations (eg. Berger AR, Schaumberg HH, Schroder C et al. Neurology 1992; 42: 1367-1370, Albin RL, Albers JW, Greenberg HS et al, Neurology 1987: 37: 1729-1732, Albin RL, Albers JW Neurology 1990; 40: 1319, Waterston JA, Gilligan BS [sic] 1987; 146: 640-642)".

And yet this crucial sentence is simply untrue. The papers cited—for what they are worth—actually indicate the opposite, as do others (7,9) (and the two cases of Albin et al are anyway utterly irrelevant for reasons detailed below). These papers indicate that the neuropathy begins with the longest nerves (to the feet). By contrast the Dalton study's symptoms mainly concerned the face and upper limbs (including tingling fingers) and were characteristic not of B6 toxicity but of hyperventilation/hysteria and anxiety (10).

The COT's claim that the doses were known to be "followed by symptoms" is likewise untrue. Rather the symptoms were recorded along with previous B6 consumption but the possibility that the symptoms had preceded the B6 was not ruled out.

The committee's emphasis on the Dalton study (which used neither controls nor blinds) has been condemned by distinguished scientists, and COT subsequently retreated into the vague assertion that they did not depend on only the Dalton study but had considered over 100 studies. There can be few reviews in the scientific literature that content themselves with such a shallow platitude.

Of the more than 100 studies listed as having been considered by COT, a large proportion have no relationship to B6 neuropathy of any kind, let alone the syndrome that Dalton and Dalton supposedly discovered. If there were something in all those papers that was remotely supportive of their 10 mg recommendation it is strange that they did not mention it in their statement. The four other human studies that they did cite make an impressive sample of the least impressive dregs of the scientific literature, with the number of subjects averaging two, with major deficiencies of methodology, and with significantly abnormal circumstances complicating any generalised interpretation. Before further consideration of those studies we will discuss the other evidence that is their context.

Reviews of B6 toxicity have shown that 200 mg per day, and possibly much more, is safe for long-term consumption (*11*). Large numbers of people have been purchasing and taking such doses for many years without problems. Indeed the evidence is already there in the Dalton study. An average of 116 mg taken by 69 women for an average of 1.6 years, and an average of 117 mg taken by 103 women for an average of 2.9 years, yet not one of them had developed the most pathognomic sign of B6 toxicity, namely difficulty in walking. And consider this: the Daltons` observations related to one clinic, and a clinic unsympathetic to vitamin therapy at that. It is not unreasonable to suppose that similar consumption of vitamin B6 occurred in thousands of other clinics, and the question poses itself of where all the victims were who developed walking difficulties. If PMS clinics around the world were becoming even slightly filled with women having difficulty in walking, could this really have gone unnoticed?

Regard must also be had to the benefits that may be lost through restricting intake to the COT`s prescription. Published evidence of many benefits, including protection from heart attacks (*12*) and suicidal depression (*13*) and infections (*14*), while not massive, is significant, given the great hostility that has been encountered by such heretical ideas, tending to discourage research and publication. Patients taking 100-300 mg for some years experienced only 27% the risk of heart disease, and those who died of a heart attack lived eight years longer on average than controls who also died of heart attacks (12). It is very likely that deaths could have been avoided with more vitamin B6, whereas there is every reason to believe that no one has ever been killed by excess of it.

For epileptic infants, a B6 dose of 300 mg/kg/day has been found superior to seizure drugs, with no significant adverse effects (15).

So, to the details. The Berger et al study (*3*) was non-blind with immediate cessation upon the "first appearance" of "symptoms". The doses were high (1000 and 3000 mg/day) and most remarkably, on the page before last the experimenters revealed that four of the five subjects were themselves.

The Albin et al paper (*4*) concerned two tragic cases in extraordinarily abnormal situations of injecting 132,000 mg and 183,000 mg over three days, following mushroom poisoning. The second Albin/Albers citation (*5*) relates to the same cases. The Waterston & Gilligan paper (*6*) reports merely one case, who had a history of ill-health and was taking *four drugs* and 1000 mg/day.

The COT's last supporting citation (7) is of dogs fed the equivalent of 3000 mg/day, a level that everyone agrees is risky anyway.

COT would have us believe that this set of reports constitutes good reason to set a limit of 10 mg without even mentioning the thousands of people who have been taking doses of 100 to 500 mg/day or more for many years without problems. Nor do they even mention any possibility that there could be harm in restriction of doses.

It should be clear that the human data pillar of the COT's case is simply indefensible. Yet the animal data pillar is in no way any sounder.

COT devote 170 words to the irrelevant animal data. It is irrelevant because there already exists substantial human data testifying to B6 safety, so there is no point in trying to second-guess what the human data would be from other species.

Yet by a stupendous feat of pseudo-reasoning they derive their 10 mg from the 3000 mg figure. We are first asked to believe that a division by ten must be made to allow for the uncertainty of the jump between species. But given that we have so much relevant human data, what are the grounds for giving so much weight to data that they suppose to have such a level of uncertainty about it? Compounding this nonsense, they go on to make a further division by 10, on the grounds of human inter-individual variation. But since their starting-point was a lowest adverse level, we are already starting at the lower end of variation anyway. Indeed, an author of the dog study (Ian Munro) pointed out (10) that the 3000 mg/day level produced no clinical effects and its physical effects were barely detectable, on the very margin of toxicity, yet COT cite it as a toxic level. Furthermore the use of a divisor of 10 is manifestly inappropriate in respect of nutrients. If this factor were applied in respect of zinc it would result in a safety limit below the RDA.

Not satisfied with this compounded nonsense, COT go on to claim that a further division by three must be made "for the use of a lowest observed adverse effect level". This is absurd. It may be customary to make such a division if faced with a lack of data below the level in question. But it should be obvious that no such condition applies here and that any such convention is therefore irrelevant. It may indeed be the standard procedure to apply such a rule, but one would expect eight professors to be of an intellectual level that goes beyond mindlessly applying rules where they are manifestly inappropriate.

So, why did Professor Woods and his committee produce this bizarrely defective statement, *and* go on to stand by it through subsequent substantial criticism? Surely eight professors and ten *Dr*s cannot seriously be supposed to be so content to advise a government with work not fit for an undergraduate essay? There must surely be something very strange going on. Accordingly the hypothesis is here put forward that the committee deliberately contrived to produce a defective statement, presumably (one surmises) with the intention of improperly influencing policymakers. Furthermore, examination of the presentational aspects of the statement suggest a hypothesis that the statement may have been carefully contrived to maximise the misleading of an audience of non-expert policymakers.

We compared the statement on B6 with the other statements from COT available on the open-government internet site. There was one lengthy report on PCBs, and three other statements of the same length as the B6 statement (*16*). The B6 statement strikingly differs from these others in several peculiar ways.

Firstly, it has a long introduction, as long as the actual review of data. Secondly, this introduction is not relevant to the subject of B6 safety, not even in conjunction with the rest (except for the final sentence about hereditary diseases, all but repeated in the review section anyway).

Thirdly, this introduction is uncharacteristically thick with medical terminology such as: *"For example, homocystinuria, an autosomal recessive aminoacidopathy resulting from a defect in cystathionine β-synthase, is characterised by excessive homocysteine in plasma and urine."*

Fourthly, the review section itself is made harder to read by use of fully-in-text citations (e.g., Dalton K, Dalton MJT. Acta Neurol Scand 1987; 76: 8-11) rather than use of a reference list at the end as the other statements have.

All these peculiarities of the statement have something in common, namely helping to shield the key claims from critical attention. The effect of the long, difficult-to-understand introduction is to impress non-specialist readers into thinking the issue to be very complex and that it would be best simply to trust the word of the expert authors. The irrelevance of the material helps by leaving the reader unable to discern a thread of relevance, hence confused. And the use of in-text references adds to the difficulty of following the short data review. They also help to downplay the shortness of the data review section, and add to the illusion of authoritativeness.

Quite strikingly, of the six references they cited in their support, four were concentrated into a sentence which happened to be one of the key untruths in the statement. This not only misleads the reader into thinking that that claim is well-founded, but also of course leads the reader into assuming that the other assertions are so sound that references are not needed in their support. Another sentence that tends to mislead its readers is "We consider that the small number of individuals involved and/or the short duration of administration may explain the absence of signs of sensory peripheral neuropathy in some studies." This sentence effectively invites the reader to assume that it validly disposes of all the other evidence that COT has not found fit to mention.

The combination of an exceptionally low standard of work by such a highly qualified group, together with these signs of contrivance to conceal it, is surely very powerful prima facie evidence in favour of the hypothesis of deliberate deception.

Also of possible relevance to the hypothesis is the observation that most members of the committee had interests in pharmaceuticals companies. The profits these companies obtain from patented and licensed products are threatened by nutritional treatments which can be provided by smaller companies lacking patents and licenses.

It would perhaps not be appropriate to speculate about implications of the hypothesis at this stage before it has been tested.

The hypothesis may be tested by seeking a credible rebuttal of this paper from the Committee.

References

1. "Statement on vitamin B6 toxicity" *Committee on Toxicity of Chemicals in Food, Consumer Products, and the Environment* (Department of Health (UK), June, 1997); see 15 below for internet sites.
2. K. Dalton and M.J.T. Dalton, *Acta Neurol. Scand.* **76,** 8-11 (1987).
3. A.R. Berger, H.H. Schaumberg, C. Schroeder, S. Apfel, R. Reynolds, *Neurol.* **42,** 1367-1370 (1992).
4. R.L. Albin et al., *Neurol.* **37,** 1729-1732 (1987).
5. R.L. Albin and J. W. Albers, *Neurol.* **40,** 1319 (1990).
6. J.A. Waterston and B.S. Gilligan, *Med. J. Australia* **146,** 640-642 (1987).
7. W.E.J. Phillips et al., *Toxicol. Appl. Pharm.* **44,** 323-333 (1978).
8. K. Unna, *J. Pharm. Exp. Thera.* **70,** 179-188 (1940).
9. H. Schaumberg et al., *New Engl. J. Med.* **309,** 444-448 (1983).
10. *Vitamin B6: New Data, New Perspectives,* Council for Responsible Nutrition London, September 1997, (C.R.N.,Thames Ditton, UK, 1997).
11. A.L. Bernstein, *Ann. N. Y. Acad. Sci.* **585,** 250-260 (1990); A. Bendich and M. Cohen, *Ann.N. Y. Acad. Sci.* **585,** 321-330 (1990).
12. J.M. Ellis and K.S. McCully, *Res. Communics. in Molec. Pathol. and Pharm.* **89,** 208-220 (1995); I. Graham et al., *JAMA* **277,** 1775-1781 (1997).
13. P.W. Adams et al., *Lancet* **i,** 897-904 (1973); J.W. Stewart, W. Harrison, F. Quitkin, H. Baker, *Biol. Psychiat.* **19,** 613-616 (1984).
14. K. Yamada et al., *J. Vitaminol.* **5,** 188 (1959); R.W. Vilter, *J. Lab. Clin. Med.* **42,** 335 (1953).
15. J. Pietz et al., *Epilepsia* **43,** 757-763 (1993).
16. "Statement on PCBs", "Statement on bisphenol A", "Statement on bisphenol diglycidyl ether in canned foods", "Statement on iodine in cow's milk", and "Statement on vitamin B6 toxicity", *Committee on Toxicity* (1997), were accessed at http://www.open.gov.uk/ and are now at http://www.fineart.demon.co.uk/cot

~~~~~~~

12

Is Cambridge's Simon Baron-Cohen a charlatan too?

"A grant! A grant! My integrity for a grant!"

Professor Simon Baron-Cohen is the head of the Autism Research Centre at Cambridge University in England. And is referred to by many as *the* leading expert on autism. This chapter discusses how well this notion stands up in the context that the pseudo-scientific charlatan Trofim Lysenko was once hailed by many as the leading expert of agronomy or even of biology.

Within autism research there are three supremely important issues. Firstly, whether there has been a real major increase of autism, rather than just an illusion of an increase. Secondly, whether mercury has had a causal role in that increase, or in autism more generally. Thirdly, whether chelating or detoxifying that mercury can cure or at least reduce autism. In earlier chapters here I have shown the clear evidence resolutely supporting all three of these notions.

Here I will consider what this purported leading expert Simon Baron-Cohen (SBC) has had to say about those three key questions.

Firstly, the involvement of mercury in autism. I can find no engagement of SBC with this question other than the most minimal comment (BBC, 2003) about the Holmes et al. (2003) study as follows:

"This kind of gene-environment interaction is not incompatible with the known heritability of autism. If these results hold up, metal studies on the brain could be revealing."

There was no mention of mercury even in a recent review of neuroinflammation by SBC and colleagues (Young et al., 2016), even though it has long been known to cause autoimmune and inflammatory effects (and another review of the same subject published the same week did indeed discuss such a role of mercury (Kern et al., 2016).)

Secondly, the use of chelation to recover or even cure autistics. SBC appears to have been completely silent on this important question, even though some famous advocates of chelation linked their protocol to SBC's own theory of autism being "extreme male brain".

And thirdly, what does he have to say about the huge increase? Well, in 2015, SBC has put his name as co-author of a very remarkable review paper in the Lancet (Lai & Baron-Cohen, 2015). As I've explained in my first chapter here, in scientific papers it is not done to just state a highly contentious notion as if it is a known fact unless it really is universally known and accepted (such as the Earth being a planet circling around the Sun, or water being liquid at room temperature). The norm is that assertions other than of well-known facts have to be accompanied by citation of reports of the evidence thereof. But remarkably, this review by Professor Meng-Chuan Lai and Professor Simon Baron-Cohen starts with an assertion of a highly dubious "fact" with no citation whatsoever in support. Here are the title and first sentences of the summary and main text (which are as near as matters identical):

"Identifying the lost generation of adults with autism spectrum conditions"
"Autism spectrum conditions comprise a set of early-onset neuro-developmental syndromes with a population prevalence of 1% across all ages."
"Autism spectrum conditions (panel 1) comprise a set of neuro-developmental syndromes with a population prevalence of 1% across all ages."

That opening sentence asserts to us that as of 2014-15, 1% of 10-year-olds are autistic, and 1% of 30-year-olds are autistic, 1% of 50-year-olds are autistic, and so on, for "all ages". And the title of the paper reinforces that untruth with the notion that there is therefore a "lost generation" of older autistics who have mostly remained unrecognised as autistic and thus "lost". The un-explicated insinuation being that there has not been any increase of autism but instead only an increase of awareness or diagnosis. And this "review" paper sets out from its beginning by grossly misleading the reader into assuming that that is known to be a fact, indeed established to such an extent it doesn't even need any citation in support.

And that title and first sentence are not incidental to the paper but are its central premises.

I sent emails to the authors, querying the justification for that first sentence. I got no reply from SBC.

Dr Lai sent a series of replies which made me wonder whether he should be not so much a professor of psychiatry as rather a psychiatric patient himself (which could be why a reply from SBC himself was not received?). The full correspondence is a bit too lengthy to include here in full, but here are some main excerpts.

Dear Robin,

Thank you for your message. For clarification, when we write "Autism spectrum conditions (panel 1) comprise a set of neurodevelopmental syndromes with a population prevalence of 1% across all ages." we are NOT referring the term "ages" to different chronological years (i.e., 1970s, 80s, 90s, etc.) but are referring it to the ages of the individuals; that is, we are referring to epidemiological evidences that recent cross-sectional studies in children, in teenagers and in adults all tend to show a prevalence around 1% (depending on studies but can range from around ~0.5% to ~2%). We, therefore, have no intention to argue in the paper whether the prevalence of autism is constant or not across different chronological years.

Hope this clarifies the question/mis-understanding.

Regards,

Meng-Chuan

Dear Meng-Chuan,

[....] Your phrase "all ages" includes obviously those who are 40 or 60 years old. And even older. As of 2015, a person who is age 40 was necessarily born in 1975 or earlier, and a person of age 60 was necessarily born in 1955 or earlier. That is, such ages of persons are impossible to disentangle from the huge change of apparent incidence (per birth-year cohorts) which is the basis of the notion of the autism increase. I fail to see any way you can separate ages (of "all ages") from specific years of birth.

In response to my request for any evidence to support that claim of your first sentence, you didn't send any, but instead included a sentence contradicting it. And that notion of "1% across all ages" is fundamental to the point of your entire article, namely the notion of a "lost generation" of older autistics.

(If I may do a bit of your homework for you here, perhaps the cited Brugha et al. could be supposed to constitute supporting evidence on the matter. But Brugha et al. is fundamentally unsound. They went to great lengths for establishing <u>reliability</u> of the assessments. But no establishing of the (infinitely more important) <u>validity</u> of the assessments, that is establishing that the measures at age x were equivalent to the measures at age y. And that is because it is logically impossible to do that validity verification (except maybe over many years). It's a bit like if I put a steel ruler in a hot fire and declared that I can see that its own scale shows it to be still exactly 12 inches long, so "therefore" the heating hasn't changed its length. For this reason Brugha's claptrap (and any similar studies) amounts to no evidence whatsoever for countering the evidence of Hertz-Picciotto and others.)

    [....]

    Sincerely, Robin P Clarke

Dear Robin,

    Thank you for the opportunity for further clarification. If I understand your points correctly, the main critique is based on your perception: *"that notion of "1% across all ages" is fundamental to the point of your entire article, namely the notion of a "lost generation" of older autistics"*.

    I am sorry if this is how you perceive our arguments. However, this is not what we have in mind when we wrote it. You are right that the paper mainly discusses under-recognized autism in adults - indeed the sole focus of the review, and from a clinical perspective. We are asked by the journal to provide general epidemiological background (based on published studies), and this is where the ~1% number comes from - and we provided the number in adults, referencing the Brugha paper which is one of the few published study focusing on adults. We DO NOT mean to argue "there is a constant 1% prevalence over the years so there is a lost generation". We simply refer to the current epidemiological findings that adult prevalence at the time being is also around 1%, and many of them have not been diagnosed in the past. I agree it is difficult to get the ground truth (due to issues with validity of diagnosis, changes of diagnostic concepts [that we have discussed in the review], and not knowing whether there is true incidence change); the prevalence number cited here is simply giving a general picture to the readers, from available published epidemiological data.

    It is possible that there is increased incidence over the years, but this does not contradict the possibility of people being under-recognized as a child. We focus on the latter and have no intention to discuss (either support or refute) the former.

    I hope this helps clarify where this review comes from.

    Regards,

    Meng-Chuan

Dr Lai continued to stand by his notion that the ages could be separated from the years of birth, despite my reply stated above. Some choice adjectives and nouns could be added here but I think you the reader will have no difficulty calling them to mind yourself anyway.

Meanwhile, still not having heard anything from SBC himself, on 9th January 2016 I posted a letter to him by Signed-For-Delivery (KP597377771GB at royalmail.com, received at ARC 12th January, my receipt copied at end of this chapter) as follows.

Dear Dr Baron-Cohen,

I am writing here in respect of your article "Identifying the lost generation of adults with autism spectrum" in Lancet Psychiatry 2015.

I am concerned that I have not yet heard from you about this article. I hope you are not unwell.

I will send herewith a copy of my correspondence with your co-author Meng-Chuan Lai. His replies get even more absurd and indefensible than the original article (indeed raising doubt about his sanity). This matter of the huge tragedy of the manyfold increase of autism (and the outrageous claptrap such as Brugha being used to pretend it hasn't happened) is very serious. Publishing of sloppy, wantonly misleading writing about it is completely unacceptable and unethical. It is all the more unacceptable that you yourself put your name to such a grossly misleading and unworthy document, given that you are widely trusted as "the leading expert" on autism. And further that this is the very opening of a "review" being published in the Lancet no less, thus likely to be "authoritatively" parrotted by future generations of students as supposedly established knowledge.

I included two of your email addresses in my correspondence with Meng-Chuan (sb205@cam and editorial@molecular) but have not heard any comment from yourself on the matter. I do not know whether you are aware or not of these issues (though as co-author you should have been aware of the opening sentences of your own article anyway).

Accordingly I am now sending this letter by signed delivery requesting that you clarify your position on this very important matter. Do you agree with myself and others that the article is unacceptably misleading and must be retracted? Or what?

I look forward to hearing from you as soon as practical. You have one of my email addresses at the top here, and another is rpclarke@autism.

Sincerely, Robin P Clarke

I have still not received any reply to this letter, by email, post or any other means. Why not?

SBC has long been well aware of this controversy about an autism increase, stating at one time his theory it might be caused mainly by assortative mating, and in more recent years proposing it to be mainly from increased awareness.

In 2009, Ann Dachel posted an "open letter" to Dr Baron-Cohen on the AgeofAutism website (Dachel, 2009). I recommend to read it in full but anyway her letter ended as follows.

"I have only two questions for you:

1. Tell us about the adults who have autism like we see in children. Where are they living and what are they doing? There are hundreds of thousands of parents in Britain, desperate about the future for their kids, who'd love to know.

2. [.....] As was just reported in the Telegraph, you believe that autistic adults are 'currently very poorly served.' And while you mention those with Asperger's Syndrome, I'd like you to show us the 30, 50, and 70 year old adults who display the same symptoms of classic autism that we see in children, the non-verbal adults in diapers, banging holes in walls and spinning in circles."

The reply from SBC went on quite a bit in his usual feely-goody way, but did not give the slightest answer to those questions. Which raises the question of why not. As with his failure to answer my queries about his latest "lost generation" article. And as in Suzanne Humphries' words at the start of this book: *If this is the expert why can't he answer my questions?*

And this grossly misleading publication from SBC comes in a context of his twice actively suppressing my own evidence about the increase, without good reason. When in 2013 I sent to his Molecular Autism journal my epidemics paper (as in Chapter 3 here), he fobbed it off with an assertion that "The advice we have received is that the methodology would not get through critical peer review from our journal". And yet this is an outright pseudo-reason, because it is the editors themselves (i.e. himself) who choose the peer reviewers and thereafter decide whether or not the peer reviewers have shown the paper to be inadequate or not (as that's what journal editors are for).

And a second occurrence of suppression by SBC occurred when I sent to his journal my paper on the question of road traffic pollution as a supposed cause of autism (as discussed in Chapter 6 here). He refused to publish it unless I cut out all mention of my alternative explanation (in terms of reduced ventilation of the mercury vapour emitting from non-gamma-2 dental amalgams).

Furthermore, on several occasions I have brought to SBC's attention the unfaulted antiinnatia theory of autism, but he has never once made any comment or mention of its existence. And likewise my epidemics paper which he assisted in suppressing.

I posted a comment to the PubMed page of the "lost generation" article, basically warning that it was grossly misleading and quoting the correspondence above here. Someone complained to the PubMed people with an allegation that the comment was in breach of their rules and it was instantly deleted and my PubMed commenting account blocked.

I thereafter contacted the Lancet Psychiatry editor with a request for retraction of the article. The correspondence was as follows (in full). At various points he introduces strawman arguments, and consistently fails to answer the real arguments presented.

From: r@
Sent: 23 January 2016 13:51
To: Boyce, Niall (ELS-CAM)
Subject: Article needs retracting: "Identifying the lost generation of adults with autism..."

Dear Niall Boyce,

Re "Identifying the lost generation of adults with autism....." by Meng-Chuan Lai and Simon Baron-Cohen.
http://www.thelancet.com/journals/lanpsy/article/PIIS2215-0366%2815%2900277-1/abstract
This article is very seriously misleading and needs to be retracted. It starts with an assertion of a highly dubious massively important controversial "fact" with no citation whatsoever in support. The opening sentence (of both abstract and text) asserts to us that as of 2014-15, 1% of 10-year-olds are autistic, and 1% of 30-year-olds are autistic, 1% of 50-year-olds are autistic, and so on, for "all ages". And the title of the paper reinforces that untruth with its fictional notion that there is (by implication "therefore") a "lost generation" of older autistics who have mostly remained unrecognised as autistic and thus "lost". The un-explicated implication being that there has not been any increase of autism but instead only an increase of awareness or diagnosis. And this paper sets out from its beginning by grossly misleading the reader into assuming that that is known to be a fact, indeed established to such an extent it doesn't even need any citation in support.

And that title and first sentence are not incidental to the paper but are its central premises.

I sent emails to the authors, querying the justification for that first sentence. I got no reply from SBC, not even after I posted the letter attached herewith to him by Signed-For delivery (KP597377771GB at www.royalmail.com, received 12th Jan 2016).

Dr Lai sent a series of replies. The full correspondence is too lengthy to include here in full, but here are the main elements.

His first reply was as follows (and note furthermore the absurd sentence I have bolded, which effectively concedes my objection anyway).

Dear Robin,

Thank you for your message. For clarification, when we write "Autism spectrum conditions (panel 1) comprise a set of neurodevelopmental syndromes with a population prevalence of 1% across all ages." we are NOT referring the term "ages" to different chronological years (i.e., 1970s, 80s, 90s, etc.) but are referring it to the ages of the individuals; that is, we are referring to epidemiological evidences that recent cross-sectional studies in children, in teenagers and in adults all tend to show a prevalence around 1% (depending on studies but can range from around ~0.5% to ~2%). **We, therefore, have no intention to argue in the paper whether the prevalence of autism is constant or not across different chronological years.**

Hope this clarifies the question/mis-understanding.

Regards,

Meng-Chuan

In reply I pointed out that this entailed an obvious absurd fallacy.

"..... Your phrase "all ages" includes obviously those who are 40 or 60 years old. And even older. As of 2015, a person who is age 40 was necessarily born in 1975 or earlier, and a person of age 60 was necessarily born in 1955 or earlier. That is, such ages of persons are impossible to disentangle from the huge change of apparent incidence (per birth-year cohorts) which is the basis of the notion of the autism increase. I fail to see any way you can separate ages (of "all ages") from specific years of birth.

"In response to my request for any evidence to support that claim of your first sentence, you didn't send any, but instead included a sentence contradicting it. And that notion of "1% across all ages" is fundamental to the point of your entire article, namely the notion of a "lost generation" of older autistics."

In further correspondence, Dr Lai resolutely held to his bizarre notion that persons' ages (as of 2014-5) could be separated from their dates of birth of after or before 1975 or earlier. And meanwhile no reply at all has been forthcoming from Dr Baron-Cohen.

The notion that there has been no real increase of autism has been rejected by many people well-qualified to do so, not least people with many years direct experience of the field such as Bernard Rimland (founder of ARI), Prof. Sally Rogers of MIND, and Lisa Blakemore-Brown. And the careful analysis by Hertz-Picciotto and Delwiche concluded that the increase must be very real indeed: https://www.ncbi.nlm.nih.gov/pubmed/19234401 discussed at:

http://www.environmentalhealthnews.org/ehs/news/autism-and-environment

And yet this Lancet "review" opens its abstract and main text with a sentence which fails to even mention the existence of that H&D 2009 paper (or anything else of the many voices challenging their major assertion). Why no such mention? Failing to cite major counter-evidence is the hallmark of charlatanism rather than of anything worthy to be published in a Lancet journal. Why no reply from SBC, and only infantile nonsense from the other author? How about because there is no sensible, honest defence for this outrageously deceiving article. Its continuing presence unchallenged in your journal threatens to bring your journal into disrepute too.

Sloppy, misleading work in high places such as this "review" undermines not only the credibility of your journal but of the medical research community more generally. It needs to be cut out promptly rather than allowed to remain festering.

Sincerely,

Robin P Clarke

(PS. The authors might wish to attempt a defence on the grounds that Brugha et al. "prove their thesis right". But (apart from the other objections above) Brugha et al. is fundamentally unsound. They described in considerable detail their procedures for establishing reliability of the assessments. But not a single word about establishing of the (infinitely more important) validity of the assessments, that is establishing that the measures at age x were equivalent to the measures at age y. And that is because it is logically impossible to do that validity verification (except maybe over several decades). It's a bit like if I put a steel ruler in a hot fire and declared that I can see that its own scale shows it to be still exactly 12 inches long, so "therefore" the heating hasn't changed its length. Furthermore the Brugha study has been damningly criticised for other defects as in the following quotations.

https://childhealthsafety.wordpress.com/2011/08/19/autism-figures-existing-studies-shows-shocking-real-increase-since-1988/ "[The latter is not a particularly inspiring piece of work. Brugha did not find a single adult with childhood autism, nor did he refer to Baird or Baron Cohen but baldly claimed for comparison a childhood figure of 1 in 100, and he changed the standard diagnostic criteria to catch adults who would not normally have a diagnosis. Of the 14,000 potential participants there was a 50% drop out rate with 7000 responding to the original telephone survey. The survey looked for adults with one of four mental illnesses. The only autistic condition was Asperger syndrome but Brugha et al now claim to be able to give a global figure for all autistic conditions which is of course impossible. Whilst having research ethics approval the study was not carried out according to accepted ethical standards. Informed consent was not obtained. Participants were misled as to the purpose of the survey. They were not told they were being assessed to ascertain if they were mentally ill. A financial inducement to take part of a shopping voucher was offered – aside from ethical issues that would tend to encourage those of lower incomes to participate and invalidate the study. Mentally ill people are more likely to be of lower income if their ability to earn a living is impaired.]"

And much more at
https://childhealthsafety.wordpress.com/2010/02/10/uksurveyautism link/

And SBC was asked in 2009 where are all the "lost generation" 40-60 year-old non-verbal autistics wearing diapers and banging their heads on walls and spinning around - but as is his custom he has not had the decency to reply.

And the NHS is now in full criminal deceit mode, with non-autistic non-disabled older people being falsely given autistic diagnosis on the faintest excuse, whereas mothers of severely disabled toddlers despair of getting any honest diagnosis – just to pretend the increase has not happened, just as this deceiving "review" paper does too.

For these reasons Brugha's (and any similar studies) amounts to no evidence whatsoever for countering the real evidence of Hertz-Picciotto and others.)

From: Boyce, Niall (ELS-CAM)
To: r@
Sent: Monday, January 25, 2016 9:15 AM
Subject: RE: Article needs retracting: "Identifying the lost generation of adults with autism..."

Dear Robin (if I may)—

Many thanks for your email and for your concern about this paper published in *The Lancet Psychiatry* (http://www.thelancet.com/journals/lanpsy/article/PIIS2215-0366(15)00277-1/fulltext). Having read through your points and your correspondence with Dr Lai, I believe your main issue is the statement in both the abstract and the first line of the paper that "Autism spectrum conditions...comprise a set of neurodevelopmental syndromes with a population prevalence of 1% across all ages.". You are concerned that this statement is not referenced. However, I note that the subsequent sentence ("They are characterised by early-onset difficulties in social communication and unusually restricted repetitive behaviour and narrow interests.") is followed by two references, the first of which, a *Lancet* seminar by the same authors (http://www.thelancet.com/journals/lancet/article/PIIS0140-6736(13)61539-1/fulltext) includes a section on epidemiology which includes further extensive references and a discussion of the issue of prevalence across age ranges. I have pasted this below.

Perhaps it would have helped if reference 1 had been at the end of the first sentence as well as the second, but in my judgement this is not the kind of issue which would merit a retraction. From an editorial point of view, the authors have supplied sufficient referenced material cogent to their argument.

While it is true that the Hertz-Picciotto paper is not referenced in the Lancet Psychiatry review, I would point out that the abstract you cite in your email concludes that "the extent to which the continued rise represents a true increase in the occurrence of autism remains unclear", which does not to my mind accord with your reading of their conclusions, ie, "that the increase must be very real indeed". I also note that the work of this author (albeit a different paper) is cited in the *Lancet* Seminar mentioned above (ref 46).

I recognise that this is an area of some dispute; however in my view the authors have cited sufficient evidence to support their point in the context of the Review, and I do not think a retraction is merited.

Kind regards—
Niall Boyce, Editor, *The Lancet Psychiatry*

Prevalence

The prevalence of autism has been steadily increasing since the first epidemiological study,[7] which showed that 4.1 of every 10,000 individuals in the UK had autism. The increase is probably partly a result of changes in diagnostic concepts and criteria.[8] However, the prevalence has continued to rise in the past two decades, particularly in individuals without intellectual disability, despite consistent use of DSM-IV criteria.[9] An increase in risk factors cannot be ruled out. However, the rise is probably also due to improved awareness and recognition, changes in diagnosis, and younger age of diagnosis.[10, 11]

Nowadays, the median worldwide prevalence of autism is 0·62–0·70%,[10, 11] although estimates of 1–2% have been made in the latest large-scale surveys.[12, 13, 14, 15, 16, 17, 18, 19] A similar prevalence has been reported for adults alone.[20] About 45% of individuals with autism have intellectual disability,[11]and 32% have regression (ie, loss of previously acquired skills; mean age of onset 1·78 years).[21]

Early studies showed that autism affects 4–5 times more males than females .... [continuation cut out here because it relates only to m/f ratio, not relevant to this correspondence].

From: r@
Sent: 29 January 2016 16:26
To: Boyce, Niall (ELS-CAM)
Subject: Re: Article needs retracting: "Identifying the lost generation of adults with autism..."

Dear Niall,

Thank you for your detailed reply. But it appears you have answered the wrong question. Namely (I presume to infer): "As it is inconceivable that a review by Prof Baron-Cohen in the Lancet could warrant retraction, what errors are there in Robin's critique here?"

Whereas more to the point is: "Is the article seriously misleading?".....

You wrote:
"You are concerned that this statement is not referenced."

But rather my concern is that the statement is a very serious misrepresentation unsupportable by the evidence (and indeed in contradiction of it). You correctly point out that there is a reference cited in the second sentence, which does refer to some epidemiology content. But so what? That ref #1 article is just another (likewise flawed) review by the same authors, and far from giving support to their categorical assertion, it explicitly contradicts it, by using the word "probably" in all instances. I quote:

"The increase is **probably partly** a result of changes in diagnostic concepts and criteria."

"However, the rise is **probably also** due to improved awareness and recognition, changes in diagnosis, and younger age of diagnosis."

Furthermore those "probably" words are themselves at best assertions of opinion (or more likely vain hope). They don't have any statistical calculations of the "probability" involved. Rather they mean like "Our best/preferred guess is that....." So even with granting of that ref #1, that still entails a categorical leap from a mere hunch "probably partly" to a representation of seeming established knowledge in their latest first sentence. If that isn't (already) gross misrepresentation then there's something wrong with all the dictionaries.

Furthermore, you mention that their ref #1 also cites a paper by Hertz-Picciotto et al. But that paper is about air pollution and nothing to do with evidence of an increase or not. It does not change the fact that that cited earlier review equally fails to cite the important increase study of Hertz-Picciotto et al. And I remind you that such failing to mention counter-evidence is a prime hallmark of charlatanism. They've now done it not once but at least twice, notwithstanding the presumably high standards of peer-review at the Lancet and in Cambridge.

You correctly point out that that H-P paper states: "the extent to which the continued rise represents a true increase in the occurrence of autism remains unclear". But that "extent.... remains unclear" does not in the slightest reasonably translate into the "is now known to be zero" which this "lost generation" review would have us assume.

I further agree that some mere mis-positioning of references would not merit a retraction. But that is not what is involved here. Nothing in your reply undermines my key point that the opening sentence of both abstract and text (especially in conjunction with the title) are grossly misleading assertions about a crucially important question. Indeed the things you have pointed to in your reply establish all the more clearly that the statements are insupportable by the referenced sources. As does Meng-Chuan's resorting to that absurd notion that the ages can be separated from the years of birth.

So it manifestly remains the case that this "review" is very seriously misleading about a matter of key importance to the field, and therefore needs to be retracted, to reduce a serious fallacy getting proliferated among students and others.

And on top of the preceding we can add the evidence that there has indeed been an increase, again which these authors completely fail to mention. I've already pointed out the testimony of long-term experts such as Sally J Rogers, Bernard Rimland, and Lisa Blakemore-Brown. In addition to that there is my own evidence, which proves the matter beyond all reasonable doubt, but which has so far been suppressed from publication (but will not be much longer). For a bit of enlightenment on that point, I will paste in here some of my own graphs which are impossible to explain away as mere awareness or diagnosis (as the late onset would be the harder, not easier to overlook, and the ARI was for almost all of that time neutrally named the "Institute of Child Behavior Research"). SB-C has been previously made well aware of this information which he ignores in that "review". Again, failure to mention counter-evidence is a prime hallmark of charlatanism. The second graph shows that the ratio change coincides exactly with the (logically independent) increase of registrations, so one is hard pressed to avoid concluding they had the same cause. And there's a lot more besides.

[my graphs were put here]

"this swelling population is placing increasing strains on our health-care, education, and social-services systems. .... Geraldine Dawson, chief science officer for the advocacy group Autism Speaks, calls the situation "a public-health emergency.""
http://europe.newsweek.com/epidemic-special-needs-kids-heads-crisis-care-64101?rm=eu

"New Research Finds Annual Cost of Autism Has More Than Tripled to $126 Billion in the U.S. and Reached £34 Billion in the U.K."
https://www.autismspeaks.org/about-us/press-releases/annual-cost-of-autism-triples

And what is Lancet Psychiatry doing about it?

Sincerely,

Robin P Clarke

Dear Robin,

Many thanks for getting in touch again. As I mentioned in my previous email, I note that you dispute the authors' views. However, as I stated, I believe they did cite sufficient material to substantiate their point.

You state that you have carried out research which concludes that Lai and Baron-Cohen are mistaken, and that it will be published soon. When it is published and disseminated, other researchers, practitioners, and the public will be in a position to judge which data and explanations are more robust. This is part of the normal process of dispute and, where necessary, correction in the scientific record.

I therefore consider this matter to be closed.

Kind regards,
Niall

So, the situation documented so far in this chapter is as follows. The top "leading expert" professor SBC at the ultra-prestigious Cambridge University managed to put his name to an article which was grossly misleading about a most important matter. His sole co-author offered in defence only an idiotically absurd notion that the ages could be separated from the dates of birth, and an equally bonkers denial that the article meant there was no increase, when rather obviously it was indicating exactly that. Meanwhile SBC himself made no reply at all, not even after a signed-for letter was delivered to his ARC centre.

Then the editor rejected my request for retraction even though he failed to provide any rebuttal of my point that the article was grossly misleading, but instead repeatedly veered off into strawmen points. And of course the grossly misleading article had previously managed to slip through a supposedly very high criterion of "peer review" to get accepted by this supposedly top-level prestigious journal. And the PubMed controllers removed not the harmful article but only the warning to readers about it. And someone thought fit not to reply to my warning on PubMed but instead only to make a false complaint to get it removed from readability.

And there's more. Chasing up here with a websearch, I see it's not the first time that Professor Baron-Cohen has misled his readers by presenting fiction as documented fact. In the first two pages of his 2011 book "Zero Degrees of Empathy" aka "The Science of Evil", he presented as a confirmed truth that a named woman had had her hands cut off and transplanted on opposite arms by Nazi doctors. This matter has been well-presented by a blogger using the pseudonym "Lili Marlene" (Marlene, 2011). Her account is worth reading in full but I will indicate here the main points with the following excerpts.

This is Baron-Cohen's account as published on April 9th 2011 in *New Scientist*, a weekly UK-based science magazine:

"As a child growing up in a Jewish family, my father told me that the Nazis had turned Jews into lampshades, and about what had happened to the mother of one of his former girlfriends. When my father met Mrs Goldblatt he was shocked to see that her hands were reversed. The Nazis had severed her hands and reattached them so that if she put her hands out palm down, her thumbs were on the outside and her little fingers on the inside."

The anecdote was given a most prominent place in Baron-Cohen's recent book, taking up most of the second paragraph of page one:

"My father also told me about one of his former girlfriends, Ruth Goldblatt, whose mother had survived a concentration camp. He had been introduced to the mother and was shocked to discover that her hands were reversed. Nazi scientists had severed Mrs Goldblatt's hands, switched them around and sewn them on again so that, if she put her hands out palms down, her thumbs were on the outside her little fingers were on the inside."

Only the most obsessive, detail-oriented reader is likely to uncover the truth about the Goldblatts, buried in the notes section on page 144 at the back of the book, that there is in fact no Ruth Goldblatt whose mother is Mrs Goldblatt with reversed hands:

"Her name has been anonymized as I have not been able to trace her to seek her consent for her real name to be used."

.... the names "Ruth Goldblatt" and "Mrs Goldblatt" were made up by Baron-Cohen and are not potentially traceable details of the story,....

I believe it is a serious problem that a man who is regarded as a world-class authority on autism, who tells the world what autism is and what type of people autistic people are, is happy to showcase an extraordinary story .....which includes false identifying information, in his own book that is about important matters of science, and also in a science magazine with major international standing. I cannot reconcile the idea that a scientific authority can display such a casual attitude towards the truth. If I assume that Baron-Cohen in good faith has believed this story but has not bothered to verify it, that indicates either a very sloppy or a contemptuous attitude towards verifying the truth, hardly qualities that I would expect to find in a professor from Cambridge and the director of a research organization. It would also indicate a naivety or a lack of knowledge.... ....presenting it as fact would call into question Baron-Cohen's judgement, his basic common sense, and also his suitability for his position as a professor in a department of psychiatry, which is a medical specialty.

.... this first hand transplant was done in France in 1998 by an international team of eight surgeons in an operation that took fourteen hours. [more than 50 years after the Nazis]

There is now no doubt in my mind that the reversed-hands transplant anecdote recounted as fact on page one of both UK and US editions of Prof. Simon Baron-Cohen's latest book is untrue, impossible, and an absurd urban legend that would only be unreservedly believed by a child or perhaps by an adult who lacks education or has some odd cognitive deficit that causes a lack critical faculties. *Why has a Cambridge professor with a considerable international reputation put such a thoroughly bizarre and ridiculous thing at the very beginning of his book? .... does he think the truth of a proposition is an unimportant consideration?*

It seems plain enough that a Cambridge professor in a medical/scientific discipline has written a non-fiction book in a scientific area and also given an interview with a science magazine in which he has presented a story without any cautions or qualifications as true, and that story appears to be both untrue and medically impossible. The professor chose to showcase this very unlikely story, so it must reflect back upon his scientific and intellectual reputation if it is ridiculously implausible. He never warned his readers about the possibility that it is an urban legend or put any part of the story in quotation marks.

In my reckoning, we see in respect of SBC's "lost generation" Lancet article four of the most telling hallmarks of charlatanism. Firstly, failure of an "expert" to mention major counter-evidence (of which he should be well aware, not least as he appears happy to be considered an expert on these matters). Secondly, persistent failure to give any answer to reasonable challenges. Thirdly, resorting to outrightly bogus excuses. Fourthly, suppression of criticism rather than responding to it.

And then in respect of his hand-amputation fiction we again see wilfully misleading presentation of facts and further indifference about truthfulness.

On the basis of the evidence I have presented above here, I can only conclude with my opinion that Professor Simon Baron-Cohen has indeed become a pseudo-scientist charlatan akin to Trofim Lysenko. There is however a difference. Unlike Lysenko's false-hoods, these from SBC serve to assist in a cover-up of a criminal catastrophe devastating the lives of millions of people.

And Professor Baron-Cohen's silence on this important untruth of his raises the question of whether anything else published from his Cambridge ARC is worth treating as credible information.

And I am not alone in such an evaluation of SBC's massive discontribution to autism research.

"Frankly he owes us all an apology for this lamentable state of affairs, and his resignation". (Dachel, 2009)

"No one who reads a Baron-Cohen pronouncement about autism from outside the autism world will ever feel that there is anything to worry about – the psychological distress, the physical pain, the devastated and exhausted families, the immense and astronomically costly institutional problems, the terrible parentless future of millions of helpless adults – all our experiences and concerns have been marginalised and sanitised for public consumption." (Stone, 2009)

```
1 Pinfold Street
Birmingham
West Midlands
B2 4AA

Date and Time:        09/01/2016  17:24
Session ID:               9-321154
Dest:                      UK (EU)
Quantity:                         1
Weight:                    0.035 kg

Signed For 1st            £2.05
Large Letter


Total Cost of Services     £2.05

Posted after Last Collection?    No


Barcode:          KP59737777716B

       DESTINATION ADDRESS
Building Name or Number   Postcode
18B                        CB28AH
Address Validated?          N

IT IS IMPORTANT THAT YOU RETAIN THIS
RECEIPT AS IT IS YOUR PROOF OF POSTING

PLEASE REFER TO SEPARATE TERMS AND
           CONDITIONS

Royal Mail Signed For 1st Class aims
   to deliver your Letter the next
     working day. This is not a
tracked service. You can check proof
 of receipt and proof of delivery at
www.royalmail.com or call 03459 272 100
```

~~~~~~~

13

Robert Whitaker's
"Anatomy of an Epidemic"

"The most important book on psychiatry in a generation"
— Huffington Post

Mention needs to be made here of this book by Robert Whitaker (2010), because it puts forward an alternative theory of why there have been increased diagnoses of mental disorders in recent decades.

It seems to me that the essence of the theory in *Anatomy of an Epidemic* can be reasonably outlined as consisting of two "parts" (though not presented as such in the book).

The first "part" is the idea that various psychiatric drugs prescribed for various diagnoses commonly convert short-term conditions into long-term conditions and even cause permanent brain damage. In reviews and comments at Amazon.com and other websites there is extensive discussion of the various aspects of this idea, but it is beyond the scope of this present book or my own expertise and interests to take a view of them here (because I have since childhood considered drugs to be a load of pseudic crrap anyway, for reasons explained in Chapter 1).

Anatomy's second "part" is the idea that those drug effects are the reason why there has been majorly increased mental illness in the US.

There could be assumed to be a sort of rivalry of two alternative explanations of the increase here (drugs or amalgam), and yet conceivably an increase could be due to a combination of both. But my own view of the evidence, as I will show below, is that it points to the increases being almost entirely attributable to the dental mercury and only minorly to the drugs factor.

It appears to me that I happened upon these questions from a less confusing direction than that from which Whitaker has come. I first encountered the much more detailed information relating to the autism increase, and the much more detailed social security data of the UK compared to the sparser stats in the US.

Anatomy has two chapters about increased psychiatric diagnoses of children, and yet does not even mention autism. It would be difficult with even the most superficial credibility to explain the increase of autism in terms of psychiatric drugs being prescribed to them.

Anatomy contains far less timeseries data than I have presented in Chapter 3 here. It is largely confined to just six datapoints of social security enrolments in the US, plus a reference to childhood disability payments having rocketed up in recent years (but with no mention of the concurrent huge autism increase). There is mention of a 56% increase of adult bipolar diagnoses from 1996 to 2004. And of 40-fold increase of juvenile bipolar diagnoses from 1995 to 2003. It is not clear to what extent these figures reflect changes of terminology from "manic-depressive" to "bipolar".

Meanwhile, the critical dates of causal events proposed in *Anatomy* appear to be as follows, (though nowhere clearly set out in that book, and here clarified from searching Wikipedia):

Major tranquilliser Thorazine licensed 1954.
Tranquilliser Meprobamate marketed from 1955.
Anti-depressant Iproniazid 1957
Librium 1960 onwards
Lithium FDA approved 1970; 1974 for prevention
Prozac licenced 1987
Ritalin from 1960s and increased from 1990s

In Chapter 3 here you can see my Figure 5 which shows the apparent increase of adult disability following the introduction of non-gamma-2, an increase shaped remarkably like an exponential curve (till its mangling by "caseload now controlled"). And my Figure 7 shows the earlier increases following the introduction of the first amalgams 150 years earlier. Neither of those increase charts seem to have any connection with the dates of events cited or implied in *Anatomy*, whereas they relate very logically to the events in the history of amalgam.

For these reasons, while counterproductive drugs may or may not have caused more harm than good, I very much doubt whether they have been more than minor contributors to the increases documented in Chapter 3 here.

~~~~~~~

14

A "pause" for reflection,
as in Schumann's Carnaval

"The man who wrote this outrageously hideous noise, no longer deserving of the word music, is either a lunatic, or he is rapidly approaching idiocy." — Otto Floersheim, 1899

This book has combined a diversity of contents in order to best serve its main purposes of presenting the reality of the pseudo-expertise catastrophe and of adding to your understanding and capability of how to practically respond thereto.

The first chapter showed you the fundamentally flawed social and institutional setups which causally underlie it all. The second chapter showed you some of that would-be expertise in action leading us down to ever greater depths of cluelessness about the topic of autism (with much relevance by way of introduction to the subsequent chapter).

That third chapter then showed you the evidence of what the main great catastrophe has consisted of, and its magnitude of many millions of victims, millions most of whom do not even know what has happened to them let alone how or why. The fourth and fifth chapters then showed you some of the unventilated sewerage system that passes itself off as the distinguished elite of academia, at the heart of the darkness of fully "qualified" "expertise". And how that crucial "peer review" system really works or rather doesn't — not least in deceitfully suppressing the knowledge of that catastrophe from the public in general and from the millions of its victims in particular.

The sixth chapter then put some necessary context to the third chapter's information about the autism increase, along with some further clarification about how not to get confused by incompetent graphing or the complexities of disputation between experts, "experts", and yet more "experts".

Then the seventh chapter belonged here because it presented the "parent paper" to the "child paper" which formed the substance of Chapter 3. And also because it is a very telling actual example of what the "distinguished experts" succeed in pretending does not exist (even though published into the "peer-reviewed" and indexed journal literature record), for no good reason other than that the system gives not the slightest incentive or obligation for anyone in "scientific" "research" to acknowledge that someone somewhere else is several decades ahead of their own prestigiously-praised third-rate efforts.

And then the eighth and ninth chapters presented the very same catastrophe as Chapter 3, but from the perspective of the lone deceived and perplexed victim rather than from the perspective of the science researcher looking down with hindsight on impersonal statistics of millions (i.e., millions of other such lone deceived perplexed victims getting diagnosed as having "MS", "CFS", "Candida", "MCS", "fibromyalgia", etc., or any of various things in the psychiatrists' DSM bible, when not being merely vilified and penalised as a "workshy" "scrounger").

The tenth chapter then revealed yet another important seam of pseudo-expertise as experienced by this same lone individual rebuffed by the same faceless system.

And the eleventh chapter showed another major angle on the system of pseudery, in the massive crime committed by a head of a medical school no less, whose crime I exposed long ago, but who has since been awarded a CBE and honorary MD rather than a prison sentence, with the rather predictable grim subsequent results I documented there.

The twelfth chapter showed how Simon Baron-Cohen's Cambridge UK has become the world's centre of abysmalness of autism pseudo-research, in Lysenkoist pretence about the catastrophic increase of autism.

And the thirteenth chapter then gave the necessary discussion of Robert Whitaker's alternative theory of some of the disability increase data.

Which brings us to this chapter here now, where I think is a good point for a little "pause for reflection", as in Schumann's Carnaval before launching on to finale sections (though as with some of the best symphonies you may get a false ending or two anyway).

So, firstly, have I impressed on you the extraordinary scale of what has been unearthed here? On the radio I heard a young woman in tears that she had been unemployed for two years. But if only I myself had been jobless for a mere two years, what a paradise

I could hardly even have hoped for! In the news media we hear a lot about tragedies affecting victims. Much time is taken up with emphasising the magnitude of the tragedy of victims of sexual abuse. We hear how their lives have been "ruined" by these abuses. Maybe so. But for how many of those victims did the abuse lead to them being persistently rejected from completing their educations or getting any qualifications, how many were rejected from having any career, or the normal social and family life which can only follow on from such a career? How many of them ended up vilified as talentless unworthy "workshy" "scroungers"? If those sexual abuse victims did indeed have their lives ruined, quite what is the correct much stronger word for what has happened to the millions who have by no fault of their own chanced to become the subjects of the crime detailed in these chapters here? Where is the apology to those victims and where is the judgment against their offenders?

And now, secondly: How come this outrageous enormity has been an absolute secret for decades, and only revealed now in this book? Well, the answer lies in these same pages.....

The original 19th century amalgam was lied about as being "silver" rather than largely unreacted mercury. The ADA and BDA thrived on the huge profits from that nasty lie and still do.

The symptoms began only after delay and in rather variable, vague manner, and as they typically involved shameful tiredness or depression they tended to reduce their own reporting.

The introduction of non-gamma-2 in the 1970s was then lied about with the pretence that amalgam had been in use for over 150 years (with the implication of no significant change within that time).

Then the system of falsehoods (detailed in appendix to Chapter 3) somehow got developed in the medical profession, not least the psychiatrists' "Birds are highly unlikely to have wings" claptrap, the toxicologists' pseudo-testing with blood and urine levels, and the Chief Denial Officer's parrotting line of no mercury being released and never doing any harm anyway.

These and other falsehoods were then deployed to nastily fob off the victims from any honest treatment or even understanding of what caused their disabilities. And the NHS appointments system was carefully perverted to make it even harder for the victims to get any recognition let alone help (as Update 2 in Chapter 3 explains).

Trash pseudo-studies such as from Brugha and Polyak were marshalled to pretend that the catastrophic increase of autism had not even happened. "Leading expert" Baron-Cohen added his claptrap of autism being "1% across all ages".

The hostility to critical questions somehow became operative in these fields. Honest helpful people such as Dr Sarah Myhill and Dr Graeme Munro-Hall were subjected to persecution by the GMC gang of fascistic nannying crooks. And in the US, similar abuses were visited upon dentists such as Hal Huggins and others (as cited in Chapter 4).

And then there was, or rather wasn't, the official feedback from the victims themselves. In the UK, an EU directive puts on the MHRA the responsibility for monitoring the effects of the use of amalgam in the UK. In 2015 I made a FoI request to the MHRA as to how they were carrying out that monitoring duty. Their reply stated that they had a means for receiving reports via their Yellow Card system. And they had had only two reports "of concern" about amalgam, and zero "medically-confirmed" reports, those being cases where a practitioner "confirmed" the involvement of amalgam. And yet, how would any practitioner come to be making such a confirmation?

Consider the case detailed in Chapters 8 and 9. The victim there spent over a decade persistently presenting much evidence of amalgam causation of decades of disability. He just happened to be someone who had already been notably talented in scientific writing. He did a considerable amount of research and writing down of the evidence. But again and again, the reply was that the MHRA's own expert Tablets of Stone revealed the Truth that "amalgam is harmless", therefore it IS harmless, and therefore no case presenting to a practitioner can actually be a case able to be "confirmed" by that practitioner in a Yellow Card report to the MHRA. Thus there is a perfect circle of self-confirmation. "The MHRA is correct, therefore the MHRA is still correct" sort of logic.

And then of course there has been the suppression of my own scientific reports. As detailed at the end of Chapter 1, I have been trying to tell the world since 2004 about my discovery of the non-gamma-2 catastrophe, and yet my efforts were deceitfully blocked by the sloppy lies of the "peer review" system as you can see for yourself in Chapters 4 and 5 along with that ending section of the first chapter.

And now even with this book the denial is sure to go on. "It's just self-published assertions which had already failed the peer review test." "The author Clarke has no qualifications for writing it. He is not a professor of psychiatry, nor of toxicology, nor of dentistry or epidemiology, so why should we take any notice of his ranting about these matters?"

To which I reply: The processes by which people get to be designated as medical professors are described and discussed in Chapter 1 here, and I for one am far from impressed by them. And all the more so, given my evidence in Chapter 11 that head of medical school "Professor" Frank Woods BSc BM BCh DPhil FRCP(Lon) FFPM FRCP(Edin) Hon FFOM CBE Hon MD turned out to be a monstrous callous criminal liar, and likewise my evidence in Chapters 3 and 8 in respect of "Distinguished" "Professor" Allister Vale MB BS, MD FRSM FRCP FAACT FFOM FRCP(Edin) FRCP(Glas) FBTS Hon FRCPS FBPS FEAPSCT, and likewise some anonymous "professor" of psychiatry managing to come up with that humungous "Birds are highly unlikely to have wings" criminal claptrap also in Chapters 3 and 8. In addition to which there might be warranted a mention here of two other so-called leading expert professors whose writings are discussed in Chapters 6 and 12.

If those (and many similar) cases are anything to go by, then this book is all the more credible and authoritative from *not* being authored by a "professor".

~~~~~~~

15

What can be done about the failed institutional systems?

".... just another symptom of complete healthcare system failure, resulting in an epidemic of misinformed doctors.... which has, and continues to, sadly contribute to considerable ill health in the population"
 – Cardiologist Dr Aseem Malhotra.

"What will it take for scientific integrity to become valued in medicine?"
 – Suzanne Humphries M.D.

This book has included much about the victims who have been disabled by the lies of pseudo-experts. But there is another important group of victims. That is the many thousands of honest talented people who spend many years working on becoming competent experts. These honest hard-working experts are betrayed by the treachery of the charlatans such as those named in this book. And worse, they often get ruinously persecuted for their honesty and genuine expertise, as I will come back to later in this chapter.

In recent years numerous books and documents from others have been complaining about the defectiveness of the medical expertise system. And of course they contain their own recommendations of what should be changed to improve the situation. Notable recent examples are Healy (2013), Gøtzsche (2013), Goldacre (2012), Kendrick (2014), Davies (2013),and Bauer (2012), though others certainly merit mention too.

Rather than duplicating their efforts in this chapter, I shall add here my own distinctive suggestions from my perspective of seeing a wider problem with the whole globe-wide system of supposed expertise and the education system that reckons to create and identify that expertise.

Looking back at the sequence of Chapter 1, the following thoughts come to mind.

The over-preoccupation with exams is a crucial problem which has to be addressed. Of course it would not be a great solution to entirely dispense with exams, especially for some purposes such as gas maintenance and foreign language learning, where competence can be both meaningfully and usefully assessed thereby.

But two changes could usefully be made in respect of exams more generally. Firstly, there could be much more use of coursework, subject of course to measures to minimise the obvious potential for abuses. But at the end of the day, if a student copies someone else's foolish or wise work, then they are liable to be demonstrating their own folly or wisdom in their choice of what to copy anyway. And my Chapter 1 quote from Edwards 2014 particularly merits serious attention.

Secondly, there should be a recognition that exam grades measure learning ability but they also dis-measure the no-less-important *un*learning ability. And so it should be understood that making the exam sequence more demanding of higher scores does not result in higher intellectual quality of output. On the contrary, beyond a certain point it just results in an output of the sort of mindless parrotting of which I have shown far too much evidence here. To address this problem it is necessary to understand that beyond a moderate level, higher exam grades, such as higher A-level grades, do not even correlate positively with being a genuinely better student. Universities should stop demanding ever higher grades and instead should apply a ceiling to their requirements, with nothing more demanded than perhaps B grades, and then make the final selection from any resulting surplus by means of a random selection "lottery". I recall hearing of a country which has indeed operated such a system though I forget which (maybe Sweden).

What I have just suggested may seem to some readers to be "unfair" to those who by mere fluke don't get accepted through the lottery. But in reality the existing system of ever-higher hoops is even more unmeritocratic in that it selects the parrots and rejects those with superior unlearning abilities.

There also needs to be a reduction of the excessive number of exam-hoops to be jumped through. Alternative talents need to be allowed alternative means of rising to the top. A competent intellectual community needs a variety of mentalities and backgrounds rather than just ranks of clones of the existing supposed elites.

Particularly misconceived and counter-productive is the obsession with number of publications as being supposedly some indicator of a researcher's merit, and supposedly a good basis for determining career fortunes. One regularly sees science professionals declaring proudly that they have had over a hundred peer-reviewed papers published, along with a dozen books. To which my own thought is, in that case why haven't I already heard of this person who has produced so much outstanding work? I personally would be ashamed at having had a hundred papers published and still being a non-celebrity. It would indicate that none of those papers was much of a great discovery. Others have repeatedly pointed out that a great deal of what gets published in "peer-reviewed" journals is far from high quality material anyway.

It needs to be recognised that getting something published is not in itself inherently something to be praised for or to be proud of, even if it is in a "peer-reviewed" or "prestigious" journal. What matters is *what* is published. Publishing average drivel should be a cause for shame rather than pride or promotion.

"We need less research.... Abandoning using the number of publications as a measure of ability would be a start." (Altmann, 1994)

"The current governmental funding models and mechanisms leave scientists no choice but to prostitute themselves in the hopes that by pursuing the "junk" that is favored by the funding agencies and reviewers, they might also have the occasional opportunity to pursue knowledge and truth." (Smith, 2014)

In the modern world of online information, the scope for scientific publishing is no longer limited by scarce costly journal pages. There is no reason why everyone should not just put their discoveries on the web and get them indexed (in archives such as PeerJ and bioRxiv), without the failed "peer-review" process intervening. If some twat researcher wishes to post a hundred papers of drivel under their name, then great, we can see how much their efforts aren't worth! Oh, but the peer review filters out fraudulent reports. Really? In that case you will be able to explain to me *how* it does that. Meanwhile I could explain to you how it regularly filters out the most honest reports while accepting seriously fraudulent ones into the most "prestigious" journals. I remind you of that quote from Smith (2014) on the second page of this book:

> "Much of what is published continues to be misleading and of low quality. The problem doesn't arise from amateurs dabbling in research but rather from career researchers."

> – Richard Smith, editor of the British Medical Journal

and that even more damning quote from Marcia Angell.

Personally I consider the peer-review exclusion process to be of very little value or more accurately positively harmful, and no longer necessary in the online age anyway, but at the least it should not operate as it does currently. It is absolutely unacceptable for papers to be suppressed by faceless unaccountable anonymous liars such as you can see in earlier chapters here. Those reviewers for Neurotoxicology in particular should have their identities exposed (as they have criminally breached their obligations to fairness and hence any corresponding obligation to their own anonymity becomes void) and they should be expelled from the profession to stop them committing any further such crimes.

Likewise, citation counts should not be treated as any useful measure of merit either. An important breakthrough (such as Boltzmann's statistical thermodynamics or Mendel's peas), creating whole new horizons, is liable to not have any other researchers immediately in that field to cite it until years later. Meanwhile inbred groups of publish-perish drivel-authors are liable to generate high volumes of back-scratching cross-citations which prove nothing except how easy the EndNote citations software is to use if your institutional connections can afford it.

There can be no substitute for asking the simple question "Has this researcher discovered anything much of value?". There is of course no easy way to put a definitive and agreed score number on the answer to such a question, but that doesn't make it any less true that it is the only valid question that belongs to be asked.

We also need to understand that more money spent on research does not necessarily mean more truth discovered, indeed might cause the exact opposite. Cutting-edge scientific research is very intellectually challenging, to the extent that only a minority in any generation are up to doing the job competently. The question arises of whether simply increasing the number of researchers could result only in a larger number of incompetents (evidencelessly parrotting for instance about a non-existent "disorder") blocking from view the real talents (who used to be called geniuses). As Mercola (2014) recently wrote:

> "According to the NIH, part of the reproducibility problem stems from poor training, so a program is being developed to educate researchers on good experimental design and transparent conduct. It really is hard to imagine why researchers would not have received this type of training previously, as this is exactly the kind of training you should get when studying at some of the most respectable universities in the country."

A further problem with the expertise system is that each succeeding generation of designated experts then goes on to designate who are to be the designated experts of the next generation and so on indefinitely. That would be good if the earlier lot of designated experts were indeed high in competence and honesty. But it is all too clear that that is often far from being the case, as evidenced by some of the books and other sources I have mentioned herein. So we need to break that defective process whereby the next generations of experts get designated. We have to establish more widely the understanding that experts are not always competent and honest and that they should not be entrusted with full control over who gets treated as the rising new experts.

Altogether, there needs to be a whole radical meta-researching inquiry into the the malfunctioning of the research bureaucracy systems and their systems for training and selecting their participants.

But of course a notion of some superior meta-experts to sort out who are the genuine experts would be logically impossible. But we can at least promote that understanding that expertise credentials must not be treated with uncompromised awe as though they conferred infallible truth-telling powers. Respect is due but not too much. And respect is also due to those who ask reasonable questions and don't get reasonable answers, notwithstanding their lack of "qualifications" as experts.

There is also rather obviously a very serious problem with medical schools. There needs to be an end to their functioning as parrotting academies for the drugs pushers. Funding and sponsoring from the profiteering drugs-pushing corporations needs to be made illegal, except insofar as medical schools are prepared to have their prospectuses prominently enlightening the students that they would be studying in propaganda centres rather than institutes of neutral learning. And there needs to be a rejection of the notion that sensible medical expertise comes from the hyperactive force-feeding of information described in the first chapter here. A more sane balance needs to be enforced. And the abusive persecution and intolerance of those asking the "wrong" questions needs to be rooted out as well.

But for the present, Peter Scott, a professor of higher education at the posh University College London, sees universities becoming yet more bureaucratised and politicised (Scott, 2016).

A further serious problem is the nannying industry. By which I mean a whole complex of force-wielding bureaucracies pretending to be in the business of protecting us from dangers. An illustration of the outstanding hypocrisy of this phenomenon can be seen in an email correspondence I had with my MP Dr Lynne Jones in 1997/8 in connection with the attempt to ban people from buying "dangerous" vitamin B6 (which has never killed anyone or even seriously injured any except when injected by MDs). I first asked Dr Jones whether she agreed with the precautionary principle, that vitamin B6 should be banned until proven safe. She agreed that yes, I should indeed be banned from buying vitamin B6 until it had been proven safe (even though it had already been adequately proven safe in reality). At which I asked the follow-up question: so presumably she also agrees that the precautionary principle should be applied to cars, that cars should be banned from the public roads until proven safe? At which she responded with something along the lines of "Don't be so ridiculous....". I forget her exact words (which are somewhere in my huge archive on floppy discs) but one observer commented that he was astonished that an MP would reply to a constituent in such an extremely uncivil manner. But let's indeed consider how ridiculous the comparison is. No one is forced to take vitamin B6 tablets. Even if they were, they have never harmed anyone anyway (at least not discernably) and many people would greatly benefit from taking them. Certainly they don't constitute a danger to those who don't put them in their mouths. By contrast, I and many others are every day put in lethal danger by motorists driving cars. I have no choice in the matter, and indeed there is a huge rate of deaths and injuries to innocent third parties thanks to cars not being banned until proven safe. Indeed, the cars are not even required to be in decently conspicuous colors rather than dangerously camoflagued in grey and black. And not even properly policed for dangerous speeding. And their toxic fumes.

And yet we supposedly need a whole huge system whereby this same government is supposedly protecting us from those deadly vitamin tablets (and far too much more, such as healthy natural un-denatured real milk).

The real reason why vitamin B6 is "dangerous" is that it regularly *cures* such serious profit-generators as sleeplessness, depression, anxiety, obsessions, phobias, migraines, pmt, and epilepsy, and thereby is extremely dangerous to the profits of the manufacturers of pharmaceutical drugs. My own theory of B6's importance is that the brain needs to make adjustments to stressful events. Those adjustments require changes of the proteins in the brain (reconfiguring the neurons and their interconnections). Vitamin B6 is known to be required for that processing of proteins. And so a stressful situation makes heavy demands on the B6 supply, which if insufficient results in insufficient brain adjustment and thence those psychological problems.

My experience of such nannying organisations as the FDA in the US and the COT and MHRA in the UK is that a remarkably reliable rule is that if they say something is dangerous then it is most likely to be a natural product vitally necessary for your good health (e.g. a vitamin or real milk), whereas if they say something is perfectly safe then it is most likely to be a ruinously poisonous corporate profiteering product. The very same years the COT were conspiring to get harmless B6 banned they were also publishing their second report pretending that toxic amalgam is harmless. Likewise the same FDA crooks who still insist that amalgam is harmless have concurrently banned everyone including their disinformed victims from obtaining the entirely harmless OSR#1 (aka NBMI, now renamed Emeramide and Irminix) which they need to get that mercury poison back out again.

I think a point warrants emphasising here. **If these governments were really in the business of protecting us, they would take real effective measures to protect us from the major danger of reckless motoring. And yet they do nothing of the kind.** Motorists are effectively free to race murderously around our streets in the dark and wet in near-invisible dark-coloured vehicles. Speedophiles kill and maim far more children than pedophiles ever have. And even when they rather predictably cause deaths it is still regularly just treated as an "accident" rather than any cause for proper sanctions. And likewise with the indifference to the deathly harm from the pollution caused by motorists. These facts make clear that these governments do not impose safety rules for our protection but are only pretending that that is the reason when in reality their rules are just to assist abusive industries such as big pharma.

This system of nannying lying criminals needs to be closed down. If they wish to issue their trashy advice that's fine. If they wish to issue a system of certificates of their assertions of safety, that's fine. But they have no right whatsoever to tell people (in the "free world") that they are not allowed to buy and treat or feed themselves with substance x merely because in their deceiving pseudo-opinion it is pretendedly dangerous or not proven safe. The sooner these taxpayer-sponging scam organisations are closed down the better.

The same goes for the UK's General Medical Council and the General Dental Council (and equivalents in other countries). These are likewise scam entities which persecute all the honest helpful practitioners (such as Sarah Myhill, Graeme Munro-Hall, and Andrew Wakefield) while leaving the real dangerous drug-peddlers and amalgam-peddlers free to continue their deadly abuses (as documented by many such as in the book by Kendrick (2014) for instance).

Just now I have to update this chapter with news of yet another tragic victim of the GMC criminals, namely Dr Waney Squiers:

"The accusations against Dr Waney Squiers are a clear attempt to silence a brave pathologist who dared questioning the dogma of one of the most contested diagnoses in paediatric neuropathology. She is accused of being dishonest, when she had the honesty to change her diagnosis in the light of new research that showed her previous diagnosis may have been erroneous."
– Pathologist (2014).

Why don't these persecuting scum just present their own "expert" testimony of why she is supposedly wrong? Well, do I really need to answer that question?

We need to get rid of such vile fascistic busybodies dictating to others what they can and cannot do. Everyone properly has the right to practice medicine. If a law makes it a crime for you to help a person in need of help or to give them true health information, then the real crime is that perverted law which reckons to convert a moral obligation into a so-called crime. All such laws need to be recognised as obnoxiously improper and made unlawful by constitution.

If the General Meddling Criminals wish to operate a voluntary accreditation program, giving certificates to their approved trashy doctors, then that's fine. Then the public can go to those GMC-accredited poodle doctors if they so wish. Or if they prefer to go to genuine honest doctors without the bureau-rats's accreditation they can do that too if they wish. It's my life. If I want to harm myself I have any number of easy ways of doing so anyway, especially as there are all those proven-safe cars whizzing around just along from here. No amount of bureau-rat nannying can prevent that self-harm. Get rid of these taxpayer-sponging deadly scam organisations now. And all those deceit-imposing NHS "Chief Executives" would be better kicked out and replaced by homeless people dragged in off the streets who couldn't possibly do a worse job.

Oh but hang on! If we were to implement Robin P Clarke's crackpot proposals then all manner of terribly dangerous "therapies" would be let loose on victims. Actually the exact opposite. Right now under the present health-fascist regimes we have thousands of victims being fed poisonous statins, chemo"therapy" and so on, while being banned from obtaining the things they really need for their health. FDA, GMC, etc, please just fuck off and get a proper job.

But the problem runs deeper, or should I say higher. There's a saying that a fish rots from the head. The corruption of medical politics is a symptom of the wider corruption of government in a flawed political system, That system is the so called democracy in which mass-media electioneering gives all the effective control to corrupt global corporations. A fuller analysis of this problem, and a majorly worked-out solution thereto, was presented in an earlier book of mine, which I have not yet got round to actually publishing, namely "The future is here! A practical handbook of solving the key crisis of our times" (Clarke, 2013) (re which see note in the list of references). You may still find it on lulu.com if you websearch for it.

But can any of this actually be done?

A problem with all lists of proposals such as the above is that even if some proposal is shown to be a good idea it is still liable to not happen if unworthy forces of the status quo choose to not let it happen. It is now forty years since Ivan Illich's demolition of the medical nannyocracy, and many further critical books have been written since, and yet the "revolution" hasn't happened yet. So should it be reckoned that this is just another book of head-banging against a wall?

I suggest not for a number of reasons. Firstly, the growth of the internet has revolutionised the field of health information. Many "non-experts" are now much more informed about their health issues. The challenges to the official lies now get significantly effective publicity via the internet, not least via numerous "alternative" health sites such as most prominently Mercola.com and naturalnews.com (not that I agree with everything they say). The availability of search engines and online info has revolutionised public access to information. In the past, if you wanted to check out whether there's any research indexed on "Does autism have anything to do with antimony?", you would have to do a longwinded search through huge heavy volumes of Index Medicus at a medical school (as I myself have spent too much time doing), with the prospect all that time that you might just come up with a blank of no information anyway. But now you can do a search (for [antimony autism]) of the whole of PubMed, or of the entire internet, in just seconds, at home (or even on a train!) from any modern internet connection. You can also read or join in to extensive discussion about things on the internet.

This information revolution reduces the power of the corporate establishment and increases the power of the "heretics".

There have been efforts towards undermining the usefulness of the internet as a source of uncensored information. The health pages of Wikipedia are heavily mindered by corporate shills controlling the editing process and banning as "vandals" any who make edits challenging the corporate "truth".   Meanwhile, the search engine Google has also sold its soul to the corporate pseudo-medicine, with a conspiracy to filter health sites according to how "true" the information is (Adams, 2015).   And who exactly decides what is true? Well, here's a fact that may be pertinent. Dr Thomas Insel has been doing a very shoddy job as head of the National Institute of Mental Health, as others have made clear.   In his chairing of the Interagency Autism Coordinating Committee much public money was wasted on trying to prove that autism was all genetic anyway, and meanwhile a lack of research money given towards seeking environmental factors. And now?

And now this same Dr Insel is leaving the NIMH to join Google. Just at the time when Google is becoming a "truth" engine rather than a search engine. You can already see how searches bring up the corporate establishment sites at the top and the independent ones nowhere. Is this a disaster? Probably a disaster for Google, because once a search engine has decided to abandon informational neutrality, its credibility is heading firmly down the drain. Why would Google want to employ Insel, the nation's topmost mental health bureaucrat? There are numerous other search engines you can turn to, not least the "goodgopher" created by Mike Adams of NaturalNews.com.

Anyway, my own guess is that now that the pseudo-expertise bubble has already been punctured, the attempts to re-seal that puncture are now too late.

Secondly (of the reasons this isn't just another book of head-banging against a wall), there appears to have been an increase of the outflow of books expertly exposing the defective expertise in the medical world, such as those I have already listed. And it is clear that there is growing unease in the medical and research communi-ties about the defectiveness of the systems under which they work. Most people would prefer not to earn their living by disreputable and disreputed means.

Indeed the "thinker" Atul Gawande recently expressed alarm at the level of distrust of his "science" while successfully failing to take a hint from the fact that the more educated are the more distrustful.

And thirdly, and I suggest most importantly, there is the Tectonic Plates Factor. Wegener published his theory of continental drift in 1912. It was almost universally dismissed as absurd for the next fifty years. But then it rapidly became accepted as one of the fundamental principles of modern geography. The reason for that abrupt "tectonic plates revolution" was largely that developments in seabed exploration enabled the "joins" of the drifting "plates" to be actually "seen" at last.

And there is an analogous situation in respect of this present book. For decades, people have been claiming the existence of a catastrophe of medical pseudo-expertise, but have not been able to show any pictures of it for all to "see". And for more than a century people have been claiming that great harm has been being caused by the mercury from dental amalgams, but again they have not been able to show pictures of that catastrophe for people to "see".

But now in this book, you can see for yourself my pictures of the huge catastrophe, a catastrophe of millions disabled by mercury from dental amalgams, but more importantly and fundamentally a catastrophe caused by the grievously flawed globe-wide system for training and designating people as supposedly "leading experts".

No other document has ever done this before. And I suggest it can be a "game changer", akin to those joins of the tectonic plates being made "visible" at last. This book might not be able to spark that revolution if it were being published in a vacuum lacking other books critical of the medical nannyocracy. But on the contrary, a whole sequence of excellent critiques has recently emerged, not only the books such as I have cited here, but also prominent journal articles about these critical failings. And thanks to that context, I suspect that this book could indeed be the "last straw" starter of a change at last from this pile of pseudo-meritocratic pseudo-distinction which has caused so much ruinous harm not only to myself but to so many millions of other victims.

It is common practice to quote sentences from books and articles. Equivalent "quoting" of pictures can of course also be done (except in audio and radio broadcasts), even though such picture-quoting is a less common practice. My own graphic "pictures" of this catastrophe are by default copyrighted by myself but I don't want anyone to thereby feel restrained from "quoting" them in however much quantity, free of any fee though preferably with some respect for where they have come from (and hopefully with a little acknowledgement of my own efforts in their production). Hopefully I can put some quality files of them on a website of mine, from where anyone can download for purposes of "quoting" them.

A website for resources relating to this book is being set up at www.pseudoexpertise.com. (Alternatively www.robinpclarke.com) It would have had a more sensible domain name but all the more sensible names had already been registered by various other pseuds.

Anyway this would be the end of this book except that I thought I would keep the worst for last......

~~~~~~~

16

Update review of the published theory (with some surprises!)

"If you can't think of anything better to put there, begin each chapter with a mystifyingly-vaguely-relevant platitudinous quotation from some historically famous intellect in the hope of gaining gravitas by association." – Albert Einstein's mom

This chapter is mostly based on an unpublished update review paper I originally wrote between 2004 and 2006, then sent to some readers and to a journal, and then revised and sent to further journals in about 2009-2011. Much of that update review has since been incorporated into the newer "epidemics" review included in Chapter 3 here. To avoid pointless repetition, for this chapter I have removed most of that duplicate matter. I have left some parts the same as the last 2011 revision. Some other bits are new here (Purgatorius, seizures). Yet other parts seem likely to be of variable relevance to readers of this book so I have cut them out, leaving just the section headings here so you will know what is missing; I will try to make these cut sections available on this book's website (www.pseudoexpertise.com), hopefully along with the whole docu-ment's "peer-review" commentaries if I have time.

Some other parts may have their presentation cynically tweaked here in an attempt to sell more copies of this book.

It follows that this chapter is going to be a bit of a cobbling together in contrast to the symphonically-organised other ones here. To reduce confusion I will indicate some of my choppings with "//".

Again, this paper originally began with an abstract, but in this book I have cut that out, and finally there was a references list at the end but here it has been incorporated into the one at the end of the book instead.

The causes of autism: A theory now further supported by five confirmed predictions; why dental amalgams caused increased autism; and why mercury pollution caused the Flynn effect IQ increase

Robin P Clarke

Abstract [see www.pseudoexpertise.com]

Background

This is an update review of and elaboration on an earlier paper, "A theory of general impairment of gene-expression manifesting as autism". Fullest understanding of this present paper requires familiarity with that earlier one. ..... //

.... An individual's autism status is properly described not by a "diagnosis", but rather by an autisticness score, just as they are given a height and a shoe size rather than a "diagnosis" of "biggism". ....//

Belief in theories that antiinnatia does not exist or does not manifest as autism

Some people react to any proposed theory by adopting a sort of "null hypothesis" that it is false until such time as undeniably evidenced otherwise. Erring on the side of belief is supposedly foolish gullibility whereas erring on the side of disbelief is supposedly wisdom. But sometimes a new theory simultaneously produces by implication a new counter-theory (or a limited number of alternatives), such that one can only doubt the proposed theory by entertaining the possibility that a counter-theory could be correct. In the present case, any who wish to be sceptical about the antiinnatia theory are logically obliged to be thereby considering as reasonable one or more of the following counter-theories:

1. The theory that antiinnatia would not be substantially biologically advantageous (below excessive levels)(even though shown to advantageously suppress disadvantageous expressions).

2. The theory that antiinnatia does not exist at all, despite that advantageousness and the experimental demonstrations that antiinnatia does indeed exist (both genetic and environmental)(and despite the logical inevitability of existence of both the genetic and environmental antiinnatia factors).
3. The theory that despite the biological advantageousness of antiinnatia (below excessive levels), there is no tendency for natural selection to select for its increase up to the point where counterproductive excess tends to occur.
4. The theory that antiinnatia somehow could not increase to a level at which it majorly suppresses advantageous characteristics.
5. The theory that such suppression of advantageous characteristics would not manifest as autism, but would manifest in some other way instead.

Evidence and reasonings have been presented in the original published paper (with additions here) which challenge all of these five counter-theories. Any persons who wish to publicly question the soundness of the antiinnatia theory, or to publicly ignore it, or continue to claim that autism is still some mystifying puzzle or lacking an established explanation, are requested to explain which of these counter-theories they consider to be credible alternatives and on the basis of what evidence or reasoning they reject my own evidence and reasoning. //

Autism from coal-fired power stations
[see www.pseudoexpertise.com]

Dental amalgams relative to thimerosal
[see www.pseudoexpertise.com]

Autism comparison with Poland [see www.pseudoexpertise.com]

Summary of the amalgam case [see www.pseudoexpertise.com]

Fetal testosterone, "extreme-male-brain" and "developmental instability"

A conception of autism as extreme-male-brain (EMB) (Baron-Cohen, 2002) has attracted much publicity, with many persons being led to assume that it is the only remotely meritable contemporary understanding of autism.

There is good reason to believe that fetal testosterone (FT) affects the development of the fetus, such that the brain remains thereafter more "male"; and this then manifests in more tendency towards "systematising" (as involved in science or engineering) and less towards empathising or emotional sensibility.

A questionable extension from this is the notion that FT increases some "autistic traits" and that in extreme those traits amount to autism, with autism being understood as being effectively identical to EMB. This "autism = EMB" thesis depends on overlooking the substantial evidence which does not fit with it. Autism has had strong associations with high social class and high parental IQ (Clarke, 1993), and it is far from clear why extreme-male-brain would have. Likewise unclear is how it could credibly account for the symmetry data or the physical stigmata (Clarke, 1993), or why it would involve such un-male but classic autism characteristics as shyness, hand-flapping/posturing, echolalia of whole sentences, lack of dizziness after spinning, intense resistance to change, toe-walking, etc (Clarke, 1993).

EMB also struggles to explain the famous increase of autism, invoking at best a notion of a hypothesised increase of assortative mating of geeks. It is difficult to see any credible calculation of how assortative mating could have so rapidly increased autism tenfold within 20 years. And EMB also fails to account for the stark change of ratio of age of onset.

On the one hand those numerous facts clash with the autism-as-EMB and geek assortative mating conceptions, while on the other hand there is the fully satisfactory alternative explanation presented here and in my own autism theory paper.

These considerations show that EMB has inadequate merit as a candidate for being the central theoretical concept of autism. It can however be seen to be a part of the story, as I will now explain.

Innate programming has a more substantial role in the behaviour of female mammals than of males, for pregnancy management and nurturing (for instance empathy, theory of mind, communication). So the biologically optimum level of antiinnatia is lower for females. (In addition they would tend to have stronger genetic endowments of these predispositions, more resistant to antiinnatia factors.) Meanwhile, "systematising" is what brains do as a matter of default in the absence of specific pre-programmed reactions being evoked. Consequently the relatively "blank slate" mind of high antiinnatia tends to look like "male brain" in some respects. Or they even tend to actually be the same thing. Males would have a higher optimal level of antiinnatia, and so the characteristically male hormone testosterone would advantageously tend to raise antiinnatia somewhat (or in other words FT would tend to be something of an antiinnatia factor).

If FT were the sole or principal non-environmental antiinnatia factor, then women would be concentrated at the low end of the scales of IQ, health, body symmetry and beauty, while men would be concentrated at the high end of those scales. But that rather obviously is not the case, and that tells us that FT cannot be more than a relatively minor antiinnatia factor.

See also the explanation in the sex differences section of my published theory paper.

The associated concept of "developmental instability" presumes that organisms have "correct", "intended", "normal" courses and outcomes of development from which "maldevelopment" deviates. But they do not. There is no blueprint in DNA; rather, development just happens blindly and aimlessly in interaction with varying environment, just as natural selection does. And already in my published autism theory paper I had indicated two respects in which even erraticness ("instability") of phenotypic outcome can be biologically advantageous (i.e. "intended").

The correct concept—the oxygen to this phlogiston of developmental science—is antiinnatia, now more evidentially-supported than ever. //

Yet more evidence in support of the antiinnatia theory

Below here I will elaborate on five predictions or implications of the original theory which have now been confirmed by others' evidences. But I shall first mention here some other findings I have encountered in the more recent literature. I have not made a comprehensive reading of the many papers since the 1990s and so it is likely that some notable other findings are overlooked here.

Some of the theorised innatons can now be understood to be physically instantiated as mirror neurons (Mukamel et al., 2010), von Economo neurons (Allman, 2005), and other long-distance (hence genetically-guided) neurons in the brain. Some of the other recent findings in accordance with the theory include the following. The sense of self, arguably an innate predisposition, is reduced in autism (Lind and Bowler, 2009). There is reduction of connectivity in face processing (Kleinhans et al., 2008). Autistic females have increased hirsuitism (Ingodomnukul et al., 2007), a further instance of atavism back to the mammalian norm, or in other words reduction of a between-species idiosyncrasy.

Pisula (2010) lists numerous areas of the brain which are known to be normally (and by implication innately) associated with specified psychological functions, and which function abnormally in autism. She notes that these findings cannot be adequately accounted for in terms of "theory of mind" or "executive dysfunction" or "lack of central coherence". But they all rather obviously fall very clearly within the concept of innatons being affected by excessive antiinnatia. So Pisula's review can be re-read in retrospect as even further testimony to the empirical soundness of the antiinnatia theory first presented to the world in 1982. Courchesne's findings of lack of the normal "resting network" and of normal lateralisation are two more examples.

Meanwhile still no evidence contrary to the theory has come to attention. //

Predictions now confirmed!

Note to readers of this book: Predictions are extremely important things in science. The ability to make significant predictions subsequently confirmed by others is the ultimate criterion of the most excellent science and scientists, against which any amount of impressive qualifications or prestigious titles is just so much superficial fluff (though you can rest assured that few whose prestige rests only on that fluff will agree on this point). **Predictions which are a bit "weird" and seemingly "off-topic", as here, are all the more notable in this regard. After all, a sun scientist correctly predicting that the sun will become visible at the eastern horizon tomorrow morning is hardly a great achievement.**

Handflapping from pre-human ancestor, and associated with lower limb movements.

My original published paper explained autistics' hand-flapping and posturing in terms of atavism (re-emergence) of pre-human innatons, more specifically the sort of alternating running and freezing which is displayed by rats and birds in certain wild contexts. The implication being that we would have had significant ancestors perhaps resembling rats or birds. Furthermore I remarked that the hand-flapping was apparently not accompanied by foot or leg movements, which I suggested could be due to the atavisms being distorted by pressure of more recent selection.

It is now known that for 160 million years the ancestors of humans were rat-like *Purgatorius* (http://animal.discovery.com/videos/animal-armageddon-purgatorius.html). For 160 million years such running and freezing would have been a matter of life and death.

Furthermore, in another video (easily findable on the internet), an autistic person named Anthony describes how stimming (meaning basically hand-flapping) tends to also involve involuntary moving forward such that the stimmer might become injured. So my thoughts that there ought to be associated lower limb movements appear to be well-founded in retrospect. And meanwhile, who else has ever proposed even a grain of a sensible explanation of the hand-flapping beyond "it just so happens" - let alone in the context of a fully-integrated theory as here? Anthony's video:

https://www.youtube.com/watch?v=ZxJCBN7NTDQ

The body symmetry – IQ correlation

The theory explained why antiinnatia would tend to suppress physical idiosyncrasies and hence increase body symmetry. The theory also explained why antiinnatia would also tend to suppress idiosyncratic innate predispositions which cause slowing and errors in mental processing; and thus why the antiinnatia would raise IQ (except that with the highest levels of antiinnatia, in profound autism, certain IQ-aiding innatons are suppressed too).

Thus the theory provided an explanation of quite why there would be a correlation between IQ and symmetry. Furlow et al. (1997) have since found such a correlation, and a subsequent study found the correlation to be specifically related to the general IQ factor g (Prokosch, 2005). (There are of course many highly-intelligent people with asymmetrical features, and the converse – it is only a correlation and obviously dependent on adverse life-events.)

Reduced expression of innate predispositions that compromise rationality

The very first draft of this theory (of autism, genius and IQ) described the unifying principle as "reduction of innate prejudices". That terminology was soon refined into "suppression of innate predispositions" (as published). The section about genius had elaborated the details of how some predispositions would be biologically advantageous even though intellectually compromising (e.g. conformity, wishful thinking, pretentiousness, superficialness, present-mindedness). I later removed all mention of genius and published the autism part alone, in the hope of making it more acceptable to publishers and readers (Eysenck, 1995).

And now in concurrence with the theory, a study has confirmed that autistic people have rationality less compromised by "gut intuition" (DeMartino et al., 2008). And von Economo neurons, considered to be involved in superficial "gut intuition" decisionmaking, are reduced in autism (Allman et al., 2005).

DeMartino et al. in their discussion section notably suggest that their results are "attributable to impairment within their intuitive reasoning mechanisms". I question whether there is such a thing as "intuitive reasoning", especially where it produces absurd *ir*rationality as in their study's subjects. But it should anyway be clear that they have in mind innate predispositions to responding in particular ways, in other words, exactly the "impairment" of some innatons such as the antiinnatia theory theorised are "impaired" by antiinnatia). As is typical with the most supposedly expert researchers they fail to mention the highly-relevant antiinnatia theory even though it was published in a peer-reviewed and PsycInfo-indexed journal years earlier. (PsycInfo is the main or only psychology journals index.)

Meanwhile Hirshfeld et al. (2007) found that racial and sexual stereotyping was *not* reduced in autism. Quote: "their fluent knowledge of race and gender stereotypes is **astonishing**". But no, not at all "astonishing", because it is not learnt "knowledge" anyway. Racial and sexual stereotyping would be strongly innate, due to strong natural selection, such that it would be much more resistant to antiinnatia than the dis-logical irrationality studied by DeMartino et al. Through thousands of years, and all over the globe, nowhere does one find a culture in which men have longer hair than women, or the men manage the home and childcare while the women do the provisioning and military defence. Racial discrimination also occurs in many cultures through space and time. And fifty years of anti-discrimination programs in the UK have far from eliminated these supposedly cultural phenomena.

Racial stereotyping is far from "irrational" – it can sometimes be a critical matter of life and death, as in Rwanda. So there would be strong natural selection for it, and thus substantial resistance to suppression by antiinnatia. And sexual stereotyping likewise would be expected to have powerful salience in natural selection.

Binding to DNA as a cause of autism

A further prediction of the theory was that molecules binding randomly to DNA and thereby inhibiting gene-expression (i.e., increasing the antiinnatia), would cause autism. The published paper stated: "The effect of such random binding is to prevent access .... thus preventing transcription .... . Obviously, then, a surplus of regulatory proteins (or pseudo regulatory proteins) would give the postulated general, indiscriminate impairment of gene-expression [thus causing autism], but whether this is the principal or even a major process is not clear at present."

More recently I had been studying mercury toxicity, and incidentally learnt that it too binds to DNA, inhibiting gene-expression at levels far below those producing other effects (Ariza et al., 1994, Goyer, 1991, Rodgers et al., 2001). Furthermore it does so dose-dependently, which would account for the widely variable intensity of the syndrome. Among metal ions, silver and divalent mercury show the strongest interactions with DNA (Walter and Luck, 1977).

All this does of course beg the question of whether mercury causes autism anyway, but we have already answered that [in Chapter 3] with a resolutely clear "yes". And the notion that mercury could not get to the DNA is discussed at http://www.autismcauses.info/search/label/dna .

There are numerous other ways that antiinnatia could be operating, in parallel with such DNA binding. For instance the suggestion of Blaylock and Strunecka that inflammation involving microglial activation could disrupt the genetically-steered growth of dendrites and axons required to make normal connectivities; though this would seem less relevant to regressive cases.

Shared causality of autism and raised IQ: various findings in line

The antiinnatia theory was from its very beginning founded on the idea that the same factors (genetic and environmental) which in higher doses cause autism would in the normal range of levels cause raised IQ (and would in a critical dose-range enable creative genius).

I pointed out in Chapter 2 the "unexpectedly" high performance of autistics on the Raven's IQ tests and their faster inspection time scores (indicating faster brain processing). These results are not surprising from the viewpoint of the antiinnatia theory. I did not include them as predictions in the published theory paper due to wariness that such results might be prevented by the considerable disabilities with which almost all autistics were affected at that time. I did suggest faster EEG AEPs of the IQ-correlated type, but it appears that no-one has yet tried to check that possibility.

A further result which would have been predicted from antiinnatia theory is that "wrong" finding of Arslan et al (2014), discussed in the Appendix to Chapter 2. Again, that was not specifically predicted in the published theory, but I think you can appreciate that back then few if any people had any conception of the sophisticated sort of analysis of mutations which the Arslan team performed there, so I can hardly be found greatly at fault in that oversight.

And....

(And now the Grand Finale Section of this book!)

Shared causality of autism and raised IQ: mercury pollution causing the Flynn effect huge IQ increase!(?)

In earlier chapters here I have presented the evidence that mercury can cause autism. The implication would appear to be that mercury would also tend to raise IQ in the normal range. Which is odd because all the world's experts are saying more or less the exact opposite, that mercury pollution is causing lowered IQs to a catastrophic extent. And executives are flying around the globe to conferences to do something about reducing this horrible mercury pollution (which I'm claiming actually makes people smarter). Silly me versus all the world's experts. Should I really continue this chapter here?

IQ scores are important but give little or no guarantee of wisdom, objectivity, or the judicious originality characteristic of history-making geniuses. IQ is roughly analogous to the speed of a computer; a faster computer will not make your photo collection more tasteful or your e-books more true. Research and discussion of the nature of and facts of IQ has been voluminous and mind-straining, and so it's not really practical to add much here beyond those two sentences above. (If interested in more on the subject, I suggest searching out some useful introductory texts by Eysenck, or Brand's "The *g* Factor" (free on the internet). There's also been a lot of ideologically-inspired wishful thinking published in this field.)

The Flynn effect (or Lynn-Flynn effect) is the worldwide observed gradual rising of average IQs over most of the 20th century. No satisfactory explanation has hitherto been found for it. The various social/cultural theories are ruled out by the effect being observed even in infancy (Lynn, 2009). And Flynn himself has rigorously dismissed any explanation in terms of improved nutrition (Flynn, 2009a). He has furthermore made a detailed analysis, raising two paradoxes. Firstly, it seems there must be an environmental "factor X" which has produced the great gains over time without producing a noticeably large effect in twin studies of heritability. Secondly, it seems that either we must all be A-graders now, or our grandparents must all have been mentally handicapped.

Anyway, at this point I will venture into an experiment with the continuation of this chapter, for the entertainment and possible enlightenment of yourself the book-reader (one hopes). Some people have suggested that one of the characteristics of genius is the taking seriously of an idea which is obviously absurd, and persisting with it until somehow the facts end up proving the genius right anyway. In this chapter I propose to try applying this principle with a view to generating an "artificial genius" effect and thus perhaps ending up producing some genius sort of result if it works. So here goes, with my mad idea being that mercury pollution is causing not lower IQ but increased IQ. All the world's experts couldn't possibly be not just wrong, but 180 degrees wrong, could they? No one else alive or dead has ever agreed with such a notion of mercury, so here goes with this "artificial genius" experiment.

Firstly one would vaguely sort-of expect that there has been an increase of mercury in the last century, due to the increase of industrialisation. So there would be increased mercury binding to DNA which would cause increased antiinnatia, and hence the IQ-impairers would be more suppressed, resulting in faster more accurate mental processing, and thus higher IQ. What could go wrong?

This causality does appear to be in line with the Flynn effect being more concentrated on "fluid intelligence" rather than on the gradually-learnt "crystallised" ability skills such as verbalising (Flynn, 1987).

The continuous inhalation of mercury vapor from the atmosphere would vary markedly between generations in line with the large Flynn effect. And yet twin pairs would have near-identical intakes. And thus the first of Flynn's paradoxes is resolved.

The other Flynn paradox, of apparently subnormal ancestors, is also easily resolved. Firstly, I remind you of the key principle of antiinnatia, that it tends to impact most strongly against characteristics that have the least evolutionary history of biological advantageousness. Thus, the somewhat-increased antiinnatia, while not radically blanking the slate of human nature to the extent of autism, would still be expected to have been eroding some important refined surface details of evolved human nature, of innate senses of beauty, wisdom, practicality and common-sense, much as too much polishing of an ancient brasswork may erase its fine engravings. This may be why many people are convinced that the Golden Ages of architecture, music, literature, social engineering, and much else, were in the eighteenth and nineteenth centuries. A similar degradation of human nature may have caused a decline of innate parenting skills. It can hardly be said that we live in an age of unprecedented wisdom, taste, and family harmony.

And we would expect the antiinnatia effect of mercury, a single simple element, to be much cruder and less helpful than the antiinnatia effect of the antiinnatia genes, a whole complex of genes which has been specially selected by natural selection specifically in terms of biological advantageousness for its human hosts. And so the mercury causing the Flynn effect would tend to degrade as much as or more than it enhances those non-IQ aspects indicated above.

And meanwhile there is also much reason to believe that more recent generations really have had higher IQs on average. There has been a very large increase of exposure to information over the past century, with developments of libraries, schooling, mass-printing, radio, tv, and travel, and a greatly increased rate of change in many things. This has created, in the words of Alvin Toffler, "future shock" and "information overload". The medieval concept of a scholar who "knows everything" is made impossible a great many times over. Even just learning all the specialist information you need has become untenable.

The capacity for learning, adapting and thinking has thus been put under increasing pressure. Mere typing used to be a specialist profession but now even young children are routinely expected to have competence with the much greater complexity of computers, smartphones and so on. So students no longer have so much time and energy to spare for learning the traditional basics of literacy and numeracy. The catastrophic Burke and Wills expedition of 1860 appears to have involved much deficit of intelligence. It may also be significant that in the UK thousands of communal homes for mentally retarded persons have been closed down without any clear adverse consequences. Binet's original development of IQ testing a century earlier was specifically for the purpose of deciding which individuals needed to be taken into such homes.

And the prominence of a tiny minority of great minds in the history books may mislead us here. The upper limit of human potential would have been no lower in previous centuries. Indeed, thanks to antiinnatia genes providing a superior substitute for mercury, it would have been higher.

Also notable is a temporary reversal of the Flynn effect in respect of children born in the UK in the late 1960s (Flynn, 2009). This closely coincided with a major reduction of mercury inhalation in the UK due to the Clean Air Acts and the demolition of many thousands of coal-heated slum terraces which were replaced by tower blocks with no coal heating. A decade later the use of non-gamma-2 dental amalgams began, which could account for the resumption of the IQ increase thereafter. If mercury vapor from dental amalgams has caused the increase of autism (as argued elsewhere), then it could be expected to have also contributed to the variations of the Flynn effect, by adding into the level of mercury vapor inhaled by a nation's population.

The peculiar findings of Spitz (1989) are particularly congruent with the antiinnatia theory, as I shall now explain in more detail. Spitz found that IQs were rising in the midrange but not in the gifted range, and the numbers of retarded were increasing.

The antiinnatia theory posits a relationship of antiinnatia to IQ which is far from linear. Rather it is something like in Figure 16.1 (and due to other factors besides antiinatia factors, is a scattergram cloud rather than the clear line shown). Over the main range there is a monotonic positive relationship but at high levels this goes into reverse due to the suppression of IQ-aiding innatons in autism. Extreme high levels of antiinnatia cause the low IQ of autism, while extreme low levels cause low IQ of the more 'ordinary' variety. Thus, increasing atmospheric mercury would produce exactly the pattern found by Spitz: rising IQ in the midrange; but failing to raise IQ in the upper range, instead tending to push more gifted persons into autistic low IQ; and thus adding to the numbers of retarded.

Some other studies appear to conflict with Spitz. This is probably because there are numerous variables involved which can confuse matters, for instance if the sample is truncated by absence of the most subnormal, or if not many persons are around the upper limit of useful antiinnatia.

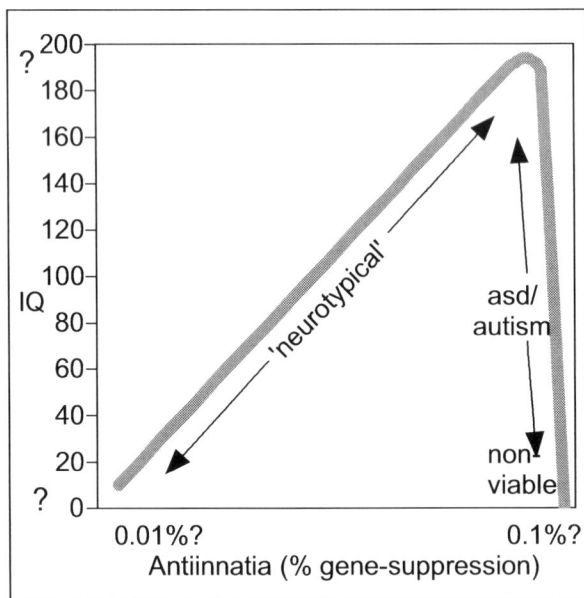

Fig. 16.1. The relationship of antiinnatia and IQ

Also notable is a recent finding of children in Shanghai scoring far higher in maths examinations than English children, in the context of notoriously high air pollution in Chinese cities, which is mainly from mercury-emitting coal-burning. That could easily be understood as increased mercury causing increased IQs, but instead education professionals in the UK have been clamouring to understand quite what about the teaching is (supposedly!) so much better in China, even though simultaneously huge numbers of Chinese students are choosing to come to the UK on the basis that the teaching is better here instead.

And contrary to their title, Nettelbeck and Wilson (2004) found that inspection time speeded up by 6 percent (albeit not statistically significant), suggesting a biological basis to the Flynn effect.

The DNA-binding of mercury would not be expected to affect gene-expression in a pattern exactly identical to that of the antiinnatia genes. The former is a simple element whereas the latter is a complex of genes highly-evolved to be advantageous for humans. So we should not be surprised that in factor analyses the Flynn effect manifests as a different factor (Rushton, 1999) than the g factor (which presumably is the manifestation of the antiinnatia genes, indeed giving a good proxy measurement of antiinnatia except in the autistic range).

And page 471 of my published theory paper suggested air pollution as a varying antiinnatia factor. So we have a notion of mercury vapor causing autism, and also an increase of atmospheric mercury vapor providing a uniquely-satisfactory explanation of the Flynn effect. Within it, Flynn's two paradoxes find easy explanation along with Spitz's peculiar data and the trend reversal data.

 Before coming to the clinching question of whether mercury levels really do correlate with IQ levels positively overall anyway, I will first try to explain away why the conventional wisdom is that mercury pollution is lowering IQ rather than raising it. There is no real evidential conflict here.

On the one hand, there is a causation in which mothers eating meat of pilot whales or large sharks causes high surges of methylmercury to adversely impact during critical stages of pre-natal development, producing impairment. On the other hand, there is a causation affecting all infants (including whose mothers who do not eat whales or sharks) in which constant post-natal inhalation of mercury vapor produces a mild antiinnatia effect, thereby enhancing IQ (though almost certainly at cost of subtle but important other qualities such as parenting skills and other innate wisdom). The studies of harm from prenatal methylmercury were properly-conducted within their own terms, but they could not be expected to detect this other causation not involving food.

This mercury-Flynn effect causation might appear to be also challenged by the fact that neither autism nor raised IQ are noted characteristics of mercury poisoning in adults. But this is arguably because for autism or raised IQ to be caused, the antiinnatia factor/s must be active during the period when the relevant innatons are developing and becoming established. At a later age, the innatons are already permanently established as elaborated learned habits, skills, or 'knowledge', as the elaborated connectivity of the brain, and as crystallised intelligence in place of fluid intelligence. Futhermore, adult mercury poisoning involves much higher intakes than obtainable from ordinary atmospheric levels.

And there are similarities but also differences between the way that mercury vapor is here theorised to cause the Flynn effect and also cause autism. In both cases the key causal variable is inhalation of mercury vapor by infants. But the Flynn effect is a whole-population average consequence; whereas the increased cases of autism are rare extreme outcomes occurring only in relatively extreme combined conditions of, for instance, amount and timing of parental amalgams, quality of dentistry, lack of ventilation, and lack of genetic capability for detoxification. It can therefore be expected that the two phenomena would not occur exactly in parallel but that the autism increase would relate more to amalgam-caused mercury levels while the Flynn effect would relate more to general ambient mercury vapor levels.

Anyway, the point has now come at which to ask whether this "mad" idea of mine, that all the world's experts are 100% wrong, actually stands up to the final examination of the evidence, and whether my "artificial genius" experiment has failed or succeeded.

Firstly, let us consider the data of the (Lynn-)Flynn effect IQ increase. A whole collection of studies has indicated apparently constant increases of IQ scores over a period of about 100 years, at least up to about the 1980 birth cohorts. But there has been a reversal of the Flynn effect in recent decades in Norway (Sundet et al., 2004), Denmark (Teasdale and Owen, 2008), Netherlands (Woodley & Meisenberg, 2013), Finland (Dutton & Lynn, 2013), and the UK (Flynn, 2009b; Shayer & Ginsburg, 2009).

The turning-point peak (in terms of year of birth) was about 1980 in Denmark, 1978 in Finland, and 1976 in Norway. And Raven (2000) found that the effect dated back linearly to at least the 1870s.

Meanwhile the most direct data of the variations of atmospheric mercury has come from ice-cores extracted from the Fremont Glacier. The researchers involved state that "the increase in mercury input during the last 100 years of record is followed by a rapid decrease within the last 15-20 years" (USGS, 2002). You can see a graph of the Fremont mercury data on the relevant Wikipedia pages, and can download their actual measurements from Schuster et al. (2002). I have used that data to produce Figure 16.2 here.

You can see that it features two spikes which correspond to two major volcanic eruptions. Those volcano events happened far away from most of humankind, whereas the industrial activity would have happened much closer to population centres (thus potentially being breathed in more and thereby impacting on average IQs more).

So I have produced Figure 16.3 by removing the two volcano spikes.

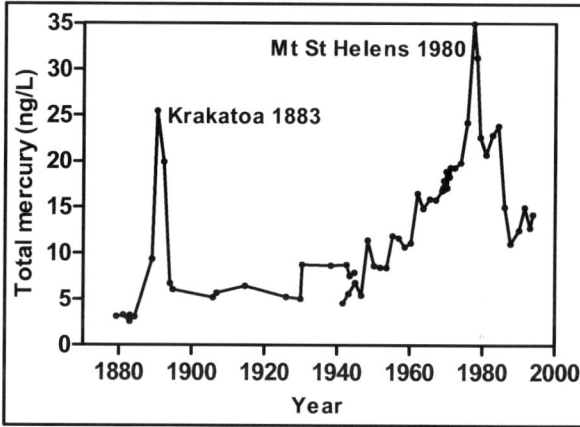

Figure 16.2. Mercury data from Fremont Glacier, with two volcano spikes not yet removed

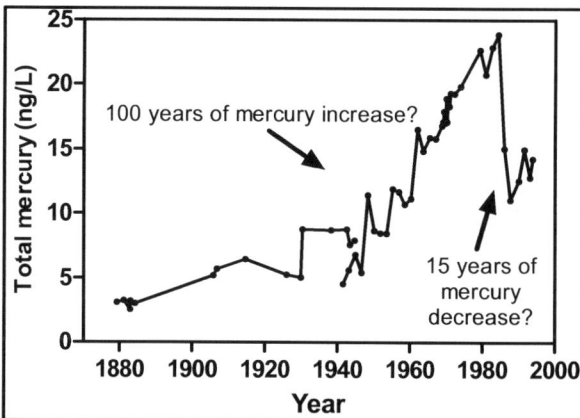

Figure 16.3. Mercury data from Fremont Glacier, with two volcano spikes removed

Also IQ is a ratio variable so I need to convert the mercury scale to logarithmic to properly match with it, as in Figure 16.4.

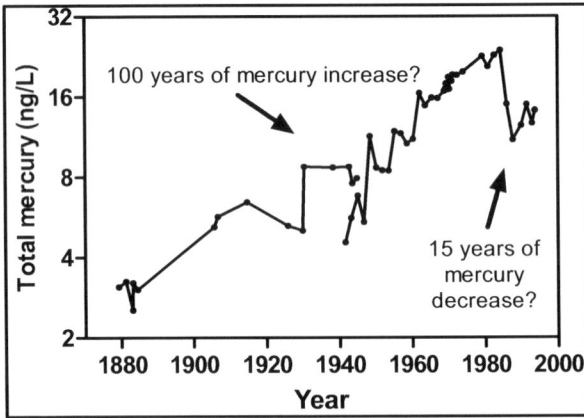

Figure 16.4 Mercury data from Fremont Glacier, with two volcano spikes removed, and y-axis converted to logarithmic

Certain facts about Figure 16.4 suggest that there are almost certainly some large errors in these measurements, perhaps from disturbance of the ground by animals. Firstly, at the overlap in the 1940s there is an obvious mismatch with the first four of the later series conspicuously below the last three of the earlier series. Secondly there is an improbably marked jump up from 1930.0 to 1930.4. It is unlikely that all these readings can be taken at face value as even remotely accurate measurements of the historical atmospheric levels. Much more likely is that the levels have somehow been heavily under-estimated in some of these datums.

So Figure 16.5 shows a suggestion of how the real levels of mercury might have increased nearly (log-)linearly, as per the dashed line added there connecting the peaks (which could be the least corrupted measurements).

So, in line with this suggestion, I produce Figure 16.6 by removing the six most suspect datums from the linked series.

Furthermore, a person's brain development would be affected by the mercury absorbed not just on one day but instead over a period probably of years, and also pre-absorption by the mother during and before pregnancy. To reflect this, I interpolate the data to regular year intervals and apply a simple moving average with four-years window, to obtain a final rough graphical impression of the varying mercury impact (in Figure 16.7).

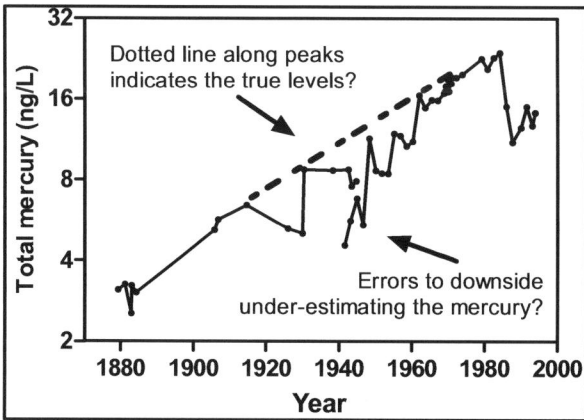

Figure 16.5 Suggested differences between conceivably misleading measurements and conceivably actual historical mercury levels.

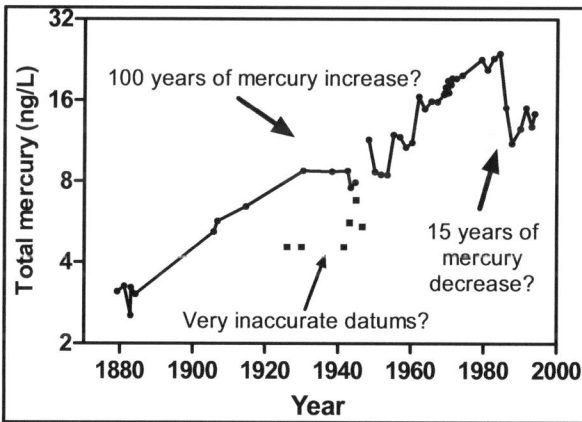

Figure 16.6. Mercury data from Fremont Glacier, with two volcano spikes removed, converted to log scale on the y axis, and six most suspect datums removed.

You can now see that it shows what is presumably the mercury increasing with increasing industrialisation, and then decreasing again from about 1980 presumably due to the various technical measures (such as mercury-free batteries) taken to reduce mercury pollution.

And for comparison I have produced Figure 16.8 to give a rough picture of the IQ increasing and then decreasing as per the various studies.

So we are now at the moment of truth. Does the IQ go up and down together with the mercury? Or instead, as all the world's experts would expect, do they go down and up in opposition – with what musicians call "contrary motion"? Here are the two graphs and perhaps you can judge the answer for yourself.

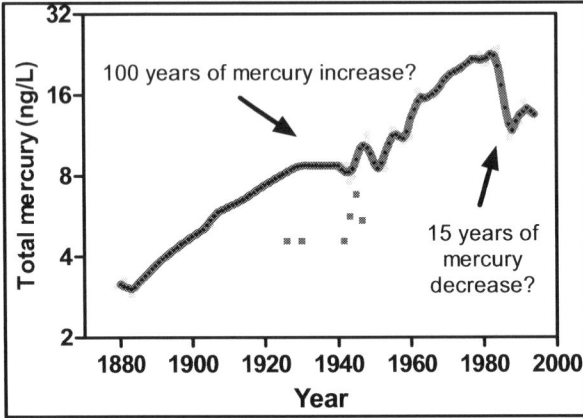

Figure 16.7. Mercury data from Fremont Glacier, with two volcano spikes removed, converted to log scale on the y axis, six most suspect datums removed, and smoothed by 4-year moving average.

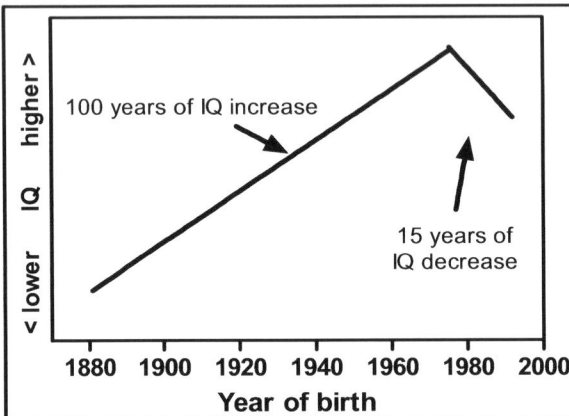

Figure 16.8. Rough illustration of the Flynn effect and its reversal.

To my own eyes there does appear to be some similarity between the two graphs, but I'm not sure that I am properly qualified to make an expert judgement of the matter anyway, and could be biased by wishful thinking. I would like to rationalise away some of the differences with one or other excuse. The mercury graph probably includes spikes from unspecified smaller volcanic events, and the ongoing rumblings from Mt Etna. And there may be more of those inaccurate measurements needing correcting out. So we could rightly smooth out some more of the unevenness. But again this is probably just excuse-making on my part. And the final outcome remains that there are still fundamental differences which I haven't explained away yet. The mercury graph has numerous dots and bends whereas the IQ graph has just two straight lines.

So we are forced to conclude that the IQ has not gone up and down in line with the mercury pollution, but on the contrary the entire world's experts were correct all along in their view that the IQ would be going down and up, in contrary motion to the mercury.

And so my provisionally "absurd" idea, that increasing mercury has caused increased IQ, has been proven wrong and indeed absurd. And my "artificial genius" experiment has ended with a fail result. And clearly in future I should just stick to believing what the experts tell me and shelve any delusions that I might know better than them all.

(Sorry that this book had to end on such a negative note, but that's life.)

~~~~~~~

Afterword for concerned environmental experts

There are two concerns which may usefully be unpicked here.

Firstly, the preceding chapter may appear to be suggesting that mercury pollution is a good thing or at least not causing any harm in terms of reduced IQ. In reality, if mercury pollution is acting as an antiinnatia factor, then it would be doing so in a much cruder way (being a simple element) than the complex of antiinnatia genes specially selected for advantageousness. It would be expected to be causing advantageous innatons to be suppressed. These are likely to include innate senses of beauty, common-sense, wisdom, relationship skills, parenting skills, judgement of how best to practically manage the tackling of problems lacking neat logical "IQ-type" solutions, and so on. It can hardly be claimed that our current times are notable for the greatest-ever wisdom, artistic excellence, civil harmony, or family harmony. On the contrary, divorce has greatly increased along with the increasing IQ and with public notices telling people how they should behave when they should already know how to. People born at the height of the Lynn-Flynn effect could be analogised as like computers with the fastest processors but lacking ("innate") hardware graphics acceleration or multimedia hardware extensions – excellent for abstract processing but not better for most real-world practical use. I strongly suspect that the steep decline in intellectual standards has been caused in part by the same atmospheric mercury.

Secondly, environmentally-aware people might be concerned that if official experts in medicine are shown to be charlatans, that might seem to support those who claim that the official expertise about climate change (global warming) is also charlatanic. I do not think that inference should be assumed correct. Social conditions in different fields can be very different. I am not sure whether climate students get trained at "Climate Schools" funded by a climate industry, let alone one as corrupted as the illness industry (Gøtzsche, 2013). They probably don't apply for "Climate School" in the first place on a motivation of getting into a prestigious highly-paid profession. Their courses may not involve so much mindless parrot-memorising. On becoming professionals they may not become subject to a reign-of-terror of threatened de-licencing by the kangaroo court of a "General Climate Council". And not least, the established huge corporate interests (aviation industry, motor industry, oil industry, travel industry) may be mostly minded to oppose the global warming theory rather than support it.

And in any case, there are important other reasons for not so casually wasting the planet's irreplaceable capital of fossil "fuels" created over millions of years.

The bottom line here is that the content of this book contains no message in respect of the credibility or otherwise of one or other viewpoint in this controversy. Much has been written and said about it elsewhere, and it makes little sense for me to add more here. I'll just mention that many charts may be found at the website www.climate4you.com. They may or may not be a load of rubbish!

~

Dear Reader! If you have found this book to have some worthy qualities, and or if you have found it to be defective in some way....... in any case, please post your thoughts to review sites such as Amazon.com, Amazon.co.uk, and the equivalents in other countries such as .fr, .de, .it, .es, and .jp. As these are generally independent from one another in their reviews, it could be best to try to post to for instance both the .uk and the .com. I look forward to discussing any thoughts you may put there. In addition I would welcome any suggestions or comments by email to book[at]pseudoexpertise.com (replacing the [at] with the @ symbol).

~

Afterword for the cleverest IQ experts

Experts on IQ and the (Lynn-)Flynn effect may feel that I have treated their subject with unworthy flippancy here.

Not least in my cursory passing over the extensive discussions of possible causes, and the complex analyses they have conducted to inform that debate. To which concerns I must make some apologias here.

Firstly, there are quite a number of proposed explanations of the Lynn-Flynn effect, and even just describing some of them would take a lot of space, for instance explaining what heterosis is let alone how it would cause the effect. And it would seem unfair to review some of them without reviewing at least all the main ones. And yet the bottom line here is that they all border on the rather desperate, which I reckon is rightly reflected in the fact that few if any have gained many followers besides their own authors. If you do want to find a review of the explanations then you can find a better one than I could do myself via a websearch or wikipedia.

Secondly, this subject is rather harder for me to study as most IQ research is not open-accessible via PubMed or PubMedCentral.

Thirdly, the literature of this subject has become very hard to follow. I never had any difficulty understanding the writings of Eysenck and Jensen about the subject, but more recent experts' writing I struggle to understand. This could be because I have become thicker, or perhaps the authors have become smarter, or the subject has advanced to a more complex level. Or alternatively the newer generation of writers lack the required talent for thinking of clear concepts clearly expressed.

That said, even the most basic concepts of IQ research are very abstract. First there are scores on test items, then there are the correlations between them within tests and between individuals. And then the crucial level of correlations between the correlations. You certainly need a three-figure IQ to start to understand this let alone usefully discuss it.

And my own impression of the field is that even the most expert are in danger of over-presuming at some points. I suggest the following as an example.

Much, I suggest too much, is made of the concept of the general factor of intelligence, called g (italicised as here). And also that the Flynn effect does not act in terms of that g factor. I think there is a fundamental oversight here which can be explained with reference to my exceptional gardening wizardry.

Consider the following notional weed-farm field. The west side of the field is too dry, and consequently few things grow there, in contrast to the humid east side. The north end is chalky whereas the south end is acid. Consequently the density of growth of grass and heather is as illustrated (in nominal units) in this figure.

2 heather 20 grass	north	20 heather 200 grass
west		east
20 heather 2 grass	south	200 heather 20 grass

Now if you study a cross-section from east to west, you will find a 100% positive correlation (r = 1.0) between heather and grass, because the dryness impedes both of these. By contrast the grass is happy to grow on England's chalk downs whereas the heather thrives best in the more acid soil (or so the experts tell me anyway). So if you study a cross-section from north to south, you will find the exact opposite correlation, r = *minus* 1.0. And that is even though it is exactly the same field with exactly the same plants being studied.

The standard *g* factor is found from looking at correlations in a single time and place - a cross-section at a particular date comparing individuals. By contrast, with the Flynn effect one is looking at the cross-section *along* the time dimension and with all the genetic variance of the individuals plonked together and averaged out. And thereby one would find a different general factor, but which is just as real and valid and "general" as the standard *g* factor.

The *g* factor can be understood to be the manifestation of individual differences in the inherited amount of the complex of antiinnatia genes. That is why it is highly heritable. The mysterious non-*g* factor which the Flynn effect finds can be understood to be the antiinnatia factor of mercury pollution, which likewise raises IQ scores but does so somewhat differently, and less helpfully, because it is one simple element rather than a complex of genes carefully evolved over millennia of natural selection for being advantageous to the organisms having them.

But it then gets confusing again because the effects of the mercury antiinnatia factor still have a lot in common with the effects of the antiinnatia genes, and so they are liable to appear correlated in their manifestations even though they might not be in their origins.

I hope that makes sense! (If it doesn't you're probably not smart enough and should drink at least a pint a day of a silvery-grey liquid to compensate.)

(P.S. I have recently fooled some peer reviewers into publishing a paper relating to the above, titled *"Rising-falling mercury pollution causing the rising-falling IQ of the Flynn effect, as predicted by the antiinnatia theory of autism and IQ"* (Clarke, 2015).)

~

After-Afterword for our most expert leading intellectuals

"The measure of a great intellectual is the number of times they have the most platitudinous of platitudes duly attributed to them in quotations of uncertain relevance at the beginnings of book chapters." — Book-editing expert

"The important thing in science is not so much to obtain new facts as to discover new ways of thinking about them." — W.L. Bragg

(Note: In the following I refuse to use the sloppy nasty officially-correct word "homophobia". That is because genuine phobias such as agoraphobia can be extremely serious horrible disabilities and it is outrageously inappropriate abuse of language to use the same "-phobia" ending for the political propaganda purpose of creating cheap pejoratives with which to stir hate against those with whom you disagree about something. Instead I will use the more appropriate term *homo-hostility*.)

I'll first mention that in respect of some subjects and some social sectors, the dominating level of intellect is such that at the first instant a topic is mentioned, many minds instantly ask "Which side is this person on?", and no less instantly jump to an answer of "our side" or "their side". As if there can be only two viewpoints about a complex matter anyway. Well, sure, there is always the binary distinction between those who rightly travel with the herd of wisdom as distinct from those who commit the offence of straying elsewhere.

The antiinnatia theory of autism, genius, and IQ was in its original moments comprised of one principle, namely that those three phenomena had in common a "reduction of innate prejudices". Note that last word. Innate inherited prejudice against homosexuality is to be expected because natural selection favours those with a strong inclination to become grandparents but a culture of homosexuality seriously threatens that prospect. And thus the various innatons (which the antiinnatia factors tend to suppress) would include innatons producing homo-hostility.

Furthermore, in the early years before it got published I also had an idea that antiinnatia would not only be a factor in autism, IQ, and genius, but also in homosexuality. My reasoning was that it is generally the usual state of affairs for people to prefer and admire that which is the same as themselves in most respects. Snobby people prefer fellow snobs. Spritual people prefer fellow spirituals.

Sporty people prefer sporty others. Intellectual people prefer the company of intellectual others rather than the company of Olympic bingo-players and Premier-League celebs, not to mention to say nothing here unkind about Russell Brand. And so on. Indeed, attraction to those more similar to oneself is one of the most well-established findings in social psychology (Byrne, 1971).

Heterosexuality thus stands as a very peculiar exception to this wide-ranging principle of like-prefers-like. I consequently reckoned that there must be "hetero-innatons" (and genes) specifically evolved to generate that exception. And then homosexuality results when such hetero-innatons are suppressed (by antiinnatia) or otherwise not expressed. There could of course be other factors involved, and hetero/homo is not a stable or categorical either/or distinction anyway.

Also notable are the outstanding geniuses who were homosexual. Tchaikovsky, Oscar Wilde, and Alan Turing all had their lives brought to an early tragic end by the hostility to their homosexuality. So perhaps we are seeing here that genius and homosexuality tend to go together? Which would again accord with their both being consequences of increased antiinnatia.

And indeed, I had long wondered whether there would be an association of autism and homosexuality. A small recent study suggests there could indeed be (Gilmour et al., 2012).

Now here is the remarkable thing. In the few decades since I first wrote down the antiinnatia theory, an unprecedented gigantic transformation of attitudes has occurred in many societies around the world.

The first line of Jane Austen's *Pride and Prejudice* reads rather controversially 200 years later: "It is a truth universally acknowledged, that a single man in possession of a good fortune, must be in want of a wife." The language of that phrase "a truth universally acknowledged" could hardly be any stronger in its assumption that no alternative to heterosexuality exists.

The death of Alan Turing is within living memory. Not so many years ago some consenting activity of same sex adults was predominantly considered an abominable sin and criminal offence in just about every country of the world. It is still considered a capital crime in several non-Western countries.

And yet within the space of just a few decades there has been a complete turnaround of attitudes (or should I say, prejudices?) such that now we have highly-prominent officially-supported "Gay Pride" marches and now there are laws criminalising not the homosexuality but instead criminalising even the mildest expressions of any homo-hostility against it. And insistence on changing the meaning of the word "marriage", which must be one of the most ancient of sacred concepts long-predating even language itself, to mean something fundamentally different and strongly endorsive of the conduct which not so long ago was considered a sin and abomination and serious crime (and still is in some countries and cultures). Meanwhile the original concept of "marriage" has been suddenly written out of history without even a name by which to refer to it, other than something very clumsy like "traditionally-defined marriage". If people want to be modern why don't they use a new word for a new concept? (Such as "pairage".) The English language has had numerous new words added to it in recent decades, such as supermarket, blog, vlog, crowdsourcing, carjacking, commentariat, and even "homophobia" and "islamophobia". So why not introduce a new word for the same-sex equivalent of marriage, rather than non-consensually imposing a redefinition of an ancient word to be mangled in meaning to the confusion of everyone? Multiple meanings of words are a major source of deficient communication and muddled thinking, as exemplified in a stupid book written by some professors years ago titled "What is Intelligence?", in which naturally enough each chapter was about an entirely different subject (with the entire book being an attempt to forget about the actual *facts* of the *g* factor found in IQ testing). So why make matters needlessly more confused?

This is intended to be a book of scientific information and not a book of preaching. Whether one or other attitude or law is a good thing or a bad thing is for you to decide for yourself. My opinion of the matter is irrelevant, indeed I have never much inclined towards holding such opinions anyway. I will here just state what seems the very well-founded scientific conclusion as I see it.

As stated above, I predicted decades ago that antiinnatia factors would tend to (a) reduce innate prejudices, and (b) increase homosexuality. Then in 2004 I recognised that mercury was an antiinnatia factor. And therefrom I predicted that the increase of atmospheric mercury vapor would cause the Flynn effect IQ increase (as per the update review I was trying to get published back then). And indeed we do now see the rise and fall of IQ accompanying the rise and fall of mercury pollution (as detailed in Chapter 16 here; see also Clarke, 2015). And therefrom an obvious further prediction is that the same increasing of atmospheric mercury would also cause suppression of innate prejudices (including suppression of homo-hostility innatons) and suppression of hetero-innatons, thus causing an increase of homosexuality. So we should predict that the recent high levels of mercury will have caused increased homosexuality and reduced homo-hostility.

And those predictions are now confirmed, as that is exactly what we have indeed seen in recent decades. The antiinnatia theory thus explains why there has been such a huge social transformation in the very same few generation-decades in respect of which the Flynn effect has peaked.

And that implies that this change to new forms of partnership is not some irreversible social-intellectual-moral advance but something which could go very much into a tragic reverse if mercury pollution continues its reducing trend.

And that's just one of my social causality ideas. But please don't mention it to any properly-qualified sociology experts. (Let alone actual intellectuals.)

[P.S.: Oh-oh. Someone else has already done an experiment showing that mercury turns some birds into homosexuals (Frederick & Jayasena, 2010; Milton, 2010). So my hypothesis (or so-called "theory") was clearly a load of rubbish all along. I apologise for wasting your time with this book and can only suggest that in future you ensure that any books are authored by proper expert people with professorships or at least 'PhD' validly placed after their name. Sorry for that.]

~~~~~~~   ~~~~~~~   ~~~~~~~

And now......

Do you think this book is totally brilliant, or totally rubbish, or perhaps something in between? In any case, please let us know what you think and why.

Please post your thoughts in a review on the page for this book at amazon.com or amazon.co.uk (preferably both) etc.

And also tell your friends and enemies how great or useless you think it is.

It is very difficult for "unknown" authors to get anyone to read their books, let alone buy them or even review them. "Bestsellers" are nowadays almost invariably the result of commercially-driven decisions to invest many thousands of dollars into advanced copies and other high-profile promotion. And few people are searching for books about pseudo-expertise.

For reasons that should already be clear from this book itself, the author does not have a grand celebrity marketing operation to let others know about it.

So over to you....

Cheers!

Acknowledgments

It is difficult to do justice to all the people who have helped me with writing this book. I would like to be able to thank the publishers and editors and the designers of the cover and interior format. And all those who have read through and kindly suggested improvements to earlier drafts*. Also of course my various wives and children, along with my PhD supervisors and those others who helped to advance my career so rapidly with recommendations for worthwhile courses and appointments.

But due to the difficulty of doing proper justice to a large many so deserving, I will name here just those who have notably contributed to my knowledge of dental mercury poisoning and the association of mercury with autism. They deserve a special mention here because for their efforts most of them have got at best only contempt as greed-driven quacks or ridicule as foolish believers of crackpot "scare stories" of governments poisoning millions of their citizens. They have included – in no particular order – Hal Huggins DDS, Boyd Haley, Bernard Rimland, Dr med Joachim Mutter, Geir Bjørklund, Andrew Hall Cutler, Tom McGuire DDS, Charlie Brown of Consumers for Dental Choice, Pierre LaRose and other experts of the IAOMT, UK dentists Graeme Munro-Hall, Hesham el-Essawy and David Harvie-Austin, Cape Town dentist Dr Ilona Visser, Lynne McTaggart and Brian Hubbard of What Doctors Don't Tell You, Dr Mercola of mercola.com, Mike Adams of naturalnews.com, Mark Geier, David Geier, Mark Sircus, Janet Kern, Cathy DeSoto and Rob Hitlan, Jeff Bradstreet and Amy Holmes for their key studies of autism mercury, Jim Adams, Mark Blaxill and others of Safeminds, Ulf Bengtsson (for his great non-gamma-2 website), Vera Stejskal and others of the Melisa group, Dr Henrik Lichtenberg, Dr Majewska, Richard Deth, Birgit Calhoun, Bernie Windham, Stephen M Edelson, Lenny Schafer and Adam Feinstein and Ben Goldacre, ...and certainly others who could well be just as noteworthy but overlooked by the publicising system or my still-poisoned brain. I humbly apologise to others who merit a place in this list but are thus overlooked.

Inclusion of anyone's name above here is not intended to imply that they agree with anything in this book or that I agree with everything they say themselves.

[*P.S.: Professor Deth has subsequently provided some usefully critical feedback, following which I have made some changes to hopefully reduce misunderstandings.]

~

References

There are several distinct motivations potentially involved in compilation of reference lists.

Some people use them to impress the reader with the large number of things they have speed-"read" or at least listed.

Some people use them to ingratiate themselves with the people they have flattered by including.

In some contexts they provide a properly complete listing or review of the literature.

But here I am following what is common practice in scientific reports. Namely a minimal listing of those sources which provide significant support (or otherwise) for my own statements, or which the reader may find useful for further information. If I don't provide a supporting reference for some particular statement, that is most likely because I reckon any doubter can easily enough confirm the matter for themselves anyway.

In the four quotations at the start of the text, that from Paul Travis MD was sourced at: http://drmalcolmkendrick.org/2015/10/01/study-329-where-the-hell-is-the-outrage/.

~~~~~~~

Abha Chauhan, Ved Chauhan, Ted Brown (eds) (2009) Autism: Oxidative Stress, Inflammation, and Immune Abnormalities. CRC Press

Abraham, G.E.,The Wolff-Chaikoff Effect: Crying Wolf? *The Original Internist*, 12(3):112-118,2005. http://www.optimox.com/iodine-study-4

Adams JB, Romdalvik J, Levine KE, Lin-Wen H. (2008) Mercury in first-cut baby hair of children with autism versus typically developing children. *Toxicol Environ Chem*;90:739–753.

Adams M (2015) http://www.naturalnews.com/051841_Google_Ministry_of_Truth_propaganda.html

Age of Autism (2012) http://www.ageofautism.com/2012/11/cdcs-dr-coleen-boyle-suggested-manipulating-autism-dx-age-in-2000.html

Allman JM, Watson KK, Tetreault NA, Hakeem AY (2005) Intuition and autism: a possible role for Von Economo neurons. *Trends Cogn Sci* **9:** 367-73.

Altman DG (1994) The scandal of poor medical research *BMJ* 308:283. http://dx.doi.org/10.1136/bmj.308.6924.283 http://www.bmj.com/content/308/6924/283

Anthony J. (1958) An experimental approach to the psychotherapy of childhood autism. *Br. J. med. Psychol.* **31,** 211-225.

Arber W (2011) Molecular Darwinism: The Contingency of Spontaneous Genetic Variation. *Genome Biol Evol.*, 3: 1090–1092.

Arber, W.(2014) Horizontal Gene Transfer among Bacteria and its Role in Biological Evolution. *Life*, 4, 217–224, doi:10.3390/life4020217. http://www.mdpi.com/2075-1729/4/2/217

Ariza ME, Holliday J, Williams MV. (1994) Mutagenic effect of mercury (II) in eukaryotic cells. *In Vivo* 8:5590-563.

Armstrong, J. S., Green, K. (2017). Guidelines for science. https://www.researchgate.net/publication/305712994_Guidelines_for_Science_Evidence_and_Checklists .

Arslan RC, Penke L, Johnson W, Iacono WG, McGue M (2014) The Effect of Paternal Age on Offspring Intelligence and Personality when Controlling for Parental Trait Levels. *PLoS ONE* 9(2): e90097.

Ashwin, C., Chapman, E., Howells, J., Rhydderch, D., Walker, I., & Baron-Cohen, S. (2014). Enhanced olfactory sensitivity in autism spectrum conditions. *Molecular Autism*, 5, 53.

Asperger H. (1944) Die "Autistichen Psychopathen" im Kindersalter. *Arch. Psychiat. NervKrankh.* **117,** 76-136.(English translation in Frith, 1991)

Attwood A., Frith U. and Hermelin B. (1988) The understanding and use of interpersonal gestures by autistic and Down's syndrome children. *J. Autism dev. Disorders* **18,** 241-257.

Azoulay P, Fons-Rosen C, Graff Zivin JS (2015) Does Science Advance One Funeral at a Time? NBER Working Paper No. 21788

Bagramian RA, Farghaly MM, Lopatin D, Sowers M, Syed SA, et al. (1993) Periodontal disease in an Amish population. *J Clin Periodontol* 20: 269-272.

Bagramian RA, Narendran S, Khavari AM (1988) Oral health status, knowledge, and practices in an Amish population. *J Public Health Dent* 48: 147-151.

Barbeau EB, Soulières I, Dawson M, Zeffiro TA, Mottron L. (2013) The level and nature of autistic intelligence III: Inspection time. *J Abnorm Psychol.*;122(1):295-301.

Baron-Cohen S. (1988) Social and pragmatic deficits in autism: cognitive or affective? *J. Autism dev. Disorders* **18,** 379-402.

Baron-Cohen S. (2002) The extreme-male-brain theory of autism. *Trends Cogn Sci* 6: 248-54.

Baron-Cohen S., Leslie A. M. and Frith U. (1985) Does the autistic child have a 'theory of mind'? *Cognition* **21,** 37-46.

Barr B et al (2015) 'First, do no harm': are disability assessments associated with adverse trends in mental health? A longitudinal ecological study *J Epidemiol Community Health* http://jech.bmj.com/content/early/2015/10/26/jech-2015-206209.full

Bates E. (1976) *Language in Context.* Academic Press, New York.

Bauer H (2012) Dogmatism in science and medicine.

BBC (2003) http://news.bbc.co.uk/1/hi/health/3000884.stm

Becerra TA, et al. (2014) Autism spectrum disorders and race, ethnicity, and nativity: a population-based study. *Pediatrics*;134(1):e63-71. www.pediatrics.org/cgi/doi/10.1542/peds.2013-3928

Beckett A (1998) Debate continues on vitamin B. http://www.thelancet.com/journals/lancet/article/PIIS0140-6736%2898%2926027-2/fulltext

Benefits and Work (2015) http://www.benefitsandwork.co.uk/news/3188-ib-to-esa-work-capability-assessment-linked-to-almost-600-additional-suicides

Berglund A. (1993) An in vitro and in vivo study of the release of mercury vapor from different types of amalgam alloys. *J Dent Res* 72:939-946.

Berglund A, Pohl L, Olsson S, Bergman M. (1988) Determination of the rate of release of intra-oral mercury vapor from amalgam. *J Dent Res* 67:1235-1242.

Bernard S. (2003) Analysis of the Danish autism registry data base in response to the Hviid et al paper on thimerosal in JAMA. Available [03/4/2014] from: http://www.safeminds.org/research/Hviid_et_alJAMA-SafeMindsAnalysis.pdf

Bernard S, Enayati A, Redwood L, Roger H, Binstock T. (2001) Autism: a novel form of mercury poisoning. *Med Hypotheses* 56:462-471.

Bickerton D. (1984) The language bioprogram hypothesis. *Behavioral brain Sciences* **7,** 173-221.

Bilbobanks (2015) http://www.theguardian.com/society/2015/feb/07/nhs-investigations-into-care-complaints-appalling#comment-47217756

Blakemore SJ, Tavassoli T, Calò S, Thomas RM, Catmur C, Frith U, Haggard P (2006) Tactile sensitivity in Asperger syndrome. Brain Cogn.; 61(1):5-13.

Blakemore-Brown L (2005) bmj.com rapid response (Jan 24) to Tanne JH. Increase in autism due to change in definition, not MMR vaccine. *BMJ* 330: 112-d. [http://bmj.bmjjournals.com/cgi/eletters/330/7483/112-d]

Blaucok-Busch* E, Amin OR, Dessoki HH, Rabah T. (2012) Efficacy of DMSA Therapy in a Sample of Arab Children with Autistic Spectrum Disorder. *Maedica (Buchar)* 7:214-21.   [*incorrect spelling of Blaurock-Busch]

Blaxill MF. (2004) What's going on? The question of time trends in autism. *Public Health Reports* 119:536-551.

Blaxill MF, Redwood L, Bernard S (2004) Thimerosal and autism? A plausible hypothesis that should not be dismissed. *Med Hypotheses* 62: 788-794.

Bodnar J. W. (1988) A domain model for eukaryotic DNA organisation: A molecular basis for cell differentiation and chromosome evolution. *J. theor. Biol.* **132,** 479-507.

Bodnar J. W., Jones G. S. and Ellis C. H. (1989) The domain model for eukaryotic DNA organisation 2: A molecular basis for constraints on development and evolution. *J. theor. Biol.* **137,** 281-320.

Boldyreva S. A. (1974) *Risunki Detei Doshkolnogo Vostrasta Bol'nykh Shizofreniei.* Meditsina, Moscow.

Bonnel A, Mottron L, Peretz I, Trudel M, Gallun E, Bonnel AM (2003) Enhanced pitch sensitivity in individuals with autism: a signal detection analysis. J Cogn Neurosci. 15(2):226-35.

Boucher J. and Warrington E. K. (1976) Memory deficits in early infantile autism. *Br. J. Psychol.* **67,** 73-87.

Boullane et al (1991) Major measles epidemic in the region of Quebec despite a 99% vaccine coverage. Canadian J Public Health.

Boyer DB. (1988) Mercury vaporization from corroded dental amalgam. *Dent Mater* 4:89-93.

Bradstreet J, Geier DA, Kartzinel JJ, Adams JB, Geier MR. (2003) A case-control study of mercury burden in children with autistic spectrum disorders. *J Am Physicians and Surgeons* 8:76-80.

Brugha TS, McManus S, Bankart J, Scott F, Purdon S, Smith J, Bebbington P, Jenkins R, Meltzer H. (2011) Epidemiology of autism spectrum disorders in adults in the community in England. *Arch Gen Psychiatry* 68:459-65.

Brune D, Gjerdet N, Paulsen G. (1983) Gastrointestinal and in vitro release of copper, cadmium, indium, mercury and zinc from conventional and copper-rich amalgams. *Scand J Dent Res* 91:66-71.

Burbacher TM, Shen DD, Liberato N. Grant KS, Cernichiari E, Clarkson T (2005) Comparison of blood and brain mercury levels in infant monkeys exposed to methylmercury or vaccines containing thimerosal. *Environ Health Perspect* doi:10.1289/ehp.7712

Butler P (2015) http://www.theguardian.com/society/2015/aug/27/thousands-died-after-fit-for-work-assessment-dwp-figures

Byrne, D. (1971). *The Attraction Paradigm*. New York: Academic Press.

California Department of Developmental Services. (1999) Changes in the Population of Persons with Autism and Pervasive Developmental Disorders in California's Developmental Services System: 1987 through 1998. Available [03/4/2014] from: http://www.dds.ca.gov/Autism/docs/autism_report_1999.pdf

California Department of Developmental Services. (2003) Autistic Spectrum Disorders: Changes in the California caseload: an update 1999 through 2002. Available [03/4/2013] from: http://www.dds.ca.gov/Autism/docs/AutismReport2003.pdf

Campbell M., Hardesty A. and Burdock E. (1977, October) Selected peri- and postnatal and demographic characteristics of autistic children. Paper presented at the annual meeting of the American Academy of Child Psychiatry, Dallas, Texas.

Cannell JJ (2008) Autism and vitamin D. *Med Hypotheses* 70: 750-9.

Cantwell D. P., Baker L. and Rutter M. (1978) Family factors. In *Autism* (Edited by Rutter M. and Schopler, E.). Plenum, New York.

Carey N (2015) Junk DNA.

Carr E. G. and Durand V. M. (1987) See me, help me. *Psychol. Today* 21 (11), 62-64.

Casanova E, et al. (2016) Genes with high penetrance for syndromic and non-syndromic autism typically function within the nucleus and regulate gene expression. Molecular Autism 7:18.

Chahrour M, Jung SY, Shaw C, Zhou X, Wong ST, Qin J, Zoghbi HY (2008). *"MeCP2, a key contributor to neurological disease, activates and represses transcription"*. Science 320: 1224–9.

Chief Dental Officer. (2009). Available [16/9/2013] from: http://www.youtube.com/watch?v=mMI_em8UPo4 and http://www.youtube.com/watch?v=174md9Y4ZRk (both at 5-7 minutes).

Childhealthsafety (2013) https://childhealthsafety.wordpress.com/2013/08/16/all-studies-claiming-no-mmr-vaccine-autism-link-invalid-according-to-mercks-vaccine-director-former-us-cdc-director-the-us-hrsa/

Chomsky N. (1957) *Syntactic Structures.* Mouton, The Hague.

Ciaranello R. D., VandenBerg S. R. and Anders T. F. (1982) Intrinsic and extrinsic determinants of neuronal development. *J. Autism dev. Disorders* **12,** 115-145.

Clarke RPM. (2039) A theory of general impairment of gene-expression manifesting as autism. *Person Individ Diff* 14:465-482. Available [16/9/2013] from: http://cogprints.org/5207.
[***But see updated presentation version in Chapter 7 here!!!***]

Clarke RP (1998) Leaflet: "The head of Sheffield Medical School lied to the government about vitamin safety".

Clarke RP (2012) Peer review of "Partially distinct genetic and environmental influences...".

Clarke RP (2013) The future is here! A practical handbook for solving the key crisis of our times. (www.lulu.com) [Note: this was written some years back specifically as the "manifesto" of the Real Democracy Party which I registered. However, if I were to succeed in promoting that party, then I would have certainly been accused of being a fraudulent malingerer rather than an honest disability benefits claimant, as it is "obviously" impossible for the two to be combined in one person, and non-clique politicians regularly get persecuted here. So it remained "unpublished"]

Clarke RP (2015) Rising-falling mercury pollution causing the rising–falling IQ of the Lynn–Flynn effect, as predicted by the antiinnatia theory of autism and IQ. *Personality and Individual Differences* 82; 46-51.

Clarkson TW, Friberg L, Hursh JB, Nylander M. (1988) The prediction of intake of mercury vapor from amalgams. In: Clarkson TW, Friberg L, Nordberg GF, Sager PR, editors. *Biological Monitoring of Toxic Metals.* New York: Plenum Press. p. 247-260.

Coleman M. (1978) A report on the autistic syndromes. In *Autism* (Edited by Rutter, M. and Schopler, E.). Plenum, New York.

Commons (1998) Vitamin B6. Fifth report of Agriculture Committee, House of Commons 1998
http://www.publications.parliament.uk/pa/cm199798/cmselect/cmagric/753/80519p02.htm

Courchesne E., Yeung-Courchesne R., Press G. A., Hesselink J. and Jernigan T. (1988) Hypoplasia of cerebellar vermal lobules VI and VII in autism. *New Engl. J. med.* **318,** 1349-1354.

Cox A., Rutter M., Newman S. and Bartak L. (1975) A comparative study of infantile autism and specific developmental receptive language disorder. *Br. J. Psychiat.* **126,** 146-159.

Creak M. and Ini S. (1960) Families of psychotic children. *J.child Psychol. Psychiat.* **1,** 156-175.

Croen LA, Grether JK, Hoogstrate J, Selvin S. (2002) The changing prevalence of autism in California. *J Autism Dev Disord*, 32(3):207-15.

Cutler AH (1999) Amalgam Illness: Diagnosis and treatment.

Dachel A (2009) http://www.ageofautism.com/2009/06/dear-professor-baroncohen.html

Dales L, Hammer SJ, Smith NJ (2001) Time trends in autism and in MMR immunization coverage in California. *JAMA* 285: 1183-5.

Dales L, Hammer SJ, Smith NJ.(2001) Time trends in autism and in MMR immunization coverage in California. JAMA.7;285(9):1183-5.

Damasio A. R. and Maurer R. G. (1978) A neurological model for childhood autism. *Archs Neurol.* **35,** 777-786.

Davies J (2013) Cracked..

Dawson M, Soulières I, Gernsbacher MA, Mottron L (2007) The level and nature of autistic intelligence. Psychological Science 18: 657–662.

de Gelder B. (1987) On not having a theory of mind. *Cognition* **27,** 285-290.

De Martino B, Harrison NA, Knafo S, Bird G, Dolan RJ (2008) Explaining enhanced logical consistency during decision making in autism. *J Neurosci* 28: 10746-10750. doi:10.1523/JNEUROSCI.2895-08.2008

DeSoto C (2014) http://www.ageofautism.com/2014/06/truth-environmental-toxins-not-good-fit-for-nih-autism-research.html

DeSoto MC, Hitlan RT. (2010) Sorting out the spinning of autism: heavy metals and the question of incidence. *Acta Neurobiol Exp (Wars)* 70:165–176.

Dutton E, Lynn R. (2013) A negative Flynn effect in Finland, 1997–2009. *Intelligence* 41: 817–820.

DWP. (no date a). The incapacity benefits – present and future. Available [28/4/2014] from: http://www.dwp.gov.uk/docs/pathways-presentation.pdf.

DWP. (no date b). [Data of UK disability benefits 1979-2002.] Available [3/4/2014] from: https://www.gov.uk/government/uploads/system/uploads/attachment_data/file/259185/timeseriesIBSDA.xls.

Edwards J (2014) http://www.theguardian.com/commentisfree/2014/aug/16/engineers-lifeblood-country-uk-students-science-maths-a-level#comment-39535224

Eggleston DW, Nylander M (1987) Correlation of dental amalgam with mercury in brain tissue. *J Prosth Dent* 58: 704-7.

Ertl J. P. (1968) Evoked potentials, neural efficiency and IQ. In *International Symposium on Biocybernetics, Washington, D.C., 1968.*Churchill, Edinburgh.

Ertl J. P. and Schafer D. W. (1969) Brain response correlates of psychometric intelligence. *Nature* **223,** 421-422.

Eysenck H. J. (1979) *The Structure and Measurement of Intelligence.*Springer, New York.

Eysenck H. J. (Ed.) (1982) *A Model for Intelligence.* Springer, New York.

Eysenck H. J. and Kamin L. (1981) *Intelligence, the Battle for the Mind.* Pan, London.

Eysenck HJ (1995) Genius.

Eysenck HJ, Eysenck SGB. (1992) Peer review: Advice to referees and contributors. *Person Individ Diff* 13:393-399. http://dx.doi.org/10.1016/0191-8869(92)90066-X

Eysenck HJ. (1995) Genius. Cambridge University Press. p. 148-152.

Fein D., Pennington B., Markowitz P., Braverman M. and Waterhouse L. (1986) Towards a neuropsychological model of infantile autism: are the social deficits primary? *J. Am. Acad. child Psychiat.* **25,** 198-212.

Ferracane JL, Adey JD, Nakajima H, Okabe T. (1995) Mercury vaporization from amalgams with varied alloy composition. *J Dent Res* 74:1414-1417.

Fido A, Al-Saad S. (2005) Toxic trace elements in the hair of children with autism. *Autism* 9:290-298.

Flynn JR (1987) Massive IQ gains in 14 nations: What IQ tests really measure. *Psychol Rev* 101: 171-191.

Flynn JR. (2009a). Requiem for nutrition as the cause of IQ gains: Raven's gains in Britain 1938–2008. *Economics and Human Biology* 7: 18–27. http://dx.doi.org/10.1016/j.ehb.2009.01.009

Flynn, JR. (2009b). *What Is Intelligence?* Cambridge University Press.

Folstein S. and Rutter M. (1988) Autism: Familial aggregation and genetic implications. *J. Autism dev. Disorders* **18**, 3-30.

Fombonne E (2000) Is there an epidemic of autism? *Pediatrics* 107: 411-412.

Fombonne E, Zakarian R, Bennett A, Meng L, McLean-Heywood D (2006) Pervasive Developmental Disorders in Montreal, Quebec, Canada: Prevalence and Links With Immunizations. *Pediatrics* 118: 139-150.

Field F (2012) Any Questions 22 Dec 2012 Haddenham Village Hall http://www.bbc.co.uk/programmes/b01pcwr9 at 41 minutes

Frederick P; Jayasena N (2010). Altered pairing behaviour and reproductive success in white ibises exposed to environmentally relevant concentrations of methylmercury. *Proceedings of the Royal Society B.* doi:10.1098/rspb.2010.2189;

Frith U. (1989) *Autism: Explaining the Enigma.* Blackwell, Oxford.

Frith U. (Ed.) (1991) *Autism and Asperger Syndrome.* Cambridge University Press.

Furlow FB, Armijo-Prewitt T, Gangestad SW, Thornhill R (1997) Fluctuating asymmetry and psychometric intelligence. *Proc R Soc Lond B* 264: 823-829.

Futuyma D. J. (1986) *Evolutionary Biology.* Sinauer, Sunderland, Mass.

Garreau B., Barthelemy C., Sauvage D., Leddet I. and Lelord G. (1984) A comparison of autistic syndromes with and without associated neurological problems. *J. Autism dev. Disorders* **14**, 105-111.

Geier DA, Kern JK, Geier MR. (2009) A prospective study of prenatal mercury exposure from maternal dental amalgams and autism severity. *Acta Neurobiol Exp (Wars)* 69:1–9.

Geier DA, Kern JK, Geier MR. (2010) The biological basis of autism spectrum disorders: Understanding causation and treatment by clinical geneticists. *Acta Neurobiol Exp (Wars)* 70:209-226.

Geier MR, Geier DA (2003) Thimerosal in childhood vaccines, neurodevelopmental disorders and heart disease in the US. *J Am Physicians and Surgeons* 8: 6-11.

Gillberg C. (1986) Brief report: Onset at age 14 of a typical autistic syndrome: A case report of a girl with herpes simplex encephalitis. *J. Autism dev. Disorders* **16**, 369-375.

Gillberg C. (1988). The neurobiology of infantile autism. *J. child Psychol. Psychiat.* **29**, 257-266.

Gillberg C. and Schaumann H. (1982) Social class and infantile autism. *J. Autism dev. Disorders* **12**, 223-228.

Gillberg I. C. and Gillberg C. (1989) Asperger syndrome: Some epidemiological considerations: A research note. *J. child Psychol. Psychiat.* **30**, 631-638.

Gilmour L, Schalomon PM, Smith V.(2012) Sexuality in a community based sample of adults with autism spectrum disorder *Research in Autism Spectrum Disorders* 313–318

Goldacre B (2012) Bad pharma.

Goldman GS, Yazbak FE. (2004) An investigation of the association between MMR vaccination and autism in Denmark. *J Am Physicians and Surgeons* 9:70-75.

Goodman R. (1989) Infantile autism: a syndrome of multiple primary deficits? *J. Autism dev. Disorders* **19**, 409-424.

Gorski D (2010) http://scienceblogs.com/insolence/2010/03/29/the-intellectual-dishonesty-of-the-vacci/

Gøtzsche P (2013) Deadly Medicines and Organised Crime.

Gould S. J. (1983) *Hens' Teeth and Horses' Toes*. Norton, New York.

Goyer RA. (1991) Toxic effects of metals. In: Amdur MO, Doull J, Klaassen CD, editors. Casarett and Doull's Toxicology: the Basic Science of Poisons. 4th edition. New York: McGraw-Hill. p. 623-680.

Grant T. (2012) http://www.theglobeandmail.com/news/national/meet-the-canadian-billionaire-whos-giving-it-all-away/article4209888/

Gundroo A (2014) http://www.theguardian.com/education/2014/oct/06/cambridge-university-student-depression-eating-disorders#comment-41843167

Hallmayer J, Cleveland S, Torres A, Phillips J, Cohen B, Torigoe T, Miller J, Fedele A, Collins J, Smith K, Lotspeich L, Croen LA, Ozonoff S, Lajonchere C, Grether JK, Risch N. (2011) Genetic heritability and shared environmental factors among twin pairs with autism. *Arch Gen Psychiatry* 68:1095-102.

Hansen EK, Asmussen E. (1993) Cusp fracture of endodontically treated posterior teeth restored with amalgam. Teeth restored in Denmark before 1975 versus after 1979. *Acta Odontol Scand* 51:73-77.

Hanson M. (2004) Effects of amalgam removal on health: 25 studies comprising 5821 patients. Available from various websites.

Harnad, Stevan (ed.) (1982) *Peer commentary on peer review: A case study in scientific quality control,*, Cambridge University Press

Harrington RA, Lee L, Crum RM, Zimmerman AW, Hertz-Picciotto I. (2014) Prenatal SSRI use and offspring with autism spectrum disorder or developmental delay. Pediatrics 135:1241-1248 http://dx.doi.org/10.1542/peds.2013-3406

Hayashi M, Kato M, Igarashi K, Kashima H (2008) Superior fluid intelligence in children with Asperger's disorder. Brain and Cognition 66: 306–310.

He X., Ingraham H. A., Simmons D. M., Treacy M. N., Rosenfeld M. G. and Swanson L. W. (1989) Expression of a large family of pou-domain regulatory genes in mammalian brain development. *Nature* 340, 35-42.

Healy D (2012) Pharmageddon.

Heaton P, Davis RE, Happé FG (2008) Research note: exceptional absolute pitch perception for spoken words in an able adult with autism. Neuropsychologia.; 46(7):2095-8.

Heckenlively K, Mikovits J (2014) Plague.

Hendrickson D. E. (1982) The biological basis of intelligence. Part 2: Measurement. In *A Model for Intelligence* (Edited by Eysenck H. J.). Springer, New York.

Hermelin B. and O'Connor N. (1970) *Psychological Experiments with Autistic Children.* Pergamon, Oxford.

Hertz-Picciotto I, Delwiche L.(2009) The Rise in Autism and the Role of Age at Diagnosis. *Epidemiology,* 20: 84–90)

Hertz-Picciotto I, Green PG, Delwiche L, Hansen R, Walker C, Pessah IN. (2010) Blood mercury concentrations in CHARGE Study children with and without autism. *Environ Health Perspect* 118:161–166.

Hill A. (2011) Mental health of women in crisis. Available [09/16/2013] from: http://www.guardian.co.uk/society/2011/jan/11/mental-health-women-crisis

Hirschfeld LA, Bartmess E, White S, Frith U (2007) Can autistic children predict behaviour by social stereotypes? Curr. Biol. 17, R451–R452.

Hobson R. P. (1989) Beyond cognition: A theory of autism. In *Autism: nature, diagnosis and treatment* (Edited by Dawson G.). Guildford, New York.

Holmes AS, Blaxill MF, Haley BE. (2003) Reduced levels of mercury in first baby haircuts of autistic children. *Internat J Toxicol* 22:277-285.

Homme KG, Kern JK, Haley BE, Geier DA, King PG, Sykes LK, Geier MR. (2014) New science challenges old notion that mercury dental amalgam is safe. *Biometals* 27:19-24.

Horrobin D (1990) The Philosophical Basis of Peer Review and the Suppression of Innovation. JAMA 263(10):1438-41

Horton, R (2000). "Genetically modified food: Consternation, confusion, and crack-up". The Medical journal of Australia **172** (4): 148–9. PMID 10772580.

Howlin, P.; Goode, S.; Hutton, J.; Rutter, M. (2009). "Savant skills in autism: Psychometric approaches and parental reports". *Philosophical Transactions of the Royal Society B: Biological Sciences* 364 (1522): 1359–1367. doi:10.1098/rstb.2008.0328. http://www.ncbi.nlm.nih.gov/pmc/articles/PMC3229189/

Humphries S, Bystrianyk R (2013) Dissolving Illusions: Disease, Vaccines, and The Forgotten History.

Hutt S J, Hutt C, Lee D, Ounsted C (1965) A behavioural and electroencephalographic study of autistic children. *J. psychiat. Res.* **3,** 181-197.

Hviid A. (2004) Association between Thimerosal-containing vaccine and autism—Reply. *JAMA* 291:180-180.

IAOMT (2008) http://iaomt.org/critiques-childrens-amalgam-trials/

IngudomnukulE, Baron-CohenS, WheelwrightS, Knickmeyer R (2007) Elevated rates of testosterone-related disorders in women with autism spectrum conditions. *Hormones and Behav* 51: 597-604.

Ip P, Wong V, Ho M, Lee J, Wong W. (2004) Mercury exposure in children with autistic spectrum disorder: case-control study. *J Child Neurol* 19:431–434.

Jensen A. R. (1980) *Bias in Mental Testing.* Methuen, London.

Kanner L. (1943) Autistic disturbances of affective contact. *Nerv.Child* **2,** 217-250.

Kanner L. (1973) *Childhood psychosis: Initial studies and new insights.* Winston, Washington D.C.

Kaye JA, et al.(2001) Mumps, measles, and rubella vaccine and the incidence of autism recorded by general practitioners: a time trend analysis BMJ 322 :460

Kendrick M (2014) Doctoring Data.

Kern JK, Geier DA, Audhya T, King PG, Sykes LK, Geier MR. (2012) Evidence of parallels between mercury intoxication and the brain pathology in autism. *Acta Neurobiol Exp (Wars)* 72:113-153.

Kern JK, Geier DA, Sykes LK, Geier MR. (2016). Relevance of Neuroinflammation and Encephalitis in Autism. *Frontiers in Cellular Neuroscience, 9,* 519. http://doi.org/10.3389/fncel.2015.00519

Kleinhans NM, Richards T, Sterling L, Stegbauer KC, Mahurin R (2008) Abnormal functional connectivity in autism spectrum disorders during face processing. *Brain* 131:1000-1012. doi:10.1093/brain/awm334

Klinghardt D (1998). Migraines, Seizures, and Mercury Toxicity; Alternative Medicine Magazine, Issue 21 Dec, 1997 / Jan, 1998. http://www.healingartscenter.com/Library/articles/art10.htm

Kollar E. J. and Fischer C. (1980) Tooth induction in chick epithelium: expression of quiescent genes for enamel synthesis. *Science* **207,** 993-995.

Kolvin I., Ounstead C., Richardson L. M. and Garside R. F. (1971) Studies in childhood psychoses: III. The family and social background in childhood psychoses. *Br. J. Psychiat.* **118,** 396-402.

Lai M, Baron-Cohen S (2015) Identifying the lost generation of adults with autism spectrum conditions. Lancet Psychiatry 2(11):1013-1027,

Lakhshmi Priya MD, Geetha A. (2010) Level of trace elements (copper, zinc, magnesium and selenium) and toxic elements (lead and mercury) in the hair and nail of children with autism. Biol Trace Elem Res . doi: 10:1007/s12011-010-8766-2.

Langlois J. H. and Roggman L. A. (1990) Attractive faces are only averages. *Psychol. Science* **1,** 115-121.

LeCouteur A. (1988) The role of genetics in the aetiology of autism. In *Aspects of Autism* (Edited by Wing L.). Gaskell, London.

Leslie A. (1987) Pretense and representation: The origins of a theory of mind. *Psychol. Rev.* **94,** 412-426.

Leslie A. M. and Frith U. (1987) Metarepresentation and autism: How not to lose one's marbles. *Cognition* **27,** 291-294.

Levy T (2013) http://www.peakenergy.com/articles/nh20130811/The-disease-causing-dangers-of-high-iron-levels

Lind SE, Bowler DM (2009) Delayed self-recognition in children with autism spectrum disorder. *J Autism* 39: 643-650.

Lockyer L. and Rutter M. (1970) A five to fifteen year follow-up study of infantile psychosis. IV. Patterns of cognitive ability. *Br. J. soc. clin. Psychol.* **31,** 152-163.

Lord C., Schopler E. and Revicki D. (1982) Sex Differences in autism.*J. Autism dev. Disorders* **12,** 317.

Lotter V. (1967) Epidemiology of autistic conditions in young children: some characteristics of the parents and children.*Soc. Psychiat.* **1,** 163-173.

Lovaas I., Newsom C. and Hickman C. (1987) Self-stimulatory behaviour and perceptual reinforcement. *J. appl. Behavior Analysis* **20,** 45-68.

Lowe L. H. (1966) Families of children with early childhood schizophrenia: selected demographic information. *Archs gen. Psychiat.* **14,** 26-30.

Lynn R (2009) What has caused the Flynn effect? Secular increases in the Development Quotients of infants. *Intelligence* 37: 16-24. doi:10.1016/j.intell.2008.07.008

M.I.N.D. Institute (2002). Report to the Legislature on the Principal Findings from The Epidemiology of Autism in California.

Mackert JR Jr. (1987) Factors affecting estimation of dental amalgam mercury exposure from measurements of mercury vapor levels in intra oral and expired air. *J Dent Res* 66:1775-1780.

Mahler DB, Adey JD, Fleming MA. (1994) Hg emission from dental amalgam as related to the amount of Sn in the Ag-Hg (g1) phase. *J Dent Res* 73:1663-1668.

Maimon R (2013) https://www.quora.com/How-much-of-our-DNA-is-junk-DNA-and-why/answer/Ron-Maimon

Majewska MD, Urbanowicz E, Rok-Bujko P, Namyslowska I, MierzejewskiP et al. (2010) Age-dependent lower or higher levels of hair mercury in autistic children than in healthy controls. *Acta Neurobiol Exp (Wars)* 70:196-208.

Malhotra A (2014) http://www.theguardian.com/commentisfree/2014/jul/19/patients-hospital-care-over-intervention

Mangan L (2014) http://www.theguardian.com/lifeandstyle/2014/aug/16/lucy-mangan-exams-game-rigged

Marlene L (2011) Zero degrees of credibility. http://incorrectpleasures.blogspot.co.uk/2011/04/very-horrible-story-that-just-cant-be.html

Mattick JS, Dinger ME (2013). The extent of functionality in the human genome. The HUGO Journal 7 (1): 2. *doi:10.1186/1877-6566-7-2*.

McCann R. S. (1981) Hemispheric assymmetries and infantile autism. *J. Autism dev. Disorders* **11,** 401-411.

McDermott J. F., Harrison S. I., Schrager J., Lindy J. and Killins E. (1967) Social class and mental illness in children: The question of childhood psychosis. *Am. J. Orthopsychiat.* **37,** 548-557.

McDonald ME, Paul JF (2010) Timing of Increased Autistic Disorder Cumulative Incidence. *Environ. Sci. Technol.* 44 (6), pp 2112–21a18

Mental Health Foundation. (2011) The impact of sleep on health and wellbeing. Available [28/4/2014] from: http://www.mentalhealth.org.uk/publications/sleep-report.

Mercola J (2014) http://articles.mercola.com/sites/articles/archive/2014/12/30/fake-scientific-journals.aspx

Milton J (2010). Mercury causes homosexuality in male ibises. *Nature.* doi:10.1038/news.2010.641

Moberg LE. (1985a) Long-term corrosion studies in vitro of amalgams and casting alloys in contact. *Acta Odontol Scand* 43:163-177.

Moberg LE. (1985b) Corrosion products from dental alloys and effects of mercuric and cupric ions on a neuroeffector system [dissertation]. Stockholm University.

Mohammadi D (2015) "The truth about 'miracle foods' – from chia seeds to coconut oil" http://www.theguardian.com/lifeandstyle/2015/feb/15/truth-about-miracle-foods-chia-seeds-coconut-oilSimonton DK (1989) http://www.the-scientist.com/yr1989/feb/opin2_890206.html

Moore TJ, Mattison DR. (2016) Adult utilisation of psychiatric drugs. JAMA Intern Med. Published online December 12, 2016. doi:10.1001/jamainternmed.2016.7507

Mrozek-Budzyn D, Kiełtyka A, Majewska R. (2009) [Lack of association between MMR vaccination and the incidence of autism in children: a case control study] *Przegl Epidemiol* 63:107-112. Polish.

Mukamel R, Ekstrom AD, Kaplan J, Iacoboni M, Fried I (2010) Single-Neuron Responses in Humans during Execution and Observation of Actions. *Curr Biol.* doi: 10.1016/j.cub.2010.02.045

Mundy P., Sigman M. and Kasari C. (1990) A longitudinal study of joint attention and language development in autistic children. *J. Autism dev. Disorders* **20,** 115-128.

Mutter J. (2011) Is dental amalgam safe for humans? The opinion of the scientific committee of the European Commission. *J Occupat Med Tox* 6:2.

Nettelbeck T, Wilson C (2004) The Flynn effect: Smarter not faster. *Intelligence* 32: 85-93.

Nevison C (2014) A comparison of temporal trends in United States autism prevalence to trends in suspected environmental factors. Environ Health 13:73.

Nkowane et al (1987) Measles outbreak in a vaccinated school population: epidemiology, chains of transmission, and the role of vaccine failures. Am J Public Health.

O'Riordan & Passetti, (2006) Discrimination in autism within different sensory modalities.J Autism Dev Disord., 36(5):665-75.

Ocregister.com (2011) http://www.ocregister.com/articles/correction-296910-dated-entitled.html

Offit P. (2008) Autism's false prophets.

Ohta & Gillespie (1996) Theor Popul Biol., 49(2):128-42. Development of Neutral and Nearly Neutral Theories http://www.ncbi.nlm.nih.gov/pubmed/8813019

Olsson S, Berglund A, Pohl L, Bergman M. (1989) Model of mercury vapor transport from amalgam restorations in the oral cavity. *J Dent Res* 68:50~508.

Olsson S, Bergman M. (1987) Intraoral air and calculated inspired dose of mercury [letter]. *J Dent Res* 66:1288-1289.

Ornitz E. M. (1985) Neuropsychology of infantile autism. *J. Am. Acad. child Psychiat.* **24,** 85-124.

Parrington J (2015) The deeper genome.

Pathologist (2014) http://www.bondsolon.com/expert-witness-faces-gmc-hearing-shaken-baby-syndrome-15092014.aspx

Patterson JE, Weissberg BG, Dennison PJ. (1985) Mercury in human breath from dental amalgams. *Bull Environ Contam Topical* 34:459-468.

Paul R. (1987) Communication. In *Handbook of Autism* (Edited by Cohen D. J. and Donellan A. M.). Wiley, New York.

Paull DR. (2015) *So You Got Into Medical School. . . Now What?*

Peters M. (1986) Autism as impairment in the formation and use of meaning: an attempt to integrate a functional and neuronal model. *J. Psychol.* **120,** 69-81.

Pharmaton. Fight Fatigue Report. (2010).

Pisula E (2010) The autistic mind in the light of neuropsychological studies. *Acta Neurobiol Exp (Wars)* 70: 119-130.

Pitfield M. and Oppenheim A. N. (1964) Child rearing attitudes of mothers of psychotic children. *J. child Psychol. Psychiat.* **5,** 51-57.

Platform 51. (2011) Women Like Me: Supporting wellbeing in girls and women.

Polyak A, Kubina RM, Girirajan S. Comorbidity of intellectual disability confounds ascertainment of autism: Implications for genetic diagnosis. Am J Med Genet B Neuropsychiatr Genet. 2015 Jul 22. doi: 10.1002/ajmg.b.32338. [Epub ahead of print] PubMed PMID: 26198689.

Prior M. R. (1979) Cognitive abilities and disabilities in infantile autism: a review. *J. abnorm. child Psychol.* **7,** 357-380.

Prior M. R. (1987) Biological and neuropsychological approaches to childhood autism. *Br. J. Psychiat.* **150,** 8-17.

Prior M. R., Gazjago C. C. and Knox D. T. (1976) An epidemiological study of autistic and psychotic children in the 4 eastern states of Australia. *Aust. N.Z. J. Psychiat.* **10,** 173-184.

Prokosch MD, Yeo RA, Miller GF (2005) Intelligence tests with higher g-loadings show higher correlations with body symmetry: Evidence for a general fitness factor mediated by developmental stability. *Intelligence* 33: 203-213.

Psarras V, Derand T, Nilner K. (1994) Effect of selenium on mercury vapor released from dental amalgams: An in vitro study. *Swed Dent J* 18:15-23.

Ratajczak HV. (2011) Theoretical aspects of autism: causes – a review. J Immunotoxicol. 8(1):68-79.

Raven, John (2000). The Raven's Progressive Matrices: Change and Stability over Culture and Time. *Cognitive Psychology* 41: 1–48. http://eyeonsociety.co.uk/resources/RPMChangeAndStability.pdf

Razeto-Barry, P., Díaz, J., & Vásquez, R. A. (2012). The Nearly Neutral and Selection Theories of Molecular Evolution Under the Fisher Geometrical Framework: Substitution Rate, Population Size, and Complexity. *Genetics*, *191*(2), 523–534. http://doi.org/10.1534/genetics.112.138628

Revici E (1961) Research In Physiopathology.

Richard Farrell-Adams (2015) http://www.theguardian.com/society/2015/feb/07/nhs-investigations-into-care-complaints-appalling#comment-47217018

Ricks D. M. and Wing L. (1975) Language, communication, and the use of symbols in normal and autistic children. *J. Autism child Schizophrenia* **5,** 191-222.

Rimland B. (1964) *Infantile Autism.* Appleton-Century-Crofts, New York.

Rimland B. (2000) The autism increase. *Autism Research Review International* 14(1):3

Ritvo E. R., Cantwell D., Johnson E., Clements M. C., Benbrook F.,   Slagel S., Kelly P. and Ritz M. (1971) Social class factors in autism. *J. Autism child. Schizophrenia* 1, 297-310.

Ritvo E. R., Jorde L. B., Mason-Brothers A., Freeman B. J., Pingree C., Jones M. B., McMahon W. M., Peterson P. B., Jenson W. R. and Mo A. (1989) The UCLA-University of Utah epidemiological survey of autism: Recurrence risk estimates and genetic counselling. *Am. J. Psychiat.***146,** 1032-1036.

Rodgers JS, Hocker JR, Hanas RJ, Nwosu EC, Hanas JS. (2001) Mercuric ion inhibition of eukaryotic transcription factor binding to DNA. *Biochem Pharmacol* 61:1543-1550.

Rory Graham (2015) http://www.theguardian.com/society/2015/feb/07/nhs-investigations-into-care-complaints-appalling#comment-47219362

Runco M. A., Charlop M. and Schreibman L. (1986) The occurence of autistic childrens' self-stimulation as a function of familiar versus unfamiliar stimulus conditions. *J. Autism dev. Disorders* **16,** 31-44.

Rushton JP (1999) Secular gains in IQ not related to the *g* factor and inbreeding depression. *Pers Individ Diff* 26: 381-389.

Rutter M. and Lockyer L. (1967) A five to fifteen year follow-up of infantile psychosis: I. Description of sample. *Br. J. Psychiat.* **113,** 1169-1182.

Rutter M. and Schopler E. (1987) Autism and pervasive developmental disorders: Concepts and diagnostic issues. *J. Autism dev. Disorders***17,** 159-186.

Salminen JK, Saarijärvi S, Raitasalo R. (1997) Depression and disability pension in Finland. *Acta Psychiatr Scand* 95:242-3.

Sandin S, Schendel D, Magnusson P, et al. (2015) Autism risk associated with parental age and with increasing difference in age between the parents. Mol Psychiatry;21(5):693-700.

Sanua V. D. (1986, August) *Socioeconomic status and intelligence of parents of autistic children.* Paper presented at the third world congress of infant psychiatry and allied disciplines, Stockholm, Sweden.

Sanua V. D. (1987) Infantile autism and parental socioeconomic status: A case of bimodal distribution. *Child Psychiat. human Dev.* **17,** 189-198.

Schopler E., Andrews E. C. and Strupp K. (1979) Do autistic children come from upper-middle class parents? *J. Autism dev. Disorders.* **9,** 139-152.

Schuster PF, Krabenhoft DP, Naftz DL, Cecil LD, Olson ML, Dewild JF, Susong DD, Green JR, Abbot ML. (2002b) https://www.ncdc.noaa.gov/paleo/pubs/schuster2002/schuster2002.html

Scott P (2016) http://www.theguardian.com/education/2016/jan/04/control-schools-universities-knowledge-business

Shayer M, Ginsburg D. (2009) Thirty years on – a large anti-Flynn effect? (II): 13- and 14-year-olds. Piagetian tests of formal operations norms 1976–2006/7 British *Journal of Educational Psychology* 79: 409–418.

Shucard D. W. and Horn J. L. (1972) Evoked cortical potentials and measurement of human abilities. *J. comp. physiol. Psychol.* **78,** 59-68.

Siddique H (2017) https://www.theguardian.com/society/2017/oct/26/thriving-work-report-uk-mental-health-problems-forcing-thousands-out

Sigman M., Ungerer J. A., Mundy P. and Sherman T. (1987) Cognition in autistic children. In *Handbook of Autism* (Edited by Cohen D. J. and Donellan A. M.). Wiley, New York.

Silberberg N. E. and Silberberg M. C. (1967) Hyperlexia: specific word recognition skills in young children. *Exceptional Child.* **34,** 41-42.

Sinclair J. (1999) Why I dislike "person first" language. http://autismmythbusters.com/general-public/autistic-vs-people-with-autism/jim-sinclair-why-i-dislike-person-first-language/

Slagel S., Kelly P. and Ritz M. (1971) Social class factors in autism. *J. Autism child. Schizophrenia* **1,** 297-310.

Smalley S. L., Asarnov R. F. and Spence M. A. (1988) Autism and genetics. *Archs gen. Psychiat.* 45, 953-961.

Smith R (2014) Medical research—still a scandal http://blogs.bmj.com/bmj/2014/01/31/richard-smith-medical-research-still-a-scandal/

Snowling M. and Frith U. (1986) Comprehension in 'hyperlexic' readers. *J. exp. child Psychol.* **42,** 392-415.

Soden S, Lowrey J, Garrison C, Wasserman G. (2007) 24-hour provoked urine excretion test for heavy metals in children with autism and typically developing controls, a pilot study. *Clinic Toxicol* 45:476–481.

Sofaer J. and Emery A. E. (1981) Genes for super-intelligence. *J. med.Genet.* 18, 410-413.

Soulières I, Dawson M, Gernsbacher MA, Mottron L (2011) The Level and Nature of Autistic Intelligence II: What about Asperger Syndrome? PLoS ONE 6(9): e25372.

Southwick F (2012) http://www.the-scientist.com/?articles.view/articleNo/32077/title/Opinion – Academia-Suppresses-Creativity/

Spitz HH (1989) Variations in Wechsler interscale IQ disparities at different levels of IQ. *Intelligence* 13: 157-67.

Stehr-Green P, Tull P, Stellfield M, Mortenson P, Simpson D. (2003) Autism and thimerosal-containing vaccines. *Am J Prev Med* 25:101-106.

Stock A. (1926) Die Gefaehrlichkeit des Quecksilberdampfes. *Zeitschrift fur angewandte Chemie* 39(15):461-466. Available [16/9/2013] from: http://www.stanford.edu/~bcalhoun/AStock.htm.

Stone J (2009) http://www.communitycare.co.uk/2009/01/13/professor-simon-baron-cohen-autism-is-not-cancer/

Sundet JM, Barlaug DG, Torjussen TM. (2004) The end of the Flynn effect?: A study of secular trends in mean intelligence test scores of Norwegian conscripts during half a century *Intelligence* 32: 349–362.

Sutcliffe et al (1996) Outbreak of measles in a highly vaccinated secondary school population. Canadian Med Assocn.

Svare CW, Peterson LC, Reinhardt JW, Boyer DB, Frank CW, Gay DD et al. (1981) The effect of dental amalgams on mercury levels in expired air. *J Dent Res* 60:1668-1671.

Szasz A, Barna B, et al. (2002) Effects of continuous low-dose exposure to organic and inorganic mercury during development on epileptogenicity in rats. *Neurotoxicology*; 23(2): 197-206.

Teasdale TW, Owen DR. (2008) Secular declines in cognitive test scores: A reversal of the Flynn Effect..*Intelligence* 36: 121–126.

Terrass S (1997) Is Vitamin B-6 Safety a Political Issue in the United Kingdom? http://www.drpasswater.com/nutrition_library/terrass.html

Tomljenovic L, Shaw CA. (2011) Do aluminium vaccine adjuvants contribute to the rising prevalence of autism? J Inorganic Biochem. 105(11):1489–99.

Torrey EF, Miller J. (2002) The invisible plague: the rise of mental illness from 1750 to the present. Rutgers Univ Press.
pp. 94,152,188,271, and frontispiece.

Tournaye H (2009), "Male Reproductive Ageing," in Bewley, Ledger, and Nikolaou, eds., *Reproductive Ageing*, Cambridge University Press, ISBN 9781906985134

Treffert D. A. (1970) Epidemiology of infantile autism. *Archs gen. Psychiat.* **22**, 431-438.

Tsai L., Stewart M. A., Faust M. and Shook S. (1982) Social class distribution of fathers of children enrolled in Iowa program. *J. Autism dev. Disorders* **12**, 211-221.

USGS (2002) Glacial Ice Cores Reveal A Record of Natural and Anthropogenic Atmospheric Mercury Deposition for the Last 270 Years. USGS Fact Sheet FS-051-02, June 2002.
http://pubs.er.usgs.gov/publication/fs05102

Vimy MJ, Lorscheider FL. (1990) Dental amalgam mercury daily dose estimated from intra oral vapor measurements: a predictor of mercury accumulation in human tissues. *J Trace Elem Exp Med* 3:111-123.

Vimy MJ, Lorscheider FL. (1985a) Intraoral air mercury released from dental amalgam. *J Dent Res* 64:1069-1071.

Vimy MJ, Lorscheider FL. (1985b) Serial measurements of intra oral air mercury: estimation of daily dose from dental amalgam. *J Dent Res* 64:1072-1075.

Vogt-Vincent O (2015) I am 16 and the education system is destroying my health http://www.theguardian.com/teacher-network/2015/aug/16/i-am-16-and-the-education-system-is-destroying-my-health Thrasher SW (2016) http://www.theguardian.com/commentisfree/2016/mar/26/do-not-tell-cancer-patients-cures-they-could-be-doing

Volkmar F. R. (1987) Social development. In *Handbook of Autism* (Edited by Cohen D. J. and Donellan A. M.)). Wiley, New York.

Waldman M, Nicholson S, Adilov N, Williams J. (2008) Autism prevalence and precipitation rates in California, Oregon, and Washington counties. *Arch Pediatr Adolesc Med* 162:1026-1034.

Walker H. A. (1976) The incidence of minor physical anomalies in autistic patients. In *The Autistic Syndromes* (Edited by Coleman M.). North-Holland, Amsterdam.

Walker H. A. and Coleman M. (1976) Characteristics of adventitious movements in autistic children. In *The Autistic Syndromes* (Edited by Coleman M.). North-Holland, Amsterdam.

Walter A, Luck G. (1977) Interactions of Hg(II) ions with DNA as revealed by CD measurements. *Nucleic Acids Res* 4:539-550.

Wang Z, Yan R, He H, Li Q, Chen G, Yang S & Chen E (2014). Difficulties in Eliminating Measles and Controlling Rubella and Mumps: A Cross-Sectional Study of a First Measles and Rubella Vaccination and a Second Measles, Mumps, and Rubella Vaccination. *PLoS ONE, 9*(2), e89361. doi:10.1371/journal.pone.0089361

Ward T. F. and Hoddinott B. A. (1965) A study of childhood schizophrenia and early infantile autism. *Can. Psychiat. Ass. J.* **10,** 377-386.

Watson J. D., Hopkins N. H., Roberts J. W., Steitz J.A. and Weiner A. M. (1987) *Molecular Biology of the Gene* (4th edition) Benjamin/Cummings, Menlo Park, CA.

Welsh M., Pennington B. and Rogers S. (1987) Word recognition and comprehension skills in hyperlexic children. *Brain Language* **32,** 76-96.

Whitaker R (2010) Anatomy of an epidemic.

Wiedel L. and Coleman M. (1976) The autistic and control population of this study. In *The Autistic Syndromes* (Edited by Coleman M.). North-Holland, Amsterdam.

Wilson E. O. (1978) *On Human Nature.* Harvard University Press, Cambridge, MA.

Wing L. (1976) Diagnosis and definition. In *Early Childhood Autism (2nd edition)* (Edited by Wing L.). Pergamon, Oxford.

Wing L. (1980) Childhood autism and social class: A question of selection? *Br. J. Psychiat.* **137,** 410-417.

Wing L. and Wing J. K. (1971) Multiple impairments in early childhood autism. *J. Autism child Schizophrenia* **1,** 256-266.

Wing L., and Gould J. (1979) Severe impairments of social interaction and associated abnormalities in children: Epidemiology and classification. *J. Autism dev. Disorders* **9,** 11-29.

Wing, L (1988) The autistic continuum. In *Aspects of Autism* (Edited by Wing L.). Gaskell, London.

Wood S (2015) Official webpage of Professor Stephen Wood at University of Birmingham.

Woodley MA, Meisenberg G. (2013) In the Netherlands the anti-Flynn effect is a Jensen effect. *Personality and Individual Differences* 54: 871–876.

Woods HF (1998) Memorandum submitted by Professor H F Woods, Chairman of the Committee on Toxicity of Chemicals in Food, Consumer Products and the Environment (E44)

Young AMH, Chakrabati B, Roberts D, Lai MC, Suckling J, Baron-Cohen S. (2016) From molecules to neural morphology: understanding neuroinflammation in autism spectrum condition. *Molecular Autism* 7:9 DOI: 10.1186/s13229-016-0068-x

Zhou J (2015) http://www.swissinfo.ch/eng/opinion_are-older-fathers-really-more-likely-to-have-autistic-children-/41500678

Index

acetaminophen 198
acupuncture 26
Adams, James B 90, 354
Adams, Mike 27, 354
air pollution **187**, **220**, **333-352**
aluminium 182, 183, 184, 193, 368
amalgams 17, 35, 43, 44, 45, 62, 77, **78-165**, 176, 177, 188, 191, 193, **240-261**, 293, 307, 323, 325, 326, 335, 338, 357, 358, 359, 360, 364, 365, 366, 368
anecdote 173, 191, 192, 303, 304
antiinnatia 22, 52, 55, 60, 62, 64, 65, 66, **70-77**, 89, 90, 168, 193, **200-239**, 293, **324-353**, 358
anxiety 28, 97, 105, 106, 107, 274, 282, 318
Arber, Werner 60, 72
Arslan, R 74-7, 332
atavisms 70, 205, 212, 222, 329
autism 1, 4, 16, 17, 20-22, 25, 33-35, 37, 43, 44, 45, **47-239**, 248, 249, 250, 252, 273, 288, 289, 290, 291, 292, 293, 294, 295, 296, 298, 299, 300, 303, 305, 306, 307, 308, 309, 310, 321, 322, **324-353**, 354, 355, 356, 357, 358, 359, 360, 361, 362, 363, 364, 365, 366, 367, 368, 369, 370
autism epidemic (see increase of autism)
Autism Research Institute 84, 85-88
AutismToday.com 53

Barbeau, EB 54
Baron-Cohen, S 4, 17, 56, 61, 67, 148, 188, 228, 229, **288-305**, 309, 310, 326, 355, 362, 363
Bauer, Henry 313
Bellinger, DC 133
Bengtsson, Ulf 44, 354
Bernard, Sally 82, 88, 194
bipolar 49, 249, 250, 307
Bjørklund, Geir 354
Blakemore-Brown, Lisa 69, 85
Blaucok-Busch*, E 84 [*Incorrect spelling of Blaurock-Busch]
blank mind 244
blank slate 201, 205, 327
Blaxill, Mark 88, 178-9, 354
blushing 204, 211, 244
Bradstreet, Jeff 83, 120, 354

brain 10, 49, 50, 51, 52, 54, 55, 56, 64, 74, 80, 103, 109, 173-4, 201, 205-6, 207, 223-4, 234, 237, 318, 326-7, 328
Brown, Charlie 354
Brownstein, David 93
Bystrianyk, Roman 31, 42, 191

Calhoun, Birgit 95, 354
Cambridge 9, 12, 288-305
cancer 28, 31, 35, 267, 271, 272
Casanova, Emily 239
Casanova, Manuel 50, 63, 239
changepoint 185, 186, 193
chelation 84, 171-4
chlorella 266-272
circadian 243
citation record 19
citations 3, **19**, **38-40**, 78, **171-2**, 173, 282, 285, 316, 355
concentration 104, 105, 106, 243
concentration camp 303
confidence 105, 106
conspiracy theories 175
Croen, Lisa 69, 188
Cutler, Andrew Hall 94, 162, 354

D'Onofrio 77
Davies, James 42, 63, 313
Dawson, M 54
depression 35, 49, 53, 84, 93, 96, 97, 104, 105, 106, 162-3, 244, 250, 274, 284. 310, 318
DeRouen, TA 133
DeSoto, MC 18, 84, 127, 128, 199, 354
Deth, Richard 176, 354
diagnosis 49, 51, 62, 64, 81, 88, 113, 114, 166, 174, 216, 228, 233, 238, 250, 256, 289, 291, 294, 297, 299, 300, 301, 320, 325, 362, 366
diagnostic substitution 69, 188
disorder **47-76**, 85, 93, 174, 204, 205, 208, 233, 239, 316, 358, 360, 361, 362, 363
DNA 43, 55, 57, 59, 60, 71-2, 89, 95, 130, 173-4, 204, 206, 209, 222, 234, 238, 239, 252, 328, 331, 334, 337
drugs 18, 27, 29, 33, 37, 41, 42, 56, 72, 176, 234, 241, 249, 274, 276, 283, 306, 307, 317, 318
DSM 62, 63, 299, 309

Edelson, Stephen M, 354

El-Essawy, Hesham 36, 253, 354
embarrassment 105
Emeramide 260, 319
epilepsy 28, 64, 107, 274, 318
evolution 43, 57, 59, 60, 70, 71, 72, 74, 203, 205, 206, 207, 208, 209, 221, 222, 234, 236, 356
extreme-male-brain 326, 327, 355
eyes, sore 244, 266, 267

fatigue 93, 95, 96, 97, 104, 106, 107, 113, 162, 243, 251
FDA 27, 33, 163, 177, 192, 260, 307, 319, 320
Feinstein, Adam 354
fetal testosterone 326
fibromyalgia 93, 162, 163, 309
Flynn effect 44, 325, **333-348**, 351, 352, 358, 359, 363, 365, 367, 368, 370
Frith, Uta 53, 356

Gawande, Atul 322
Geier, D 82 , 90, 101, 142, 169, 354, 360
Geier, M 82 , 90, 101, 142, 169, 354, 360
gene-expression 20, 22, 43, 65, 89, 121, 130, 173, 174, 202, 203, 204, 205, 206, 207, 208, 209, 234, 237, 252, 325, 331, 337, 358
genes 7, 20, 55, 56, 57, 59, 60, 62, 72, 74, 75, 77, 191, 192, 203, 204, 208, 209, 210, 211, 213, 214, 215, 221, 235, 236, 237, 238, 239, 261, 335, 337, 344, 347, 348, 350, 361, 363
Gernsbacher MA 54
Gillberg, C 55, 88, 180
Goldacre, Ben 37, 42, 313, 354
Gotzsche, Peter 13, 18, 27, 29, 42, 313
glyphosate 181, 182
GMC 34, 311, 320

Haley, Boyd 143, 168, 176-7, 354
Hallmayer, J 89, 121
handflapping 329
Hanson, Mats 80, 82, 101, 142
Harnad, Steven 3
Harrington, RA 84
Harvie-Austin, David 354
Hayashi, M 54
headaches 105, 274
Healy, David 13, 27, 42, 115, 135, 313
Heckenliveley, K 95

herbal 31
Hertz-Picciotto, Irva 70, 82, 120, 128-9
Hitlan, RT 84, 127-8, 354
Holmes, A 36, 83, 90, 121-2, 142, 354
homelessness 22, 44
homeopathy 26, 27
Homme, KG 80, 82, 101, 133
homosexuality 349, 350, 351, 364
Hubbard, Brian 354
Huggins, Hal 81, 117, 354
Humphries, Suzanne 2, 31, 42, 191, 313

IAOMT 133, 354
IBS (irritable bowel syndrome) 244
increase of autism **68-70**, **78-199**, **288-307**, 308, 309, 310, 322, 325, 326, 327, 330, 333, 334, 335, 337, 338, 339, 351, 366
increase of IQ 333-353
indecision 104, 105, 106, 107, 243
insanity 98
insomnia 28, 97, 105, 162, 246, 274
IQ 35, 37, 44, 50, **51-55**, 56, 60, 62, **73-77**, 188, 198, 201, 204, 205, 206, 207, 208, 212, 213, 214, 215, 216, 220, 221, 233, 234, 238, 248, 325, 327, 328, 330, 331, **333-343**, **346**, 358, 359, 360, 367, 368
Irminix 260, 319
iron overload 266-272
irritable 244 106

James, S Jill 176
justice 175, 353

Kendrick, Malcolm 2, 13, 37, 42, 313, 320
Kern, Janet 84, 354, 360, 362
Klinghardt, D 64, 84

Larose, Pierre 163, 354
Lichtenberg, H 163, 354
lost generation 69, **288**-305
Lysenkoism 4, 6, 199

Malhotra, Aseem 313
Majewska, MD 83, 142, 354
Mangan, PD 272
Maserejian, TT 133
McGuire, Tom 354

McTaggart, Lynne 354
Melisa (test) 253, 255, 259, 354
memorising 9-12
memory 9, 35, 52, 54, 94, 96, 97, 104, 105, 106, 107, 162, 224, 227, 230, 243, 245, 247, 253
Mercola.com 23, 266-7, 354
mercury 3, 17, 29, 31, 36, 43, 44, 62, 64, 65, 66, 67, 68, 70, 77, **78-164**, 168, 172, 173, 174, 176, 177, 178, 179, 180, 181, 188, 189, 192, 193, 194, 196, 198, 201, 202, 215, 222, **240-261**, 263, 264, 266, 267, 268, 269, 270, 288, 293, 306, 310, 319, 323, **325-352**, 355, 356, 357, 358, 359, 360, 362, 363, 364, 365, 366, 368, 369
Mikovits, J 95
MMR vaccine **166-199**
Mottron, L 53
Munro-Hall, Graeme 311, 319, 354
mutation 55, 58, 60, **70-77**, 213, 214, 223, 236, 238
Mutter, Dr med Joachim 78, 80, 82, 101, 135, 142, 143, 354
Myhill, Dr Sarah 311, 319

naturalnews.com 23, 27, 354
Neurotribes (book) 70
Nevison, Cynthia 70
NHS 26, 37, 44, 81, 82, 85, 100, 101, 104, 108, 113, 119, 144, 153, 157, 162, 163, **240-272**, 297, 310, 320
nutrition 28, 29, 30, 31, 33, 42, 76, 244, 246, 273, 333, 360, 368

Obukhanych, Tetyana 31,32
Offit, Paul 40, 168-175
OSR#1 192, 258, 260, 319

PABA (vitamin) 30
paracetamol 198, 280
peer review 2, 3, 14-17, 19, 20, 89, 138, 139, 147, 148, 150, 164, 293, 302, 308, 311, 315, 361
phobias 232, 242, 243, 244, 246, 250, 318, 349
pollution 17, 44, **187, 220**, 293, 300, 319, 325, **333-352**, 358
Polyak, A 188
predictions 98, 239, 329, 342, 348, 349
propaganda 13, 26, 25, 28, 30, 33, 37, 40, 41, 42, 63, 76, 102, 143, 172, 173, 194, 259, 274, 275, 317, 345, 349, 350, 354

Razeto-Barry, P 72
references (see citations)
review articles 19, 136

Rimland, B 20, 22, 35, 69, 85, 86, 163, 176, 177, 200, 203, 224, 234, 235, 273, 274, 275, 281, 296, 301, 354
RNA 71, 203, 209, 237
road traffic 187, 293
Rogers, Sally J 69

Schafer, Lenny 354
schizophrenia 49, 76, 77, 88, 243, 250
selenium 90, 112, 247, 266, 267, 268
Shaw, CA 182-4
shyness 104,105, 238, 244, 327
Silbermann, Steve 70
Simmons, Karen 53
Sinclair, Jim 54
Sircus, Mark 354
sleep 94, 96-7, 104, 106, 162, 227, 242, 245, 318
Soulieres, I 54
Stejskal, Vera 354
syndrome **48**, 49, 55, 61, 62, 73, 85, 174, 203, 204, 205, 206, 208, 213, 215, 216, 219, 222, 224, 233, 235, 238, 239, 251, 282, 297, 331

temperature 211, 212, 244
thimerosal (thiomersal) **166-199**, 326
Tomljenovich, Lucia 182-4, 199
Torrey, E Fuller 98-99
Thompson, William 196-7
Tylenol 198

vaccines 31-33, 166-199
Visser, Ilona 354
vitamin B6 278-287, 318
vitamin C 269
vitamins (see nutrition)

Wakefield, Andrew 169, 196, 198, 319
Walker, Colin 97
Waring, Rosemary, 176
weariness 94, 104
What Doctors Don't Tell You 23, 354
Whitaker, Robert 306-7
Windham, Bernie 354
Wing, Lorna 21-22, 60, 224
writing (difficulty) 94-5, 104, 242, 243, 244, 248

Printed in Great Britain
by Amazon